Complementary Cancer Therapies

Combining Traditional and Alternative Approaches for the Best Possible Outcome

DAN LABRIOLA, N.D.

PRIMA HEALTH
A Division of Prima Publishing
3000 Lava Ridge Court • Roseville, California 95661
(800) 632-8676 • www.primahealth.com

DISCLAIMERS
This book is not intended to provide medical advice and is sold with the understanding that the publisher and the author are not liable for the misconception or misuse of information provided. The author and Prima Publishing shall have neither liability nor responsibility to any person or entity with respect to any loss, damage, or injury caused or alleged to be caused directly or indirectly by the information contained in this book or the use of any products mentioned. Readers should not use any of the products discussed in this book without the advice of a medical professional.

Pseudonyms are used throughout to protect the privacy of the individuals involved.
All products mentioned in this book are trademarks of their respective companies.
Prima Health and colophon are registered trademarks of Prima Communications, Inc.

Library of Congress Cataloging-in-Publication Data
Labriola, Dan.
    Complementary cancer therapies : combining traditional and alternative approaches for the best possible outcome / Dan Labriola.
        p. cm.
        Includes Index
        ISBN 0-7615-1922–X
        1. Cancer—Alternative treatment Popular works. 2. Cancer—Treatment Popular works. I. Title.
    RC271.A62L33 1999
    616.99'406—dc21   99-15123
                                                                                                        CIP

00 01 02 03 DD 10 9 8 7 6 5 4 3 2

Printed in the United States of America

How to Order
Single copies may be ordered from Prima Publishing, 3000 Lava Ridge Court, Roseville, CA 95661; telephone (800) 632-8676. Quantity discounts are also available. On your letterhead, include information concerning the intended use of the books and the number of books you wish to purchase.

Visit us online at www.primahealth.com

Family is the tie that unites all of humanity.
This book is dedicated to my parents,
Joe and Virginia, and my brother, Don,
for the many decades of encouragement
and support they have given me.

ACKNOWLEDGMENTS

John Bastyr, N.D., was my mentor, teacher, and friend. He was a scholar with an insatiable hunger for knowledge and truth who, for more than half a century, selflessly applied his wisdom and heart to advance the practice and remarkable healing philosophy of naturopathic medicine. He exemplified my belief that natural medicine is most successful when applied in concert with the best that modern science has to offer. Each day that I care for my patients, I am grateful to Dr. Bastyr.

Noted medical specialist, oncologist, and researcher, Peter Wright, M.D., taught me much of what I know about the science and application of conventional oncology. He was loved and admired by his family, patients, and peers. He showed me that chemotherapy and other standard cancer treatments can be administered with great skill, genuine compassion, and, most important, ultimate benefit to the patient. My patients and I continue to benefit from his good work. He will always have my profound appreciation.

I have had the privilege of participating in the care of thousands of cancer survivors. These marvelous individuals and their families have showed me that they can make the best possible decisions about their treatment, their lives, and their future when they have clear, credible, and unbiased information along with a straightforward method to apply it. This text is written to be such a tool. I owe a debt of gratitude to each of my patients and their families, especially those who took the time to review and critique the original manuscript. Those valuable changes were incorporated and resulted in a much more useful final product.

CONTENTS

Acknowledgments   iv

Introduction   vii

Foreword by Robert B. Livingston, M.D.   xi

1   *The Best of Both Worlds*   1

2   *A Basic Tool Kit*   11

3   *A Guide to Choosing Your Health Care Providers*   25

4   *A Primer on Choosing Treatments*   55

5   *Understanding Your Conventional Therapy*   67

6   *The Side Effects of Conventional Treatments:*
     How Alternative Medicines Can Help   93

7   *Your Personal Plan for Combining Conventional and*
     Nonconventional Care   105

8   *The ABCs of Alternative Therapies*   167

9   *Special Cases: When "Average Person" Doesn't Apply*   237

10   *Prevention Strategies*   247

11 *Quality of Life: Making Every Day As Good As It Can Be*   263

12 *The Mind-Body Connection: Relieving Stress,
Getting Support*   291

APPENDIX 1   *Caffeine-Containing Foods and Medications*   299

APPENDIX 2   *Diuretics*   300

APPENDIX 3   *Common Antioxidants*   301

APPENDIX 4   *Pressors*   302

APPENDIX 5   *Common Liver Stressors*   303

Glossary   305

Index   315

About the Author   340

INTRODUCTION

Impossible obstacles are overcome every single day. The human spirit, coupled with the best that science and tradition have to offer, can triumph over challenges that are so immense that the "experts" would only predict failure. Such miracles of achievement and survival are real and verified. They exist in literally every phase of life, and cancer is no exception. No one can guarantee you a miracle, but why not try? Miracles happen, and there is no reason one shouldn't happen to you.

Billy was a two-year-old with liver cancer. His tumors were too large and his liver too tiny for surgery. Although the cancer had been responding well to chemotherapy, Billy simply couldn't tolerate its toxic side effects. Under the best of conditions, his six-month chances for survival were a mere 5%. His parents and his caregivers were out of options and desperate.

I first met Billy and his parents in a Seattle hospital. As a naturopathic physician, I consulted with Billy's oncologist and surgeon, planning a course of care that combined conventional medicine with a program of natural therapies that I designed to help him tolerate the chemotherapy while protecting his liver and kidneys. To everyone's delight, Billy responded to the new treatments. He had fewer side effects, the tumors began to shrink, and within a few weeks they were deemed operable. The surgery removed all traces of the tumors, and today Billy is a healthy nine-year-old.

I have seen many such cases, where scientific methods were used to carefully coordinate and combine conventional oncology with natural medicine. The story of Adam is another good example. This pleasant twelve-year-old had come to Seattle to undergo a bone marrow transplant for his leukemia. He was not a good candidate for other conventional treatments, and nonconventional therapies had been ineffective.

I created a course of natural medicine designed specifically for him. My goal was to provide basic nutrition and support for his immune system without interfering with his conventional treatment or increasing his risks of other side effects, such as infection. I insisted on strict coordination with Adam's oncologists during this highly technical procedure. The bone marrow transplant went perfectly, and now, more than a decade later, our young hero remains healthy and happy.

These experiences demonstrate how the carefully coordinated use of conventional cancer therapies and natural medicine, under the supervision of knowledgeable providers, can bring results better than the sum of their individual actions.

HOW THIS BOOK CAME TO BE

While modern medicine has made great technical strides in preventing, diagnosing, and treating cancer, the very methods that provide these advances can produce confusion and doubt, thus undermining people's hope. Often, much of what a person hears about medical treatments is focused on survival statistics and toxic warnings. But there is more to winning the battle against cancer than simply relying on technology.

The missing part of modern medicine is the human component, the spirit and determination that define our humanity and make us who we are. When it comes to cancer survival, conventional medicine often ignores the body's own remarkable restorative powers. Doctors are unable to explain in scientific terms instances that can only be attributed to self-healing.

The spiritual and emotional components of healing cannot be defined by statistics and cannot be measured by sophisticated instruments. But the truth is that while conventional therapies can indeed do wonders, natural medicine can support and stimulate the body's innate healing powers in ways that are simply not part of conventional treatment. To combine both alternative therapies and conventional medicine is an idea whose time has come. Yes, both conventional and nonconventional therapies have their successes, but the most remarkable successes I've witnessed are the result of the judicious use of both therapies together.

The idea of carefully coordinating modern medicine and traditional healing in the treatment of cancer is relatively new. In fact, when my good friend and mentor, the late Peter Wright, M.D., and I first looked into this area, we could not find a single scientific study on the subject. As a medical oncologist, Dr. Wright had many patients under his care who were also treating themselves with alternative medicine. Their results, however, were inconsistent. Some did very well and others dismally. After carefully reviewing many of their histories, we concluded that while some of the natural self-treatments were supporting their conventional therapies, others were not. In fact, some of the natural self-treatments were actually interfering with the ability of such conventional treatments as chemotherapy and radiation to eliminate tumor cells.

To combine both alternative therapies and conventional medicine is an idea whose time has come.

We decided to try the unheard-of practice of coordinating treatments. Dr. Wright would determine which conventional treatment would have the best effect, and I would design a natural medicine program that would take into account every action and side effect of the conventional treatments. My goals would be to keep each patient as strong and as healthy as possible, support his or her immune system, and reduce the side effects of the conventional cancer treatments. Our small group of participants did uniformly better than statistics would have predicted, some of them quite a bit better. We knew we were on the right track.

This observational experiment demonstrated that not only could we improve outcomes, but we could also remarkably reduce those tragic situations of patients who did much worse than predicted because their conventional treatments did not work as expected or because of improbable side effects, including infection.

Since those early days when alternative medicine was first being noticed by the world, I have taught many natural and conventional physicians how this science can be used to provide the best treatment for their patients. But most important is that every day I put these important principles into action.

As a consultant to many hospitals and cancer centers, I see many cancer survivors. All too often, however, I speak with patients and family members who themselves have been combining conventional oncology and natural medicine in the worst ways, often with poor results. They were unaware that some nutrients can interfere with certain conventional cancer treatments; that side effects can be made much worse; and that improperly combined techniques can actually introduce problems more serious than the cancer itself. What surprised me the most was that many of these patients and family members had done their best to act responsibly. They had read every book they could find and had even checked with their medical specialists.

It seemed that there should be at least one practical book that would explain these principles to ordinary people. I searched through no less than forty books about cancer and alternative medicine. Many of them were well-written and presented a great deal of valuable information. None, however, took the reader by the hand and led him or her through the jungle of difficult choices that faces someone with cancer. The vital principles of treatment combination were not discussed in a useful manner. In the end, I was unable to find even a single book that dealt with combining conventional oncology and natural medicine. I realized that if I wanted such a book, I would have to create it myself.

The prospect of writing such a comprehensive book seemed daunting, but each time I saw another patient who might have benefited from these principles, I moved a little closer to this undertaking. For me to make a real difference, I knew there was simply no other way to reach enough people.

A BOOK TO BRING YOU TO YOUR DESTINATION

I wanted to write a book for those people who wished to treat their cancer (or that of a loved one) using a well-coordinated combination of conventional medicine and natural therapies. Who better to tell me what this book should be like, I thought, than the very people who would use it? I asked many of my patients and their family members, and their responses were almost always the same. They wanted a single reference that would show them, step by step, how to make sound decisions quickly and effectively. They wanted to know how to select the best health care providers, both conventional and nonconventional, and they wanted to know how to decide on their particular treatments. They all recognized that they would do better with the support of qualified health care providers but didn't wish to rely solely on the decisions of others. Instead, the cancer patients and families I questioned all wanted some control over their own destinies.

Since many providers hadn't yet learned of this new science, the people I queried also wanted to understand the all-important principles of drug-nutrient combination. What was important, they told me, was that the book pay attention to diet, to lifestyle, and to environmental, emotional, psychological, and spiritual well-being.

This book, then, is the product of their wishes and of my own experiences in the exciting new field of complementary cancer therapies. I've included all the current technology and information that I believe can help you and your loved ones. I hope that this book will guide you through your survival of cancer to good health and happiness.

FOREWORD

In *Complementary Cancer Therapies,* Dan Labriola has written a book that attempts to bridge the gap between "conventional" and "alternative" medicine for the patient with cancer. As such, this volume meets a need that has not been successfully addressed elsewhere. Most of what is written in other books for the lay reader emphasizes one approach to the exclusion (and often denigration) of the other. Yet many who have recently received a diagnosis of this dreaded disease are actively searching for all available means to relieve their suffering, prolong their lives, and (if possible) achieve a cure. I am a "conventional" practitioner, but one who is well aware that his patients uses "alternative" therapies. If such therapies are to be employed, it is important to recognize that they have biological effects. Some may be helpful, others harmful. Harm is an especially likely consequence when one agent (e.g., an antioxidant) competes with another (e.g., alkylating agents, ionizing radiation) and decreases the antitumor efficacy of the latter.

Unfortunately, most forms of alternative therapy have not been subjected to rigorous testing by the scientific method. Incentives to do this have been lacking since there is little financial reward (these remedies are generally not patentable) and the agents employed are not regulated by the government like prescription drugs are. Such testing is, however, now under way, some of it sponsored by the federal government. As more information based on randomized trials become available, it should be possible for the cancer patient to make more intelligent choices about what, if any, alternative therapies to elect.

In the meantime, Dr. Labriola offers what information exists regarding the potential usefulness of the naturopath's armamentarium. He also provides pithy, readily understood summaries of how various cancers are staged and treated according to "conventional" approaches. The toxicities of the latter are well described, but fairly.

This volume can serve as a valuable reference for practitioners on both sides of the present fence. Most important, it should act as a resource and advisor for the perplexed patient or family member who is in between.

—**ROBERT B. LIVINGSTON, M.D.,** professor of medicine, University of Washington School of Medicine, and chief of the Division of Oncology, University of Washington Medical Center

The Best of Both Worlds

Discovering you have cancer is a terrible shock. One day you are carrying on with life as usual and then, after a few words from your doctor, everything changes. You suddenly find yourself on an emotional roller coaster. A woman who had cancer described it most eloquently. "It passes over me in horrible waves at unsuspecting moments," she said. "It fills me with panic and pain so overwhelming that I want to die just to make it stop." These feelings are not uncommon for someone who is battling cancer.

Even before the initial shock subsides, you realize that you must make some very important decisions—ones you do not feel prepared to make. You know that you must conquer this disease, but you don't know how. Your first step may be to visit a medical specialist such as an oncologist or a surgeon. It is here that you are told of the importance of MRIs, CAT scans, biopsies, and blood tests, just a few of the tools used to find out as much as possible about your particular situation. Depending on your particular diagnosis, you might receive recommendations for chemotherapy, surgery, radiation, or in some cases, no treatment at all.

You may not like the message, but the information-gathering process is fairly straightforward. Most competent, conventional cancer centers are fairly consistent in their recommendations and predictions. The system as a whole, however, seems to emphasize the negatives and to downplay any potential positives. Little of the medical jargon you hear is understandable, and even less of it brings you comfort.

Being told there is a 75% survival rate for treated individuals after five years does not leave you feeling reassured. You ask yourself "Who's in that 75% group?", "Why didn't the other 25% make it?", and "Which percentile group am I in?" And you want to know if there is anything you can do to improve your own chances, how you can get into that 75% group. Questions persist and the search for more satisfying answers is inevitable.

THE SEARCH FOR SOMETHING MORE

It might begin with a television report or a newspaper article. Or maybe a friend tells you about an herbal or vitamin cancer treatment. Of course, you're interested. The lure of an effective cancer cure is hard to resist. You look into it and find that numerous other herbs, vitamins, and enzymes are also recommended.

On the Internet, you find countless sites with claims of cancer cures that include detailed, plausible explanations and impressive lists of references and convincing testimonials. You wonder why your oncologist would offer only conventional treatments and neglect to tell you about a natural product that would be of benefit. Is it professional jealousy, greed, or some kind of conspiracy? Some people claim that conventional oncologists are suppressing cancer cures for financial reasons. Could this be true?

Conventional providers often support only mainstream medical treatments because they are unfamiliar with and thus suspicious of natural medicine.

The truth, however, is that conventional health care providers often support only mainstream medical treatments because they are unfamiliar with and thus suspicious of natural medicine. They may feel that alternative therapies are unproved, ineffective, or even dangerous. Natural medicine, after all, was not part of their medical school education. What you know for certain is that you are caught in the middle of a controversy.

WHAT NATURAL MEDICINE CAN DO FOR YOU

What you may not know is that many of modern medicine's successes are rooted in time-proven remedies derived from herbs and foods. In fact, the science of drugs and their actions, known as *pharmacology*, is actually based on herbal and natural remedies. For ages, natural medicines have accomplished the miracle of healing, and they continue to offer benefits that aren't available elsewhere. But what can these nonconventional therapies do for you in your battle with cancer?

As in the instance of Billy, the two-year-old with liver cancer whom I mentioned in the Introduction, natural medicine can pave the way for successful conventional therapies. Like Billy, many patients are unable to complete their chemotherapy or radiation treatments simply because they can't tolerate the difficult side effects. The careful and knowledgeable use of natural medicine can help alleviate these symptoms, making conventional treatment possible.

M any of modern medicine's successes are rooted in time-proven remedies derived from herbs and foods.

For example, in some people chemotherapy causes severe and dangerous diarrhea, which can be extremely difficult to control. Natural therapies can help control this problem and allow for the completion of the chemotherapy.

Nonconventional therapies can also help maintain a comfortable quality of life by reducing the physical discomforts caused by cancer, as well as by minimizing the side effects that result from conventional treatments. Some conventional therapies have toxic effects on the heart, liver, and kidneys that aren't noticeable until some time after the treatment. When used knowledgeably, nonconventional therapies can minimize or even prevent such damage altogether. And since many natural therapies have been shown to be valuable for the prevention of cancer, they may also be helpful in halting its further spread or recurrence.

GETTING THE BEST OF BOTH WORLDS

I've written this book to show how, with the cooperation of your oncologist and a natural medicine provider, you can make use of the best of both conventional and nonconventional therapies. I'll provide you with the tools necessary to build a health care team and to create a treatment strategy that delivers what *you* need in your fight against cancer. I'll show you how to avoid the pitfalls many cancer patients make when blindly combining conventional and natural treatments themselves. And I'll tell you what you can expect from modern medicine. You don't have to choose between conventional or natural medicine. You can get *the best of both worlds*.

Natural and conventional medicine each have much to offer in your fight against cancer. What is important is a careful coordination of both

When properly coordinated, nonconventional therapies can improve the results and reduce the adverse effects of conventional therapies.

regimens, one that is custom fit to your particular needs. When you carefully and knowledgeably combine the best that conventional and nonconventional medicine have to offer and do it with the help and supervision of experienced providers, you'll be rewarded with results that are greater than the sum of the two. Not only will these two allied specialties each do their intended work, but they also can strengthen each other. Properly coordinated, nonconventional therapies can improve the results and reduce the adverse effects of conventional therapies, while the conventional interventions can provide the time and opportunity for the gentler strategies of natural medicine to take effect.

SETTING YOUR GOALS

Deciding what you want is always the first step toward getting it, and setting attainable goals is a good way to begin. As you set your objectives, prioritize them. Decide which are the most important and which can be forfeited, if necessary. Here are some objectives worth pursuing during combined therapy:

- Allow conventional therapy to do the best job it can
- Improve tolerance for conventional therapy
- Improve quality of life
- Reduce adverse effects from conventional therapy
- Prevent metastases (the spread of cancer) or a recurrence
- Reduce symptoms caused by the cancer
- Attain a cure

As is the case for virtually all medical care, certain principles must be followed to produce the best results and to avoid creating additional problems. None of these principles is more important when dealing with cancer than to *avoid interfering with your conventional treatment.*

THE PRINCIPLE OF NONINTERFERENCE

Without question, conventional and nonconventional cancer therapies will interact in your body. Some of these interactions can be good ones, whereas others may not be. The last thing you want is for your combined therapies to interfere with each other, reducing the effectiveness of one or both. Finding treatments that won't interfere with each other must be done on an individual basis. Say that your coworker Joe has prostate cancer and is receiving radiation. The same herb that supports his cancer treatment might interfere with someone else's.

The most sensible way to begin your search for complementary cancer therapies is to discuss your situation with your conventional health care provider and to select the conventional therapy that best meets your needs. Then, working with your nonconventional provider, tailor your natural therapies to ensure that you get the best possible results from your conventional treatment while minimizing its harmful and discomforting side effects. By making the conventional treatment your priority, you allow it to eliminate as many tumor cells as possible with a minimum of toxicity, allowing your immune system to finish the job after conventional treatment has ended. This approach almost always makes the best sense, as long as the conventional therapy is working.

Whenever you make a decision about treatment combinations, you'll need to know whether or not the combination can limit your conventional therapy's ability to work effectively. The most common mistake made during combined cancer treatments is to assume that because the tumor is shrinking, you have not interfered with the conventional treatment. Except in very rare cases, it is important to carefully avoid interfering with the actions of your conventional treatment.

THE PROTECTED ZONE

Many outside factors can interfere with a conventional therapy. When this happens, the effectiveness of the treatment and final outcome may suffer. Throughout this book you will be advised not to use nonconventional medicines during the *protected zone*. The protected zone is that time period and that part of your body where your conventional treatment does its work.

The protected zone can vary from one particular organ to the entire body. The protected zone can last for hours to months, depending on the particular drug or procedure, dosage, other drugs or treatments being used, and the patient's overall condition. The protected zone also includes those times when a patient is most vulnerable to infection and other side effects.

For example, the protected zone for radiation therapy at a lumpectomy site is the local area of treatment,

The protected zone is that time period and that part of your body where your conventional treatment does its work.

for the duration of time that the radiation is actively killing tumor cells. Similarly, the protected zone for chemotherapy would be anywhere that small tumor molecules may have traveled and the length of time that the drug is killing the malignant cells. For example, the protected zone for the alkylating agent cisplatin might range from several hours to fifty days, depending on a variety of circumstances.

To be certain to avoid the protected zone, your health care providers must take into account the pharmacological actions of vitamins and minerals, the conventional procedures being used, and other nonconventional treatments used prior to your conventional treatment. As you can see, the protected zone for a particular conventional treatment is not something that you should estimate yourself, but rather it is a complex calculation requiring the expertise and clinical judgment of a physician, an oncology pharmacist, or another provider who has training in this specialized area.

HOW NATURAL AND CONVENTIONAL MEDICINES INTERACT

The correct combination of conventional and nonconventional therapies requires knowledge about the actions of both. Each type of treatment has its own individual characteristics. While some of the material I will discuss in this book may seem technical, it is important that you have at least a basic understanding of these interactions before you move on to matching your diagnosis and conventional treatment with useful alternative medicines. *I want to stress again the importance of following these procedures under the care and supervision of both a conventional and an alternative health care provider.*

When combining therapies, there are four principles for avoiding undesirable interactions:

- Use combinations that do not compete for absorption.
- Use combinations that do not interfere with the tumor-killing actions of conventional therapies.
- Use combinations that do not add combined stress to processing and elimination organs.
- Use combinations that do not add risk for complications.

Preventing Absorption Problems

Whenever you take a drug, vitamin, herb, or food by mouth, it is processed by enzymes in your digestive tract and then transported to your bloodstream. The digestive process, which involves breaking down the substance into very small particles, is necessary before the substance can get into your bloodstream. If this does not happen at precisely the right place in your digestive tract, the substance will not be absorbed but will instead pass through the body and be excreted.

The body's processing and absorption mechanisms are limited. The body can only absorb so much of a particular drug or nutrient at one time. In addition, absorption of some substances can be blocked by others. If you take two substances in the same period of time, for example, and those substances use the same enzymes or transport mechanism for absorption, they may be only partly absorbed, or perhaps they may not be absorbed at all. Depending on the drug, nutrient, and specific circumstances of the individual, this period of time can range from a few hours to a week or more.

When combining therapies, some natural treatments may interfere with the absorption of certain drugs. Such interference is possible with literally any drug that is taken orally, but some drugs are more vulnerable to this interference than others. One such example is melphalan, a chemotherapy drug used to treat a variety of cancers. The chemical structure of melphalan looks a lot like the amino acid phenylalanine. Phenylalanine is found in all protein foods and diet drinks and also in many nutritional supplements. When phenylalanine and melphalan are taken in the same time period, they compete for the same absorption mechanisms. The result can be interference of the absorption of melphalan and a disruption of the chemotherapy treatment. In effect, the phenylalanine-containing food or supplement can actually replace the drug in your body. This is why it's essential to follow your provider's instructions regarding diet and supplements during the protected zone.

Avoiding Interfering with Antitumor Actions

Our knowledge of natural medicines is growing rapidly and includes an increasing awareness of their chemical and pharmacological actions. Although our total understanding of the technical mechanisms of natural medicines is not as complete as our knowledge of conventional pharmaceuticals, it does contain much useful science that we can apply.

When radiation or chemotherapy is used in the treatment of cancer, the objective is to destroy as many tumor cells as possible. When there is good tumor response to the treatment—in other words, when the treatment is effectively killing tumor cells—the percentage of tumor cells destroyed can be very high. It may be as high as 99.99999%, but it is rarely 100%. A few tumor cells usually survive the treatment. If the conventional treatment destroys enough tumor cells, it is hoped that the remaining few will then be destroyed by your body's immune system. In some cases, however, the remaining cells can reproduce in a form that has become resistant to the conventional treatment, thus creating a recurrence. It is therefore very important that chemotherapy treatments destroy as many tumor cells as possible.

Many nonconventional therapies have actions that are exactly opposite those of certain conventional treatments and can potentially interfere with the conventional treatment's ability to destroy the maximum number of tumor cells. Unfortunately, no direct warning signs occur when this happens. In fact, if this was happening to you, you might even feel better than expected during treatment, and the short-term result, from months to five years or more, might look better because of the positive effects of the nonconventional treatment. Over the long term, however, the additional remaining tumor cells left over from an interfered-with treatment could result in a recurrence.

For example, the antitumor antibiotic doxorubicin (Adriamycin) destroys tumor cells by creating substances known as free radicals. These substances damage the DNA of the tumor cells and thus interfere with the tumor's ability to survive and reproduce. Free radicals not only attack the known tumor mass but also go after free-floating cancer cells known as *micrometastases* that years later could begin growing and multiplying into a new tumor in a new location. Antioxidant supplements are generally considered to be a positive nutritional strategy with some anticancer actions. However, the use of high levels of dietary antioxidants during chemotherapy can destroy some of Adriamycin's tumor-killing free radicals and thus interfere with the drug's ability to kill the maximum number of micrometastases.

When combining therapies, health care providers must be certain that they are not interfering with the tumor-destroying action of the conventional treatment.

Controlling Stress on Processing and Elimination Organs

Most drugs are processed and eliminated by the liver, the kidneys, or both. As this process occurs, the cells and chemicals in these organs undergo stress. In some cases, this happens to such an extent that the health and function of the organs can be threatened. Conventional physicians commonly monitor the liver and kidneys with blood tests so that they can reduce or withhold treatment if the stress level gets dangerously high.

Many nonconventional treatments can also stress the kidneys and liver. Natural treatments that are normally very supportive can have surprisingly negative effects when they stress an already-compromised body system.

Vitamin A is a good example. Normally a supportive nutrient, in high doses, especially in combination with certain drugs or prior liver damage, it can be toxic to the liver and reduce white blood cell production. This brings about increased stress on the liver and suppression of the immune system, possibly resulting in both the discontinuation of chemotherapy treatment as well as undesirable side effects.

When combining therapies, it is vital that the conventional and nonconventional treatments are not adding unbearable stress to organ systems.

Reducing Risk of Complications

Both conventional and nonconventional therapies have side effects and risks. With proper treatment, these risks can be kept at acceptably low levels. Risks associated with surgical procedures include excessive bleeding, infection, and poor healing. Infection from immune suppression is a concern with chemotherapy. Excessive fatigue, depression, and other symptoms can result from both chemotherapy and radiation. While these can be serious side effects, modern technology and competent providers can help limit them.

Both conventional and nonconventional therapies have side effects and risks. With proper treatment, these risks can be kept at acceptably low levels.

Certain botanicals and other nutrients, including aspirin (originally derived from the bark of the white willow tree) can reduce the blood's tendency to clot. This may be fine if you're trying to avoid heart disease, but using aspirin is dangerous if you're having surgery.

The use of nonsterile creams to heal surgical scars can increase the risk of infection and even interfere with healing. When applied in the area of a surgically implanted access port, as used for a patient receiving chemotherapy, nonsterile creams can result in a serious infection.

Nonconventional therapies are usually not sterile (that is, free from all germs such as bacteria, fungus, parasites, and viruses), and most are not effectively screened for potential pathogens (germs that can cause infection). No government agency, not even the U.S. Food and Drug

Administration, systematically checks these products for microbial (germ) safety. For people with normal immune function, this usually is not a problem. People have been eating foods and using plants and other traditional medicines safely for many years.

The situation changes, however, when certain conventional cancer therapies weaken your immune system. This vital system protects you from infection, and impairment of it can make you more vulnerable to infection. With some cancers, the disease itself can further increase your vulnerability to infection. During certain cancer treatments, germs that may not have been a problem under normal circumstances can overwhelm your weakened immune system.

If an infection does occur, it can usually be controlled with modern antibiotics. Your conventional medical specialist will provide a list of sanitary practices, which will do a lot to minimize these risks.

Sadly, there are verified cases in which nutritional supplements have caused overwhelming infections. If you have recently undergone chemotherapy and your immune system has been weakened, you simply cannot assume that all nutritional supplements are safe.

In many instances, nonconventional therapies can increase the risk for complications with conventional treatments. It is important to use only combinations that will not increase side effects and to avoid those about which we have inadequate information. Relying on the skills and experience of a qualified nonconventional provider will optimize the results of your conventional treatment.

Feeling overwhelmed? Don't worry. The next chapter will provide you with a basic tool kit for obtaining an overall cancer treatment that will take into account your physical, emotional, and spiritual well-being. It really is possible to get the best of both worlds.

2

A Basic Tool Kit

John, a self-employed welder, was diagnosed with prostate cancer a month before his daughter's wedding. Normally an independent, do-it-yourself kind of guy, John began having a difficult time juggling doctor appointments, finances, wedding plans, and work. He began experiencing anxiety attacks, a real shock for a man who had always prided himself on being tough and invulnerable. For the first time that he could remember, his life seemed to be spinning out of control.

For someone facing cancer, John's situation is not unusual. The implications of a cancer diagnosis are, to say the least, a distraction. The problems and situations that John might have been able to deal with effortlessly before the diagnosis now seemed to pile stress on top of confusion.

If you, like John, are finding that dealing with cancer and the everyday decisions of life is leaving you feeling overwhelmed, it is time to take a deep breath, take a few steps back, and look over your situation carefully. It's time to get organized.

If you're wondering just how this is going to happen, I offer this chapter as a basic tool kit. You aren't the first person to be in your situation, and you won't be the last. You can learn from those who have gone before you by taking things one small step at a time.

This chapter will provide you with some basic tools to help you survive your battle with cancer: how to make decisions, how to get a second opinion, what the various medical tests are and what they mean, and some general tips to help you along the path toward your goals.

THE DECISION-MAKING PROCESS

Life has its share of difficult decisions but these days things may seem worse than usual. What is important and what is not? How do you decide between treatments? How do you know whose advice to listen to? With each question, you find dramatically opposing opinions. What is the truth and what isn't? How can you sort it all out?

You have so many decisions to make you don't know where to begin. Some are simple while others are so difficult that you may feel as though you'll never make the right choice. Everyone offers advice, but only rarely does it help you make up your mind. Family, friends, the media, books, health food stores, the Internet, and coworkers all have an opinion about what you should do. While much of this advice is well-intentioned, it's also often incomplete, inaccurate, conflicting, or simply not applicable. Whether the question is choosing chemotherapy or shark cartilage, you can find dramatically opposite opinions, each with *credible* supporters and *proof,* and you are expected to decide which is right for you.

As if this weren't enough to deal with, this isn't your best time for making complex, difficult decisions. The implications of your diagnosis and treatment have added a new, distracting burden to your decision-making processes. Problems that you might ordinarily solve without much stress or strain are now competing with all the extra activities and considerations in your life.

Consider, for example, the Internet. If you type in *cancer* and *alternative medicine* you will find tens of thousands of sites. I often scroll through the results and visit some sites that look interesting, and the result is always the same. I find claims for cures that are simply not true, advice that is inaccurate, and promises that could never be kept, often at great costs to the patient, financial and otherwise. I rarely find more than one believable site for every twenty that I visit. What distresses me even more is that many of these offerings have the potential to worsen rather than improve the patient's condition. So, how does one get through this maze of promises, choosing the best answer in a reasonable length of time with confidence and without the remorse that comes with having made an important deci-

> Whether the question is choosing chemotherapy or shark cartilage, you can find dramatically opposite opinions, each with *credible* supporters and *proof.*

sion about which you are uncertain? The answer is to adopt and use a decision-making process that takes the emotions and distractions out of the process, allowing you to spend your energy instead on the solution. During those vulnerable times when you feel that you can only operate on autopilot, you need a guide that will take you to the right place without having to agonize over every step.

If you take the time to learn this process, and the time to use it, you'll be able to regain a sense of control over your life.

Three Easy Steps for Making Decisions

Using this technique for making decisions will provide you with a basic survival tool. The decision-making process has three simple steps:

1. Defining the problem
2. Deciding on objectives
3. Evaluating potential solutions

Each of these steps seems simple enough, perhaps even obvious. But taken one at a time and done deliberately, they will help considerably. You'll get a much clearer picture of your situation, be able to exercise decision making when you need it, and be able to make decisions that you will feel confident about and comfortable with. Once you get started with this simple process, decision making will become second nature to you.

An Important Tip: Write It All Down

A useful tip in applying this technique is to use pen and paper to write down all of the important factors. Make a list of the problems that face you, what you wish to achieve, and those possible ways to reach your goals. Things will look clearer and seem more objective once you get them down on paper.

Step One: Defining the Problem

This first step will provide the clarity you need to move on to the next steps. By clearly identifying the challenge, you will make the solution (or solutions) more accessible. In order to make good decisions, you need to start with a reliable evaluation of the problem.

If you were crossing a mountain range, you'd want an accurate map of where you were going. It's that simple. Without a clear picture of the challenges that face you, you will feel lost.

Once you've made your list, look it over and then list everything again in order of importance: which problems need to be dealt with soonest, which bother you the most, and so forth. It's what is important to you that matters. Start with your highest priorities at the top of the page and work your way down to your lowest.

Step Two: Deciding on Objectives

An objective is your final goal, the outcome you wish to reach. Now that you've made a list of the problems that face you and set your priorities with them, it is time to describe your objectives for each challenge. If your first objective is not immediately obtainable, list some intermediate goals as well. If you are making decisions about cancer, your final goal may be a cure. A good intermediate objective might be remission. Other intermediate goals could be tumor response (either stops growing or shrinks) with treatment, maintaining good nutrition, strengthening the immune system, controlling hot flashes, etc.

Don't limit yourself. Your objectives can be anything you choose. They are what you want, not what others say is possible. Include both objectives that are easily achieved as well as those in your heart even though other people may not understand or agree. Keep in mind that this is a living, adaptable process where you can add or subtract objectives at any time without asking anyone's permission. You can put this powerful process to work on any subject you choose.

Your highest objectives help you to remember that all things are possible. Some are more difficult to achieve than others, but no one has the right to take away your hope. While most of us in health care must deal with stark statistics and communicate with you in ways prescribed by insurance companies and lawyers, this doesn't mean that you can't reach for the brass ring. Wonderful, unexplainable events occur every day and there's no reason why you shouldn't experience one of them. So let your heart soar; take your best shot. Reach for the stars.

You can't always reach your highest goals immediately. Intermediate objectives are important because they give you more immediately attainable goals as well as force you to recognize that there is more than one useful objective. Even Sammy Sosa can't hit a home run every time at bat. Many times getting on first base is the best way to start the journey to home plate. List all of the positive goals you wish, both large and small.

Once you've completed your list of objectives, prioritize them again in order of time (that is, what can be accomplished first), not importance.

You will still be addressing all of your objectives, but in this way you can deal with first things first.

Step Three: Evaluating Potential Solutions

The solution is the way you choose to reach the goals you've set for yourself. Evaluating the potential solutions means examining every possible means for achieving your objectives. If you are dealing with cancer, you aren't limited to the proven solutions. A potential solution can be a drug, an herb, an enzyme, or anything else that could possibly help.

Potential solutions are available from many sources. In dealing with cancer, consult with both your conventional and nonconventional providers. Look over both chapter 4 and chapter 8. If your challenge is not medical, try contacting an expert. If the issue is financial, perhaps the hospital social worker can help. When looking for potential solutions, it is wise to draw on the wealth of experience of experts.

At our first visit, John the welder and I discussed the decision-making process. He went home and that evening he made a prioritized list of what challenges he thought confronted him. Two weeks later, he returned to my office and told me that his life seemed once again in order. His anxiety attacks had stopped and he felt some sense of control.

Most of the problems, he told me, were still there. Now, however, he at least had a plan for each situation. Every time something changed, he would take out his sheet of paper and redefine the challenges, the objectives, and the solutions. He had learned that decision making is a living and adaptable process, one that changes as life goes on. Eventually, he resolved all the problems on his original list, and he now concentrates on a newer, much shorter one.

GETTING A SECOND OPINION

Mrs. B., a pleasant forty-year-old woman living in Europe, contacted my office to investigate the benefits of natural medicine prior to and during her upcoming cancer surgery. She told me how she was scheduled to undergo a complete hysterectomy for ovarian cancer, followed by a bilateral mastectomy (removal of both breasts) as a preventive measure against further cancer.

Her diagnosis and treatment plan came from a well-recognized cancer center but, when we reviewed her records, our clinic was not completely convinced that adequate diagnostic studies had been done to conclusively determine ovarian cancer.

I discussed my feelings with her and we arranged for an outstanding Seattle surgeon to conduct additional tests, so that we could fully understand the diagnosis. A few days prior to her planned surgery, she flew to Seattle and spent two days at a local hospital.

The tests showed, without a doubt, that Mrs. B. had ovarian cysts, not ovarian cancer. Of course, she was very happy that she would not be needing the operations. Without this second opinion, though, she may well have undergone both unnecessary surgery and months of recovery.

Why a Second Opinion?

While most stories may not end as dramatically as Mrs. B.'s, a second opinion is necessary for more reasons than simply to confirm whether or not you really have cancer.

One of the most important benefits of a second opinion is to provide you with the assurance and peace of mind that you are proceeding on the right path, the one that you must take. This journey is best made unencumbered by doubts.

Another important benefit is to ensure that you have undergone all the tests necessary to provide an accurate diagnosis. Getting the most information will provide the best diagnosis, which in turn will provide the most appropriate course of treatment.

One of the most important benefits of a second opinion is to provide you with the assurance that you are proceeding on the right path.

Second opinions are an accepted part of modern medicine. Even the most difficult insurance company will normally pay for one. Despite the fact that conventional diagnosis of cancer is improving at an amazing rate, errors still occasionally occur. Diagnostic procedures such as MRIs, CAT scans, ultrasounds, and even routine lab work all depend on technicians to perform them correctly and specialists to interpret them accurately. Even automated diagnostics, such as blood tests, depend on numerous factors to ensure accurate results: proper collection of blood specimens, adequate storage of samples, and calibration of complex equipment are just a few. The health care system, despite being under the great financial pressures of managed care, is accurate most of the time, but it is not perfect.

Even a partially correct diagnosis can lead to significant problems. Consider some of the possibilities:

Despite the fact that conventional diagnosis is improving at an amazing rate, errors still occasionally occur.

- If the diagnosis is correct but the staging of your cancer is incorrect, this could result in less-than-optimum treatment. In other words, if an improper diagnosis tells your conventional provider that your disease is in one stage and it is in another, you may be given the wrong treatment altogether.
- If the diagnosis is incomplete or lacking relevant (but available) information, such as tumor markers, this too could lead to an incorrect or ineffective treatment plan.
- If the diagnosis incorrectly tells you that you do not have cancer when you do, you may inadvertently be ignoring a problem now that will be significantly more difficult to deal with later.

How to Get a Second Opinion

A referral from your primary care provider (your family doctor) would be an excellent way to get a second opinion. Friends, family, even colleagues may be helpful as well. Other sources include your local medical association, your local oncology association, and such help groups as Cancer Lifeline.

Ideally, the specialist who will provide you with a second opinion should have the following qualifications:

1. Training, skill, and experience in what you believe is your diagnosis. The physician needs to understand and have access to all of the available diagnostic tools, test research data, and other specialists in order to confirm or disagree with your diagnosis.
2. Willingness to review your case in a reasonable period of time. If you have to wait a few weeks for the right person, that may be fine. But waiting four to six weeks is too long for you to be less than 100% certain.
3. Willingness to spend time with you and answer your questions. You may need an hour or two of quality time with this physician to be satisfied with your understanding of the results of your tests and their implications. You may also wish to ensure the availability of this physician if other questions arise.
4. Independence from your principal oncologist. Your second opinion should not come from someone in the same group as your

oncologist. It may even be worthwhile to travel to another town to seek your second opinion.

Once you've gotten some recommendations, make a list of the names and check them against the four qualifications above. If you are left with more than one name on your list, make an appointment to speak to each of them, either in person or by telephone, to determine with whom you feel most comfortable. Plan your questions ahead of time and be brief. Most physicians are very busy.

After you have chosen an oncologist for a second opinion, discuss the basis of the original diagnosis at your first meeting and determine which records will be needed from your primary oncologist. If you wish certain tests to be repeated, this is the time to make your feelings clear. If you are not comfortable with your prior diagnosis, try to articulate why you feel this way. Your gut feelings are important.

Y our gut feelings are important.

You don't have to speak medical language to communicate with the physician, but the more you try to define the physical twinges or doubts that are troubling you, the better the chance the physician will have to confirm them and make you a satisfied customer.

After getting your second opinion, you should feel satisfied that you know precisely what kind of problem you are dealing with. If you still have doubts or questions, talk with the physician again for clarification.

Be sure that you are asking the right questions. If men are from Mars and women from Venus, then some oncologists can be from Pluto. Perhaps the physician simply doesn't understand your question. It may be worth asking a friend, your primary oncologist, or your family doctor if the questions are clear to them.

If you remain unsatisfied with your second opinion, you may need to consider a third or even fourth opinion. It is rare, however, to need more than one confirming opinion.

Getting Satisfaction

You'll know when you have the right answer. When you, your principle oncologist, and your second opinion all agree, you should feel confident that you have the best information available. If you, personally, can't agree or accept the diagnosis, this needs to be resolved before you take any irrevocable steps. If you suspect that your disbelief may be linked to your own denial, you need to address this as well. It is very important that you believe your diagnosis is accurate without lingering doubts.

A GUIDE TO UNDERSTANDING COMMON DIAGNOSTIC TESTS

In many ways, a trip to the hospital is like a trip to another country: it's very expensive and everybody there seems to be speaking a foreign language. It's easy for health care workers to assume that everyone understands the most basic medical terminology. But the truth is that not everyone knows what an IV is, or what a catheter does, or what *invasive procedure* means.

It is not only helpful but necessary to have a basic knowledge of some of the diagnostic tests that you may already have had or will have in the future. For additional information and terminology, see the glossary at the end of this book.

The Basic Tests

Initial diagnosis is usually from such diagnostic screening procedures as X rays (also known as radiography), various examinations of the blood, a physical exam, and often, a scoping procedure—a process whereby the physician inserts a viewing device through a small incision to gather information visually.

In cancer, a final diagnosis is usually made by examining the actual cells of a mass. This is usually the result of some form of biopsy procedure.

Radiography

Radiographs include X rays of every sort, including mammograms, as well as the more sophisticated techniques such as ultrasound, CAT and PET scans, and MRI. Although these studies all produce an image that provides a good look *inside* you, the information they give is not always conclusive.

Each radiographic technique has specific advantages and disadvantages, depending on where the suspected tumor is and what type it may be. It takes a skilled radiologist to select the correct method and to interpret the results properly.

In general, radiography does not provide absolute diagnosis but, in some cases, it can provide enough information to make a presumptive diagnosis.

CAT SCAN

Short for computerized axial tomography, this technique produces a series of X rays, taken at different angles, that provide the skilled interpreter with a three-dimensional view of the body, its contents, and any abnormal structures present. The advantage of a CAT scan is that it can show the shape and general dimensions of a suspicious mass from any angle.

PET SCAN

PET scan is short for positron emission tomography. It observes gamma rays emitted by the body following an administration of a chemical substance known as an isotope. Physicians use these scans to detect solid objects, such as tumors. Often, PET scans provide information that's different, and sometimes better, than that provided by CATs or MRIs.

MRI

This radiographic technique, known as magnetic resonance imaging, creates a magnetic field in the body and then measures how your body parts disrupt that field just as a magnet causes metal shavings to align at its poles. The MRI technology uses a powerful computer and an elaborate display system to convert this data into a meaningful report about what is going on inside your body.

ULTRASOUND

This technique operates on the principle that sound reflects off solid objects. Since sound bounces off different substances in different ways, ultrasound can provide a real-time picture of what is happening inside your body.

Blood Tests

The general screening of blood can reveal an amazing number of things, and, in some instances, it can even suggest a diagnosis. The most common screening tests of the blood include hematology and blood chemistries. Hematology examines white blood cells, red blood cells, and platelets. Blood chemistries look at a variety of enzymes, hormones, and other biochemicals present in the blood.

Blood tests also include checking for circulating tumor markers, which are biological substances that are either produced by a tumor or produced by the body in response to a tumor. Only in some cases can elevated tumor markers suggest a cancer diagnosis. On occasion, they may also indicate a statistical genetic increase in vulnerability to a particular kind of cancer and even a relative measure of the progress of the disease. Both tumor-marker and genetic research are rapidly evolving and promise to provide increasingly accurate guidelines in diagnosis and in treatment selection.

Tumor Grade

Tumor grade is an indication of how fast a tumor grows. The grade is given from a biopsy test. The lower the grade, the slower the growth. Variations in grade will often determine treatment options.

Lymph Node Biopsy

The lymph system serves to remove bacteria and certain proteins from tissues. When microscopic tumor cells leave the primary tumor, they are often trapped in the lymph nodes, which act much like filters.

A biopsy means the obtaining of a tissue sample for analysis and diagnosis. This can be done either surgically or with a needle. A lymph node biopsy will indicate whether or not the primary tumor has spread into the lymphatic system.

> Lymph node involvement does not determine whether the tumor has spread beyond the nodes.

With certain kinds of tumors, the lack of lymph node involvement (often referred to as nodes negative) indicates that tumor spread is either minimal or nonexistent. Positive lymph nodes, on the other hand, indicate that cancer cells have reached the lymph nodes and have, therefore, left the primary site.

Lymph node involvement does not, however, determine whether the tumor has spread beyond the nodes. Metastatic spread (beyond the lymph nodes) can be estimated, based on the number of nodes involved and the tumor grade. Conclusive evidence, however, usually depends on finding a distant metastatic site.

Flow Cytometry

Flow cytometry, a powerful diagnostic tool that uses laser, examines individual cells as they pass through a complex detector system. This technique has many clinical and research applications. Through a series of detailed individual measurements, flow cytometry can determine how cancer cells reproduce and act, thus allowing more accurate prediction of how the cancer cells will respond to treatment.

Understanding Your Basic Tests

Diagnostic tests often mean different things under different conditions. This introduction to oncological diagnostics should give you the basic tools needed to understand what the tests are about. Remember that the most current and the most accurate data about your specific tests can be had by simply asking either your physician or the laboratory.

MISCELLANEOUS TIPS TO HELP YOU REACH YOUR GOALS

Here are a couple of suggestions that should help you along the path to successful treatment and recovery.

Keep a Journal

I cannot emphasize enough how important it is to be able to recognize and identify what is happening to you during the course of your disease. Being able to clearly communicate your symptoms, your pains and discomforts, and your feelings to your providers is a necessary step in getting the best care available.

I suggest that you keep a day-to-day journal. Take a few minutes, preferably at the same time each day, to review in your mind what has happened to you. Did you experience any discomfort or pain? Any new symptoms? How did you feel about yourself and about what is happening to you? Take a few minutes to reflect and I'm certain you'll know what is important to write down.

Just taking a few moments for this reflection will itself keep you in closer touch with your disease process and provide you with information to relate to your providers. In the decision-making process, you learned how important it is to identify the problem before finding a solution. Keeping a journal will be a real help with this process. It will keep you in touch with what is happening to you as well as with your own feelings, thoughts, and needs.

Read Your Own Diagnostic Reports

This can be an important step toward gaining control. There are several reasons to read your own medical records. First, you'll want to be certain that what the medical reports say is consistent with what you understand about your situation. Second, you'll want to be certain that your medical report is complete. And third, you'll want to know that you agree with the conclusions reached by your providers. This is your opportunity to understand your oncologist's assessment of your condition as well as the basis for his or her treatment recommendations. You don't have to become an accomplished diagnostician to benefit from this information. You simply want to ensure that the data is complete and that it has been properly interpreted for you.

Many people avoid reading their own medical report because they are afraid that it will upset them or perhaps because they think they won't understand the information. If you need to, find someone to read the information for you. Don't be daunted by the language. The glossary at the end of this book should help you to understand much of the terminology. If you need additional information or interpretation, ask your oncologist, his or her staff, or your primary physician, or try the local library and such books as *Taber's Cyclopedic Medical Dictionary.*

Keep notes about your diagnostic studies. Take special care to record what seems contradictory or confusing to you and ask for clarification. Make certain that you understand not only the tests but the reasons for them. If this is not explained in the report, ask your provider.

Knowing as much as possible about what is happening to you will help you to participate in your own care in a much more active way. Knowledge will help you to make better decisions and, in the end, will provide confidence and peace of mind.

A Guide to Choosing Your Health Care Providers

O ne patient who was new to my office was also being treated by an oncologist whom I had not previously met. After my first meeting with the patient and a review of her records, I needed additional technical information, so I called Dr. J. He returned my call shortly, gave me the data I had requested, and then invited me to lunch. This was an especially unusual event since the doctor offered to treat. He asked if he could bring his oncology nurse to the meeting, and I agreed.

Both Dr. J. and nurse Julie ordered the vegetarian entree (for my benefit) and then proceeded to ask me about the practice protocols at my clinic. Since neither of them had any experience with natural medicine, they were concerned about what people under their care might be doing outside the safety net of their treatment center. An hour later, I had taken only two bites of my food, having spent the remainder of meal answering detailed questions about drug–nutrient interactions, microbial risks, pharmacology, various natural substances, and research studies. The lunch was cordial and respectful. They had done their homework well. As we left the restaurant, Dr. J. politely apologized for having so many questions.

As I told Dr. J., our lunch meeting was as good as it gets. This physician was advocating for the person under his care and wanted to be absolutely certain that nothing could happen to interfere with the very best his team could do. He was not negative. He simply could not, in his heart, accept on face value issues that were critical to his patient's outcome without having some firsthand knowledge that the alternative care was being done correctly and safely. Since that meeting I have seen many patients in conjunction with Dr. J. and nurse Julie. I remain impressed with the skill and care they provide for each of their patients.

ASSEMBLING YOUR TEAM OF HEALTH CARE PROVIDERS

Not all providers are created equal, and it's not simply a matter of education and training. Other factors are at work. These include experience and personality, as well as a willingness to listen to patients. How well your health care providers are able to include *your personal goals* into their treatment plans will determine how satisfied you'll be with the care you receive.

Most people spend more time shopping for a new car than they do picking their doctors.

The unfortunate truth about selecting caregivers is that most people spend more time shopping for a new car than they do picking their doctors. Many people don't even realize that they are able to "shop around" for a health care provider.

Selecting providers who are willing and able to work together to provide the kind of care that *you* want is one of the most significant steps in your battle with cancer as well as essential to your general health and well-being. This chapter, then, is designed to help you understand how to pick both your conventional and alternative medicine providers—what to look for and how to ensure that your health care team meets *your* needs.

CHOOSING A CONVENTIONAL MEDICAL SPECIALIST

It's important to have a conventional medical specialist, such as an oncologist, on your team. Such a specialist can provide sophisticated diagnostics that can keep you informed about how well you are doing, as well as information about the latest available medical treatments. But what kind of specialists do you need and how are you going to determine which are the ones for you?

The Kinds of Medical Specialists You May Need

During the course of your cancer treatment you will probably consult with at least one medical specialist. The most common are:

Medical Oncologist

An *oncologist* is a physician who provides the broadest of medical services in the treatment of cancer, a sort of general practitioner of cancer care. Oncologists are usually best known for delivering chemotherapy treatments, but their care will almost certainly include ordering (or referring you for) a variety of important diagnostic tests and procedures.

Oncologists are usually also *hematologists,* physicians who deal with the study and treatment of blood disorders. This is particularly important for two reasons. First, many cancers, such as leukemia, are cancers of the blood. Second, chemotherapy, one of the most common conventional cancer treatments, has significant effects on your blood cells. Knowledge and experience in dealing with blood and blood disorders is an important part of being an oncologist.

Medical oncologists are well-connected with the other medical specialists and facilities you may need. They can help you plan treatment strategies and quickly put you in touch with the experts. Just as a quarterback calls the plays in football, your medical oncologist can assist you in making the best decisions and then implementing them.

Always, always, always have a medical oncologist on your team.

Some oncologists further specialize in more specific areas. You may find an oncologist whose specialty is breast cancer, or another who concentrates on cancers of the nervous system.

When dealing with cancer, always, always, *always* have a medical oncologist on your team. Even if you are not considering chemotherapy, the medical oncologist has the diagnostic tools, specialty contacts, and training to help you quarterback your plan with nearly every kind of cancer diagnosis.

Surgeon

A *surgeon* is a physician who is trained not only to repair and remove diseased and damaged body parts, but also to perform diagnostic procedures such as biopsies. Many surgical specialties and sub-specialties exist, such as neurosurgery; ear, nose, and throat; and colorectal surgery. Virtually every part of the human body has its surgical specialist.

Radiation Oncologist

Radiation therapy has become so technological and complex that it is now a separate specialty. *Radiation oncologists* provide radiation therapy for killing tumor cells by using a number of procedures that include a variety of external beams as well as implants.

Qualities to Look for in a Conventional Medical Specialist

In order to get the kind of treatment that you need, it helps to know what to look for in a doctor. The following are some of the most important qualities to seek in your medical specialist.

GOOD COMMUNICATION SKILLS

Everyone has his or her own way of giving and receiving information. Under the best of conditions, communication style, demeanor, body language, attitude, and all the other elements of interpersonal communication can make the difference between an effective exchange of information and no communication at all. Communication with medical specialists is made even more challenging because this information has a strong emotional component for you. What's more, the information undoubtedly concerns technology and language you may be unfamiliar with, and the modern world of managed care has a limited amount of time available for this communication to take place. If you are to effectively receive information from your conventional provider, that person must be a good "communication fit" for you. He or she must be able to reach you, must use language that is meaningful to you, and must present it in such a way that it does not unnecessarily generate new challenges and emotions.

EXPERIENCE AND SKILL WITH YOUR PARTICULAR DIAGNOSIS

The explosion of research and information has made it impossible for a medical specialist to be an expert in all kinds of cancers. Even though many treatment protocols for specific diagnoses are standardized, you'll still need that element of clinical judgment from a physician who is experienced with *your particular diagnosis* to ensure that you are getting the absolute best advice. If your diagnosis is a rare one, at the minimum you want a doctor who has access to all of the latest information and to other physicians and researchers who may have more experience.

CONNECTIONS WITH THE REST OF THE RESEARCH WORLD

You don't want to miss a new potential treatment or research protocol if it suggests a better result for you. Your medical specialist needs more than a subscription to computer databases. A relationship with a major research facility, such as a university or specialty facility, is an important link to what is happening currently. The medical oncology network of research and advanced treatment facilities makes this possible for both urban and rural medical specialists, but not all medical specialists are connected equally.

WILLINGNESS TO COOPERATE WITH YOUR GOALS

If you have made a rational decision to use minimum treatment (or maximum treatment, for that matter), your medical specialist must be comfortable working with you. This does not mean that you should look for a physician whom you can walk all over, someone who simply agrees with everything you say and do. You are paying to hear the truth and to reap the benefit of many years of medical training and practice. If there is new or contrary information, you want to hear it.

Once you've made an informed decision about your treatment, however, you need the support of a conventional provider who will do his or her level best to help you reach your goal. Regardless of your decisions, once you've made your choices you shouldn't have to constantly deal with philosophical resistance.

If you plan to integrate alternative therapies into your treatment plan, you must be able to discuss these freely and completely with your conventional provider.

WILLINGNESS TO INTEGRATE NONCONVENTIONAL MEDICINE

Most conventional providers have little or no training in alternative medicine, but that's okay. If your conventional physician is skeptical about alternative medicine, that's also fine. You aren't seeing this physician for alternative treatments. If you plan to integrate alternative therapies into your treatment plan, however, you must be able to discuss these freely, completely, and openly with your conventional provider.

If your conventional physician has genuine concerns about the safety or sensibility of something you are doing, you need to hear that message. But if your physician is consistently negative about your desire to use alternative medicine, without giving specific reasons, it may be difficult for you to tell the difference between that negativity and an important warning.

The Ideal Conventional Provider

The story of Dr. J. is worthwhile because he exemplifies the best qualities in a conventional physician. He is competent at what he does and as a result, delivers the best that conventional medicine has to offer. He has a healthy skepticism about treatments he does not understand and is not afraid to ask questions But once he is convinced that his patients are being treated competently by other providers, he is willing to support the wishes of the people under his care.

When you consider that many conventional physicians have had bad experiences with alternative providers (who, as you will see later in this chapter, can range from trained and licensed naturopathic physicians to untrained individuals with mail-order diplomas), it is understandable that medical specialists can and should be concerned.

Your conventional provider must be aware of everything you are doing, be willing to listen, and be supportive of your rational use of these alternatives. Your medical provider does not need to be an advocate for alternatives. What is important is that you are granted the freedom to act openly and responsibly.

When you select a conventional provider, you are also choosing that person's staff and office facility. If you are receiving chemotherapy, for example, you may see more of the staff than you will of the medical specialist. It is these people who will answer most of your questions, respond to your requests, and see to your needs during this important time.

Be certain that you can coexist with these folks. The personality and communication traits we discussed for the medical specialist apply just as much to the staff. This may not seem important at first, but after your third or fourth time in for chemotherapy, it will.

Don't overlook the office facility, either. If your doctor is in an area of town where you don't feel safe or if the office itself makes you uncomfortable, this needs to be considered in your decision.

Consider whether or not the physician and staff are available to answer questions. To be fair, not all questions need to be answered by the physician. Nurses, physician's assistants, and other staff members will often be better contact sources during treatment. Your life will be much easier if you choose a physician whose staff members are available when you need them and who are willing and able to get the physician's immediate attention for you when necessary.

Making the Selection

Referrals are the best way to find a new physician. In most cases, the best referral sources will be your primary care physician, nursing staff, and other health care providers in your area. Referrals from friends may provide some useful cues about the communication skills and bedside manner of prospective physicians but may not be a good indicator of technical skills.

Many medical societies, specialty societies, and help organizations will give you assistance as well. Your local social worker, support group, wellness center, or cancer-support organization can also furnish lists of trained professionals.

Be clear about your priorities when asking for referrals.

Here are some suggestions to help you get the best referral.

BE SPECIFIC ABOUT THE TYPE OF PROVIDER YOU NEED

If you feel that you need a surgeon, an oncologist, a urologist, a dermatologist, or another medical specialist, be certain to ask for one. If you don't know what kind of cancer doctor you need, consult your primary care provider or find a general medical oncologist. I cannot emphasize too much how important it is to consult with a medical oncologist, even if the only service you get is advice.

In conventional medicine, there are specialties within specialties. Many surgeons, oncologists, and other specialists sub-specialize on certain parts of the body, such as the breast, the liver, or the gastrointestinal system. You don't want a urologist (kidney and urinary tract specialist) if you are considering a lumpectomy for breast cancer. Finding a specialist with experience in your area of interest is important. Sub-specialists are often good choices, but I wouldn't pass by other medical specialists who have not sub-specialized if they have the training, experience, and resources to meet your needs.

Referrals are the best way to find a new physician.

KEEP YOUR OPTIONS OPEN

If you ask only for referrals in the southeast end of town, you may miss hearing about the hands-down best specialist of all time who practices just a few miles farther away. Limiting gender may also yield less than the best. Men often prefer male doctors and women often prefer female doctors, but the best doctor in town for you may not be one of your gender. If you have cultural or religious beliefs that make this a serious issue, then by all means limit your referral request accordingly. If, on the other hand, you are just a little shy or hesitant about working with a physician of the opposite sex, then this may be the time to give it a try. Whatever part of your anatomy the doctor is examining, you can be certain that he or she has examined a thousand others. A word of caution to the doctor and staff about your modesty or other concerns will usually result in them taking a little extra care to avoid making you uncomfortable.

Men often prefer male doctors and women often prefer female doctors, but the best doctor for you may not be of your gender.

Once you've reduced your choices to the two or three best, it is time to interview them. Yes, that's right. To the surprise of many people, most specialists are willing to spend a few minutes with you to determine whether your relationship will be a good fit.

The process starts by your calling the physician's office and scheduling a brief appointment. Be clear that you will take less than fifteen minutes and that this will be a friendly encounter. Since this is the physician's livelihood, do not be offended if there is a charge for the visit. It's a good value even if your insurance doesn't cover it.

Arrive at your appointment on time. While most physicians try to stay on schedule, medical specialists are often faced with unpredictable circumstances to which they must respond. If there is a delay or problem, don't write this physician off but instead pay attention to how the staff members deal with rectifying the situation. For example, if they are rude or inaccessible now, chances are you will be dealing with that attitude later, too.

Bring someone with you to the meeting, such as your spouse or significant other, a friend, or a person who can advocate on your behalf. This gives you the advantage of a second pair of eyes and ears at the meeting and the opportunity to compare impressions and answers afterward.

During the meeting, always be dignified and respectful. The prospective physician will also develop an initial impression. Besides, this physician may be your second opinion or perhaps a standby if your number one choice becomes unavailable.

Start the meeting with three statements:

1. I appreciate you taking the time to meet with me. (Even if you are paying for it.)
2. This meeting is very important to me.
3. I am prepared and will be brief.

These statements will have the effect of putting the physician at ease, which will, in turn, make your task easier.

Avoid being too familiar. Address the physician as Doctor, not Bill or Mary. Even if the doctor is comfortable with a first-name relationship, it is considered rude to use such an address at the first meeting. Keep your demeanor as friendly and as warm as possible. Doctors are not used to being asked about their competence and experience. If your questions begin to sound like a cross examination, the meeting will not be productive.

To be as accurate as possible during this first meeting, write down the answers to your questions.

Nine Questions to Ask Your Prospective Medical Specialist

1. **At which hospitals do you have privileges if I need hospitalization?**
   Normally, this is not a problem since most physicians practice close to the hospitals where they have admitting privileges. However, this bears consideration if the hospital is the worst one in town or is too far from your home.
2. **Do you have a backup for nighttime or weekend emergencies? If so, who? If not, what happens if I need you and you're not available?**
   Backup coverage is important. Sooner or later, whether for a seminar, vacation, or some other reason, your specialist will be unavailable. If Murphy's law applies, this will be the time when you most need expert help.

   In larger communities, backup coverage will normally be another physician of the same specialty, often a medical group partner. In smaller communities, it may be a local physician who is in general practice or not in the same specialty. It may even be a well-trained nurse or physician's assistant who has access to other specialists if needed.

   No backup other than the local emergency room is the lowest level of service. If this is the only game in town, you may be stuck with it. If you have the choice, however, a backup provider with access to your records is much more desirable if you need urgent care.

3. **How accessible are you and your staff when I have "dumb" questions?**

Many of your questions can wait for the next scheduled visit. Others, however, although not emergencies, should be answered more quickly if for no other reason than to give you peace of mind.

The ideal provider will tell you that you can call in at any time, preferably during business hours, and that you will, at the minimum, get a call back the same day by someone on staff. Since medical specialists, such as surgeons, sometimes cannot be interrupted for extended periods, it is not unreasonable for a trained staff person to answer your call. Most nonurgent questions can be answered by competent providers who are not physicians. If they can't answer your questions, they will know how to get expert advice.

If, on the other hand, there is no commitment to respond to your calls in a timely fashion, you may wish to look elsewhere.

4. **I have special dietary, religious, cultural, or other needs. They are . . . (be specific). Can you accommodate them?**

Most physicians will do whatever they can to honor your specific nonmedical needs. This question provides the physician with fair warning, and the response will give you a sense of how much support you will get in this area.

If a physician has sound medical reasons why your particular needs may interfere with treatment, now is the time to discuss this. Your physician should be interested in your well-being. Don't be defensive as long as the information you receive is well-intentioned. Look for different treatments or compromises that are acceptable to you. For example, many religions have dispensation mechanisms for medical necessity. Such a dispensation can alleviate many problems.

Don't despair if there is no apparent solution. If this physician cannot provide an acceptable resolution to this challenge, another physician may. Different medical specialists may have different opinions about the necessity of a particular objectionable procedure or treatment.

Although it's almost unheard of for a physician to demonstrate a bias against a patient's beliefs, if this is the case, now rather than later is the best time to know about it. If a physician is offensive or suggests his or her own religion or beliefs during the meeting, simply look for the sign marked exit.

5. **I have brand X insurance and I have my policy right here. Are you covered? Is there a charge to me?**

This question may be referred back to a staff person, but you can be certain of a quick response if the doctor is now the one asking for you. It pays to ask about insurance coverage even if you think you know the answer. In some cases, physicians who are not listed with your insurance plan may be willing and able to become part of it. Some insurers pay for providers who are not part of their plan, but only when asked.

In some cases, some nonpreferred providers may require partial payment from you personally, whereas preferred providers in the same plan may require less payment or even none at all. If this is the case, you might want to consider the physician who costs less. However, if the nonpreferred physician is your first choice, he or she may be worth the extra expense.

6. **Is there a research institution or large medical center you call when you have questions or are looking for the latest treatment protocols or technology? If yes, who?**

There is usually more than one treatment protocol available for a particular type of cancer. Often, both established and research protocols are available and worth considering, especially if your diagnosis is tough to treat. You cannot consider them, however, if you don't know about them.

Ideally, your physician will be well-connected to the nearest regional medical center with live contacts and a solid working relationship. Journals and electronic databases are useful, but the latest news and good consultative advice are often still delivered over the medical-specialty back fence. The medical continuing education system requires all medical specialists to receive regular recurrent training, but many advances and changes that could be meaningful to you can occur between these meetings.

If your prospective physician is a lone ranger, you might consider opting for a different physician or, at the least, getting a second opinion from such a center yourself.

7. **Are you board-certified in your specialty?**

Board certification is a means for everyone to know that this physician has successfully completed the specialty training, experience, and examinations designed to demonstrate that he or she is able to safely

> Ideally, your physician will be well-connected to the nearest regional medical center.

and expertly provide the special services that are beyond the training of most general practice physicians.

This question may already be answered on the doctor's business card, but if not, it should be asked. If the answer is yes, that's fine. If the answer is no, the physician may still be able to treat you effectively, but you have no way of knowing that. It is risky to receive specialty services from a physician who is not board-certified, and I recommend against doing so.

8. **I have an interest in alternative medicine. Are you willing to work with me and to review what I am doing if I work with a nonconventional provider who is trained, licensed, knowledgeable, and willing to provide regular written reports for your consensus?**

A variety of answers is possible here. Remember that your medical specialist has little or no training in alternative medicine and, as a result, is not sure what to do or say about this information.

A good answer is a demonstrated willingness to work with you with the stipulation that you will not do something that he or she feels is dangerous until the question can be satisfactorily resolved. Your future success with this physician may well depend on your ability to find a nonconventional provider who can establish some credibility with your conventional physician. If your conventional physician knows a nonconventional provider in whom he or she has confidence, it may be worth consulting with this person.

If the prospective physician has a bias against alternative medicine because it is "not scientifically proven," don't look at this as an insurmountable problem. Many conventional physicians who have not read the alternative medicine scientific literature and are therefore not current with that body of knowledge, are still willing to work with people as long as they are convinced that it is safe. Your nonconventional provider should be able to resolve this issue.

If the prospective physician says that he or she will have nothing to do with you if you use alternative therapies, then you need to either abandon the idea of combining conventional and nonconventional treatments or try another specialist.

The other possible answer you may receive, and the one I find most frustrating, is when a physician says that you can do whatever you like with nonconventional treatment since it doesn't matter. This physician may not be aware of the potential interactions that can happen when conventional and nonconventional treatments are combined. If this specialist is still willing to coordinate with a competent nonconventional provider and will apply some basic medical logic to what you are doing, the situation may still be workable. If you don't perceive any willingness to participate in your total healing process, then this may be your cue to move on.

Although the specialist doesn't need to be expert in alternative medicine, he or she must at least be a willing reviewer of your nonconventional plan.

9. **Can you give me the name of two people under your care (either current or former) that I could speak to?**

In some jurisdictions, patient confidentiality will prohibit the physician from doing so, but when the physician is willing, this can be an important insight. The names you receive will obviously be their most satisfied clients.

When you leave the meeting, write down your subjective impression in a few sentences. Ask yourself if this is someone you can connect with and talk to. Were the answers credible? Was the staff friendly, or at least civil? Did the office make you comfortable or give you the creeps?

If you were able to get the names of people treated by this doctor, call them immediately. Ask them if they were treated well by the specialist and staff, if appointments were reasonably on time, and if they would go back to the same specialist in the future if they needed more treatment. Take notes so that you will be able to refer to this information later.

Now that you have the answers, what do you do with them? Make a list of the questions you asked and the answers the specialist gave. You should be able to find a specialist(s) who answered all the questions correctly, in which case your decision will be based on your subjective impressions and perhaps comments from other people under this doctor's care.

If none of the prospects got all the answers right and you have the time and prospects to interview some more, go for it. If, on the other hand, you need to choose from these, make a two-column list for each specialist, with the positive questions and responses on the left and the negative ones on the right. Compare the answers to your notes. Your decision should be an easy one. Once again, in the event of a tie, look to your subjective feelings and comments from other people to break the deadlock.

CHOOSING A NONCONVENTIONAL PROVIDER

Nature has provided us with most of our known cures for diseases. Conventional drugs and natural medicines owe much of their success to plants and elements from the earth. Hope for new treatments continues to focus on nature, with special attention to newly discovered species of plants and constituents from previously unexplored forests and jungles.

The options available outside conventional medicine are yet another kind of jungle, however, one with more claims and information than you could possibly evaluate on your own. This is why you need a competent nonconventional provider on your team, someone to guide you through this maze of information and misinformation.

My goal is to provide you with a straightforward way to choose the right nonconventional provider. We will look at the reasons to add this vital person to your health care team, the qualities necessary for that person to be a valuable and functional part of the team, the step-by-step selection process, and how you can manage the services provided.

Naturally, this process bears some similarities to the selection process for a medical specialist, but there are also some important differences. Consider this next section a road map for choosing a friend and an adviser who will be with you for a very long time.

Why Choose a Nonconventional Provider
Before Selecting Natural Medicine Therapies?

Natural medicine is the part of your treatment where you can have the most control. While conventional therapies may come down to just a few appropriate therapy choices, nonconventional medicine offers a wide array of options. You now get to choose whether you want to make these decisions on your own or bring in an experienced provider to guide you through the selection and implementation process.

There are a number of nonconventional treatment decisions to be made, including:

- Type of therapy, such as botanical medicine, clinical nutrition, or acupuncture
- Particular treatment, such as vitamin C, taheebo, or massage therapy
- Dosage and timing
- Coordination with conventional therapies

An important element to consider is clinical judgment. A competent and trained provider can take you the final mile, showing you how to implement a nonconventional plan that is specific to your particular condition and clinical status and to the conventional treatments that you require. An expert provider of natural medicine will coordinate your care to ensure that your natural and conventional treatments are working with rather than against each other.

With the explosion of information and the growing popularity of natural medicines, you will be bombarded with speculative cancer advice, unusual opinions, and miraculous claims of cancer cures. Virtually every form of media is involved: books, magazines, talk shows, the Internet, health food stores, and direct marketing

While some of this information is valid, much of it is not. Claims from one "expert" often directly contradict claims from other "experts." At best, the situation is confusing. A competent nonconventional provider will be able to help you separate the wheat from the chaff, guiding you away from those treatments that won't help or might even make you sick.

Regardless of how strong you are, this is a vulnerable time in your life. Claims for cure are enticing, but you may not have the time or the objectivity to figure out which are valid. The right nonconventional provider can help you weed out the ineffective options and focus on the helpful ones

> While conventional therapies may come down to just a few appropriate therapy choices, nonconventional medicine offers a wide array of options.

Types of Nonconventional Providers

There are many types of providers, offering very different kinds of services. Those services will also vary with different licensing jurisdictions because of different laws. Health care licensure in most of the world is provided by the national government, whereas in North America, licensure is governed by individual states and provinces.

The most common providers offering nonconventional therapies are:

- Naturopathic physicians
- Chiropractors
- Alternative medical doctors
- Alternative osteopathic doctors
- Acupuncturists
- Licensed massage therapists
- Physician's assistants
- Nurses
- Nutritionists and Dietitians
- Homeopaths

Naturopathic Physicians

Naturopathic physicians are the most broadly trained nonconventional providers. Depending on where these physicians practice, treatments usually include botanical medicine; clinical nutrition; manipulation of the spine and extremities; Oriental medicine, including Oriental herbs and acupuncture; physical therapy; massage; and homeopathy; as well as prescription drugs and surgery. Some naturopathic doctors specialize in one or more of these modalities and even in the treatment of cancer.

Naturopathic medicine includes not only the modes of treatment but also the philosophy for using them in a way that supports the body's own healing power.

If a competent naturopathic doctor practices in your area, make the effort to get this person on your team. Even if this practitioner does not specialize in cancer treatment, she or he can consult with a specialty care clinic to provide many nonconventional cancer services. A good naturopath can also provide referrals for other services, as well as coordinate and communicate with your conventional medical specialist.

Choosing a competent naturopathic physician requires a little more attention than choosing a conventional physician because of differences in licensing laws. Some jurisdictions, such as Washington State, require naturopathic doctors to have training comparable to that of a general practice medical physician. Other jurisdictions, such as Washington, D.C., will grant a registration to practice naturopathy to anyone who walks in and pays the fee. No education or training is required (amazing, but true). Many states, provinces, and countries have no laws whatsoever governing naturopathic medicine.

> Choosing a competent naturopathic physician requires more attention than choosing a conventional physician because of differences in licensing laws.

Chiropractors

Chiropractic doctors are licensed in most jurisdictions. Nearly all *chiropractors* provide chiropractic adjustment, a form of manipulation of the spine. Some chiropractors also provide other kinds of manipulation and/or nutritional advice, depending on the area.

The training requirements for chiropractic doctors are regulated by individual jurisdiction but are fairly standardized. A competent chiropractor with training and specialization in the services you want can be a valuable team member.

Alternative Medical Doctors

Alternative medical doctors are licensed M.D.s who have received additional training in specific natural therapies. Most specialize in *chelation therapy,* but some practice broader nonconventional therapies, including nutrition and botanical medicine.

Conventional medical schools do not teach nonconventional therapies in their core curriculum. However, some medical schools now provide alternative medicine residency programs. An alternative medical doctor, depending on training and specialization, can be a good source for certain therapies and a referral and coordination point for others.

Alternative Osteopathic Doctors

In many jurisdictions, including much of North America, *osteopathic doctors* practice medicine at a level similar to conventional medical physicians, with the exception that most osteopaths also practice manipulation of the spine and extremities.

These physicians generally provide nonconventional services that are consistent with training received outside their core medical training, most commonly chelation therapy, nutrition, and botanical medicine. An alternative osteopathic doctor can be a good source for some therapies and a referral and coordination point for others.

In some jurisdictions, mostly outside North America, the term "osteopath" refers to a provider whose principal practice is manipulation of the spine and perhaps giving nutritional advice. Regulation varies broadly. A competent non-physician osteopath with training and specialization in the services you require can be a valuable team member.

Acupuncturists

Acupuncturists are regulated in many but not all jurisdictions. In general, acupuncturists are trained to provide needle acupuncture and treatment with Oriental herbal medicines. Some acupuncturists are trained in the West, others in Asia. Training requirements vary with jurisdiction. A competent and trained acupuncturist can be a good source for acupuncture and Oriental herbs.

Licensed Massage Therapists

Massage therapists are regulated in many states and unregulated in others. Unfortunately, mostly in jurisdictions that do not license massage therapists, prostitution has masqueraded as massage and dishonored this valuable profession. If you live in one of these places, do not give up on massage as an important addition to your treatment. Real massage therapists can be found.

A quality massage therapist has training in therapeutic massage, as well as some basic training in the safety of massage procedures. Historically, massage therapy has not been considered to be appropriate for people with cancer, but experience and new training have shown that this therapy, properly administered, can be both safe and comforting. A trained and qualified massage therapist can provide safe and competent massage treatments.

Physician's Assistants

Physician's assistants are providers who practice under the supervision of a physician. Once again, the laws governing their practice vary by licensing jurisdiction. Nonconventional medicine is not part of the core training for physician's assistants, but some of these providers have undertaken it as additional training. The services provided vary with the individual but often include botanical medicine, ayurvedic (a form of herbal) medicine, and homeopathy. A competent physician's assistant with training and specialization in the services you want can be a valuable team member

Nurses

Nursing has many levels, including licensed practical nurse, registered nurse, and nurse practitioner. In certain jurisdictions, *nurses* can practice independently and, in others, can practice limited nonconventional services such as nutritional advice and coordination of treatments. A competent, trained nurse can provide valuable advice and coordination services.

Nutritionists and Dietitians

Nutritionists and *dietitians* are licensed in some but not all jurisdictions. Many are involved with hospital and other institutional dietary services, while some also work as consultants. A competent trained nutritionist or dietitian can provide valuable basic nutritional advice.

Homeopaths

Homeopaths practice *homeopathic medicine*, a therapy using very weak solutions prepared by a series of dilutions and shaking (or *succussing*), as originally prescribed by German physician Samuel Hahnemann in the nineteenth century. Some homeopaths are "lay" homeopaths, having training but no licensure. Others are trained and licensed with specific requirements, and a few are physicians (medical, osteopathic, or naturopathic) who have chosen to specialize. Homeopathy is considered to be useful under certain circumstances in treating cancer. If you are interested in this therapy, a classical homeopath can provide valuable advice.

You have many options for both nonconventional providers and treatments, although your selection may be limited by the kinds of providers in your locality. The best solution is to find a local nonconventional provider who has already established a relationship with your conventional medical specialists. If this is not possible, you can arrange a consultation with a distant provider who offers the services you want.

Take advice only from a provider who has either seen you personally or is coordinating with your local health care provider.

Our clinic routinely speaks to medical specialists all over the world, using their eyes, ears, and medical records when we are not able to personally meet with the individual seeking treatment. This is not an unusual circumstance. Take advice only from a provider who has either seen you personally or is coordinating with your local health care provider.

If you are interested in a particular treatment, such as herbal medicine, look for a practitioner who is accomplished in this area. If that provider is broadly licensed, she or he will offer ideas and advice for useful treatments. If you are undecided about the kind of therapy you want, read chapters 7 and 8 for ideas or choose the broadest scope nonconventional provider in your area to help you narrow the field.

Qualities to Consider in a Nonconventional Provider

Once you've settled on the type of nonconventional practitioner you would like, consider the qualities that will make someone a good match for you. Here are some qualities to look for.

GOOD COMMUNICATION SKILLS

As with conventional providers, good communication skills are a must. Your nonconventional practitioner must possess a communication style, demeanor, body language, and attitude that will make you comfortable and help you understand information.

CREDIBILITY

This person must be credible. You will receive information about technology, concepts, and language that you may not be familiar with. Your nonconventional provider may have to tell you that the ad you saw on the Internet for a cancer cure is simply untrue. This person must be able to get through to you even if you don't want to hear the information.

EXPERIENCE WITH
YOUR DIAGNOSIS

The nonconventional provider you choose must have some experience and skill with your diagnosis, up to a point. Experience with breast cancer is important so that the provider will understand all the implications of your diagnosis and treatment, but he or she doesn't have to be familiar with the same technical details as your oncologist. Nonconventional treatments are not so sensitive to these factors as conventional therapies are.

CONNECTIONS TO THE WORLD
OF MEDICAL RESEARCH

You don't want to miss valid new treatments or research protocols that promise better results because your practitioner didn't know about them. Unlike medical specialists, nonconventional providers can get the latest information without having a relationship with a research facility. Far fewer experimental protocols exist in natural medicine and most of these are best used after they have been published in reliable, scientific journals and subject to peer review.

WILLINGNESS TO COOPERATE WITH
YOUR GOALS AND OBJECTIVES

Your nonconventional provider must also be willing to cooperate with your goals. If you have made a rational decision to either use or reject conventional treatment, your nonconventional provider must be comfortable working with you. Don't just seek out a provider who agrees with everything you say, though. You are paying to hear the truth and reap the benefit of many years of training and practice. If new or contrary information is discovered, you will want to hear it. Once you have made an informed decision about your treatment, however, you'll need the support of a nonconventional provider who will do his or her level best to get you to your goal. This is not the time to run into philosophical resistance from your provider.

SOME KNOWLEDGE OF CONVENTIONAL CANCER TREATMENTS

Conventional medicine is a subject you should be able to discuss with your nonconventional provider. Most, however, have little training in conventional oncology methods. The provider should possess either the knowledge or the resources to understand and deal with the implications of combining therapies. He or she must also be willing and able to communicate clearly and effectively with your medical specialist so that everyone on your team is up to date with your total treatment plan.

A STAFF AND FACILITY THAT SUITS YOUR NEEDS

When you select a nonconventional provider, you are also selecting staff persons, an office facility, and an office culture. Staff members will answer many of your questions, respond to your requests, and generally see to your needs. The same personality and communication traits that are desirable for the provider apply to the staff as well. This often doesn't seem important in the beginning, but after a few visits it will become so.

Don't just seek out a provider who agrees with everything you say.

Don't overlook the facility either. You need to feel safe and comfortable with the office location and function. The atmosphere may be more relaxed than your conventional doctor's office, but it should still be clean, professional, well-lit, and organized. If the incense and chanting in the waiting room are not for you, look further.

AVAILABILITY OF PROVIDER AND STAFF

Finally, the accessibility of the nonconventional provider and staff persons to answer questions is important. Staff members will often provide most of the contact you need between treatments, so you should be certain they are available when you need them and that they are willing and able to get the provider's immediate attention when necessary.

Making the Selection

Referrals are a good place to start. Check with your medical specialist, primary care physician, nursing staff, or other health care providers to see if they have any recommendations. Referrals from friends may provide useful cues about the communication skills and bedside manner of prospective providers, but they may not be the best judge of technical skills.

Be clear about your priorities when asking for referrals. Here are some cues that will help you get the best referrals.

Be Specific About the Type of Provider You Need

If you know that you want an acupuncturist, it doesn't help to interview massage therapists. If you don't know what kind of nonconventional provider you want, consult your primary care provider, your medical specialist, or a broad-scope alternative provider to help with the selection.

Finding a nonconventional provider with experience in your area of interest is important. Many nonconventional providers specialize in particular treatment methods or certain parts of the body. Others specialize in particular individuals. Someone familiar with oncology will be a better choice than a sports medicine specialist.

Keep Your Options Open

If you ask for referrals only in your neighborhood, you may miss the best nonconventional provider, one who practices across town. Limiting gender may also yield less than the best. Men often prefer male doctors and women often prefer female doctors, but the best doctor in town may not be one of your gender. Once again, cultural, religious, or other factors that are significant to you should be part of your referral request. If, on the other hand, you are just a little shy or hesitant about working with a physician of the opposite sex, then this may be the time to give it a try.

Once you have a list of potential nonconventional providers, you can interview the two or three most promising ones. Most nonconventional providers are willing to spend a few minutes with you to determine whether the relationship will be a good fit. Start by calling the provider's office and scheduling a brief appointment. Be clear that you will take less than fifteen minutes and that this will be a friendly encounter. Since this is the provider's livelihood, do not be offended if she or he charges for this visit. It is a good value even if your insurance doesn't cover it. Arrive at your appointment on time. If a delay or problem occurs, pay attention to how staff members deal with rectifying the situation. If they are rude or inaccessible now, you may deal with that attitude again. On the other hand, if they are helpful and considerate, this is a good sign. Keep in mind that we all have scheduling problems sometimes.

Bring someone with you to the meeting, such as your significant other, a friend, or a person who can advocate on your behalf. You will have the advantage of a second pair of eyes and ears at the meeting and the opportunity to compare impressions and answers after the meeting. During the meeting, always be dignified and respectful. Many providers who are not medical physicians are still well-trained, competent, and responsible. Treating your potential nonconventional provider like a second-rate citizen will undoubtedly result in your creating a negative impression and perhaps in the loss of an important option.

Begin the meeting with these three statements:

1. I appreciate your taking the time to meet with me. (Even if you are paying for it.)
2. This meeting is a great help to me.
3. I am prepared and will be brief.

These statements will put the provider at ease, which will, in turn, make your job smoother.

Avoid being too familiar. Address providers by their proper title, not George or Sue. Even if the provider is comfortable with a first-name relationship, it is considered rude to use such an address at this first meeting.

Keep your demeanor as friendly and as warm as possible. Providers are not used to being asked about their competence and experience. If the questions begin to sound like a cross examination, the meeting will not be productive.

Write down the answers during the meeting for best accuracy.

Nine Questions to Ask Your Prospective Nonconventional Provider

1. **What specific treatment modalities do you practice?**
   Be certain that you can get the treatments you want.
2. **Do you have a backup for vacations and unavailable times? If so, who? If not, what happens if I need you and you aren't available?**
   Backup is not as great an issue here as with your medical specialist. It is customary to have short-term contingency plans for your natural treatments. Urgent care issues will normally be covered by your conventional medical specialist, especially during conventional treatment. On the other hand, you don't want to wait for the end of a six- or eight-week vacation to get your questions answered.

3. **How accessible are you and your staff when I have "dumb" questions?**

Many questions can wait for the next scheduled visit while others, although not emergencies, should be answered more quickly, if for no other reason than to give you peace of mind.

The correct answer is that you can call in at any time, preferably during business hours, and that you will, at the minimum, get a call back within a few days by someone on staff. Most nonemergency questions can be answered by staff persons, and they will know when to get you more help. If, on the other hand, they are not committed to responding to your calls in a timely fashion, consider looking elsewhere.

4. **I have special dietary, religious, cultural, or other needs. They are . . . (be specific). Can you accommodate them?**

Most providers will do whatever they can to honor your specific non-medical needs. This question provides fair warning and the response will give you a sense of how much support you will get in this area.

If the provider has sound medical reasons why your particular needs may interfere with treatment, this is the time to discuss it. Look for alternatives or compromises that are acceptable to you, ones that may alleviate the problem. Don't despair if no apparent solution arises. Natural medicine includes a wide variety of treatment protocols that can be useful. If this specialty provider doesn't work for you, undoubtedly another one will.

It is almost unheard of in modern times that a licensed provider would demonstrate a bias against your beliefs, but if this happens, if the provider is offensive or suggests his or her own religion or beliefs during the meeting, simply leave.

5. **I have brand X insurance and I have my policy right here. Are you covered? Is there a charge to me?**

This question may be referred to a staff person, but you can be certain of a quick response if the provider is the one asking. It pays to ask the question even if you think you know the answer. In some cases, it may be possible to include on your insurance plan providers and treatments that are not listed with it. Some insurers make specific exemptions for alternative providers, but only when asked.

Certain nonpreferred providers can, in some cases, require partial payment from you personally, whereas preferred providers in the same plan may require less or none at all. If that is the case, you might want to look at the provider who costs less. However if the nonpreferred provider is the best, you may consider him or her worth the extra expense.

Since the cost for most nonconventional providers is modest compared with conventional oncology treatments, the best provider may be worth paying for out of pocket if insurance does not step up to the plate.

6. **Are you licensed to practice _____ (the service that you want) in this jurisdiction? If not, what jurisdictions are you licensed in? What services does your license allow you to provide in this jurisdiction?**

The licensing of nonconventional providers is inconsistent. Even professions with licensing laws in many jurisdictions, such as chiropractic, have significant differences in the services they can legally provide from one place to the next.

Your best choice is to receive services from a provider licensed and regulated in the jurisdiction where he or she practices, if that jurisdiction has a strong licensure system. If competent, well-trained providers want to practice in a jurisdiction that does not have a good licensing law, or has none at all, they will often maintain their licensure in a jurisdiction that does a better job of licensing, as evidence that they are competent. This can be a good clue that the providers were originally trained and examined when they got the license, assuming that the license came from a strong licensing jurisdiction.

The downside of providers licensed in a different jurisdiction is that they may be practicing illegally and/or not be part of an ongoing, local regulation and disciplinary system that would have protected you in the event of problems or malpractice. With only rare exceptions, it is unwise to use providers who are not licensed and regulated in the jurisdiction where they practice.

Using unlicensed providers is a risky undertaking. Some are safe and responsible while others are definitely unsafe and charlatans. You have no way of telling which is which. The worst offenders often have the best bedside manner. People's testimonials are not always reliable indicators of who is who, since these are usually based more on the persuasiveness of the provider than on actual skill and knowledge.

Referrals from licensed health care professionals in the community can be more helpful but are still far from a reliable assurance that you

I*t is unwise to use providers who are not licensed and regulated in the jurisdiction where they practice.*

will receive quality care and advice. The lack of licensure programs for nonconventional health care providers is unfortunate and, in my opinion, an irresponsible lack of public protection

7. **Are you experienced in treating cancer? If yes, describe your experience. If no, are you comfortable working with me and why?**
Treating people with cancer is different from having a general practice. If your nonconventional provider treats a lot of people with cancer, he or she will normally have more information about the usefulness and potential interactions with conventional treatment than your medical specialist. If the provider does not have experience, she or he should be willing to consult with a provider in the field who does.

    If a potential provider tells you that mixing conventional and nonconventional medicines is never a problem, you should choose another provider

8. **Are you willing to coordinate with my medical specialist(s) and provide written notes describing everything we are doing?**
The answer must be yes. Your nonconventional provider must clearly and accurately inform, in a timely fashion, your medical specialty providers of everything being done and why. This allows the medical specialists to make decisions on short notice by simply consulting the file and knowing if a particular nonconventional treatment should not be used, either in general or as a result of a change in conventional treatment.

9. **Can you give me the names of two people under your care (either current or former) I can speak to?**
In some jurisdictions, patient confidentiality will prohibit the provider from doing so, but when this is possible it can provide important insights. The names you receive will obviously be their most satisfied clients.

When you leave the meeting, write down your subjective impressions in a few quick sentences. Is this someone you can connect with and talk to? Were the answers credible? Was the staff friendly, or at least civil? Did the office make you feel comfortable or give you the creeps?

If you were able to get references from any of the people treated by the potential providers, call them immediately and take notes. Ask them if they were treated well by the provider and staff, if appointments were reasonably on time, and if they would go back to the same provider in the future if they needed more treatment.

Call your local health department to confirm that this person has a current license and to check if any disciplinary actions have been taken against this provider. The health department will also give you a copy of the licensure law with scope of practice. This is public information in all but the most backward of jurisdictions.

Now that you have the answers, what do you do with them? Make a list of the questions and the answers. You should be able to find a provider(s) who answered all the questions correctly, in which case your decision will be based on your subjective impressions and perhaps comments from other people.

If none of the prospects got all the answers right and you have the time to interview some more, go for it. If these are the only prospects in your area, the next best strategy is to look in a nearby town or farther away. If necessary, you can use a competent nonconventional provider's services over a long distance, together with those of a local provider. Your local provider can be either a nonconventional or a conventional medical doctor.

THE CARE AND FEEDING OF YOUR HEALTH CARE PROVIDERS

Once you've made your decisions, you'll want to create a relationship that will make it easy for your providers and their staffs to meet your needs. Here are a few guidelines to keep the ball rolling.

RESPECT THE TIME CONSTRAINTS OF THE PROVIDER AND STAFF

A busy practice requires serious time management in order to run smoothly. Arrive a few minutes early for all appointments. Write down your questions before the visit and provide a copy to the specialist or staff at the start of the meeting. Stay on the subject and don't make too much small talk because this takes away from the time your doctor has to care for you. If you *must* cancel an appointment, do it as early as possible. Provide an explanation when canceling or rescheduling, not because you need an excuse but so that you are not grouped with those inconsiderate people who complicate the schedule at the last minute for no good reason.

When you have questions or concerns between appointments, if possible articulate them in writing for yourself before making the call. This helps you communicate them clearly and helps the office give you an accurate and timely response.

ALWAYS BE RESPECTFUL TO EVERYONE IN THE OFFICE

Your professional and considerate behavior will identify you as someone who is caring, and this will make the office staff more willing to go beyond the norm to support you when you need it.

When you have questions between appointments, articulate them in writing for yourself before making the call.

PROVIDE BALANCED FEEDBACK

If something goes wrong, such as consistently long waits for appointments, it may be useful to bring this up. When the specialist or office has done something well, it is worth bringing this to their attention as well. In all cases, be respectful and don't exaggerate.

It is human nature to treat others as they treat us. These strategies will make it much easier for the specialist and staff to respond to your needs, even when it is beyond the normal call of duty. Remember, what goes around comes around.

IF YOU'RE NOT SATISFIED WITH THE CARE

If either of your providers do not meet your needs, this two-step plan should quickly resolve your problem:

Step 1: **Write down your concerns as completely as possible and bring them directly to the practitioner.**

If you are not able to get return calls, answers to your questions, or civil treatment on the telephone, be as specific as possible. Deliver the message in person by making a brief appointment with the specialist. You can tell the receptionist that this is a subject you can only discuss with the doctor. Keep your comments as objective as possible. If your complaint is about one of his staff, be as specific as possible.

In my experience, the problem can usually be resolved with this meeting. Most often, the physician will have realized this was a problem and will be more than willing to mend the situation to your satisfaction. If this step solves the problem, you can skip step two.

Step 2: **If, after your best efforts, you decide that this is still the wrong practitioner for you, do not despair.**

Simply change providers. This is possible in almost every circumstance other than in the middle of a procedure. People are often intimidated about changing practitioners, but it happens every day and can be accomplished professionally without an interruption of treatment, hard feelings, or burned bridges.

A Primer on Choosing Treatments

This chapter provides you with the tools for evaluating your therapeutic options. Scientific data is available for many treatments. Having a basic understanding of this data, including a knowledge of what survival statistics are and how they relate to you, will also be helpful in weighing your choices.

You'll also want to know how a treatment will meet your personal objectives. How do the therapies you are considering compare to other therapies (or even to no therapy at all)?

Since you'll be working closely with both your conventional and your alternative providers, you'll want to know what questions to ask them about the treatments they are recommending. And since it can be difficult even to know what questions to ask, I'll provide a list of questions, the answers to which will help you and your providers decide on the best course of treatment for you.

In previous chapters, you've learned how to prioritize your goals and how to choose your health care team. I've also discussed how vital it is to combine alternative medicines and your conventional cancer therapies only with the careful supervision of your skilled and knowledgeable providers. With that information and the help of your support team, you are now ready to learn how to select the treatments you'll be using.

UNDERSTANDING THE SCIENCE BEHIND
TREATMENT CHOICES

When your medical specialist recommends a treatment, this will probably be done with careful consideration of statistics from appropriate studies. (If you wish, you can ask for and read these studies, although this may be more than you want to deal with.) The conventional medical therapies have, in many cases, been the subject of considerable human testing.

Most nonconventional therapies, however, simply have not been tested as exhaustively as the newer conventional cancer treatments. Traditional nonconventional therapies have been used for generations though and, as a result, have a long safety history for humans. Thus they do not present the same safety concerns as new drugs, for which little or no human safety history has been established. Even when a drug is designed to imitate a plant or another naturally occurring substance, it is often synthetic or highly concentrated, and we cannot assume that it is as safe as the original plant or substance.

The Office of Technology Assessment for the U.S. Congress has estimated that less than one-third of conventional medical practice has been proven effective by solid scientific studies.

Much of the testing required by the Food and Drug Administration (FDA) and other government agencies is to determine human safety. New drugs, by their very nature, require more testing because we have less human experience with them. By the same token, however, this does not mean that natural medicines are automatically safe. Some, in fact, have significant toxic effects as well as serious interactions with both other natural substances and conventional medicines.

How much scientific backing is necessary for a treatment to be proved effective? To put this in perspective, consider that the Office of Technology Assessment for the U.S. Congress has estimated that less than one-third of conventional medical practice has been proven effective by solid scientific studies. Many experts believe that this figure may even be lower for nonconventional medicine.

Not scientifically studied doesn't mean that these therapies don't work, merely that they have not been tested scientifically, and, as a result, their use is based on less than stringent evidence.

How Evidence Is Gathered

The effectiveness of conventional and nonconventional therapies is confirmed by a variety of evidence:

- Conclusive scientific testing
- Suggestive but nonconclusive scientific testing
- Reliable anecdotal evidence
- Questionable anecdotal evidence
- Analysis
- Meta-analysis
- Suggestion (or testimonials)

Conclusive Scientific Testing

Conclusive scientific studies are well designed according to scientific and statistical principles. They are done on human populations, using an adequate number of test subjects (to eliminate the possibility of coincidental findings) and placebos (to determine how those who received the treatment compare to those who simply thought they did). Conclusive scientific testing must be reviewed and accepted by other scientists who are familiar with the subject of the study. That the results of the study can be duplicated by objective independently conducted tests adds considerable credence to the conclusions of the original study.

It is important to note that even conclusive scientific testing is no guarantee that a treatment or procedure will work for you, but it can give you confidence.

Suggestive but Nonconclusive Scientific Testing

Scientific testing that merely suggests a result means the studies are missing one or more of the previous elements. This doesn't mean that the treatment being tested doesn't work, merely that you cannot be as sure. Suggestive but nonconclusive scientific testing can sometimes *suggest* safety or a particular result for you, but it's a reach to assume that you can predict the safety or results with any degree of confidence.

Reliable Anecdotal Evidence

Reliable anecdotal evidence is treatment reports from credible health providers or organizations. The reports may lack some or all of the requirements for good science, but because they come from a reliable source they can indicate that a particular treatment or procedure may have value. An example of reliable anecdotal evidence is a provider known to be careful and skilled reporting that seventy-five out of eighty patients treated with a particular drug got better much faster than normal even though that drug was not approved *on the label* for treating that particular disease.

Questionable Anecdotal Evidence

Questionable anecdotal evidence is just that, a report that may not be believable. There may be a suggestion that something works, but it is hard to advise the investment of much time or energy into such a therapy, particularly when dealing with a disease as serious as cancer.

Analysis

Analysis is the review of the data and science to form a new conclusion. Such results can be valuable if the underlying data is accurate and the assumptions that connect it are fair. Conclusions drawn from analysis are usually as reliable as the logic used to form them. Analyses can provide warnings of potential problems or interactions long before comprehensive human tests can be completed.

Meta-Analysis

Meta-analysis is combining the data from a number of independent studies of the same subject to reach an overall conclusion. Meta-analysis is very controversial and considered by some to be limited in value.

Suggestion (or Testimonials)

Suggestion (as opposed to suggestive studies) is often nothing more than a testimonial that a particular treatment works with no evidence to back it up, other than the persuasiveness of the person making the suggestion. Ads are full of such testimonials—from athletes, who are likely well-paid for their endorsements, to *doctors* who own a large share of the company manufacturing the *miracle* product.

Treatment and Survival Statistics

Often conventional providers describe the success of cancer treatment in terms of the percentage of patients who survive after five, ten, or more years. This information can have an unnecessary traumatizing effect.

In the early days of medicine, the patient was often not even told the seriousness of the diagnosis. The negative psychological implications of knowing the survival risks were thought to outweigh the patient's right to know. Critics accused doctors of playing god, which may have been true. At the same time, the medical literature showed that many caring physicians felt they were providing the kindest and best service for their patients.

The presentation of survival statistics still generates a spirited debate among both physicians and patients. The world has changed and now it is lawyers who are criticized for playing god by forcing physicians to present disease and treatment information to patients in what seems to be the most negative manner possible.

In the early days of medicine, the patient was often not even told the seriousness of the diagnosis.

Survival statistics have valid scientific uses, one of them is to assist in the selection of treatment objectives. It is inevitable that you will come into contact with survival statistics so let's make the best of their positive aspects.

The statistics themselves cannot make anything happen to you. They are nothing more than an accumulation of data from patients who came before you. The information is designed to aid scientists and physicians in making technical decisions. It is not designed to provide a balanced overview for patients.

Looking for the Truth in Survival Statistics

Survival statistics are usually organized by diagnosis, stage, and type of treatment. This information is presented as the percentage of all participants who survived for five or ten years after diagnosis. Survival data does not normally address specific tumor response to a particular treatment, but instead looks at the simple reporting of how many patients were still alive at the end of a specific period of time after diagnosis. Most studies correct the data for patients who died from causes other than the disease, such as automobile accidents, but some reports do not. Some studies take only the crudest numbers, in other words, total populations of patients with a particular diagnosis, without separating out important factors such as age, tumor markers, patient condition, patient attitude, and so on. Crude studies may have little to do with your prognosis. Unfortunately, this type of presentation feeds into the human tendency to look at the negative.

People who find themselves in a treatment that had a 90% survival rate after ten years will invariably agonize over the other 10%. How, they may wonder, can they avoid being in the 10% that didn't make it? Did the patients in that group fail to do something important? Could they have saved themselves? The researchers and statisticians who accumulate and present this data in sound, scientific format do not account for that human response.

The truth about statistics is that they describe how groups of people respond, not how individuals respond. That less than 100% of those people who ride bicycles will survive for ten years may be a valid statistical statement, but in the context of cancer, similar statistics seem more threatening. The fact is that less than 100% of virtually any relatively large population will survive for ten years.

What Survival Statistics Can Tell Us

For people who have cancer, do survival statistics mean anything at all? The answer is yes, these statistics can be useful.

Survival statistics can give you a rough idea if a particular treatment can help or not. It can tell you when one treatment is better than another, and it can give you a sense of whether you are facing a serious challenge or not.

It cannot, however, predict your personal outcome. If the survival rates for your situation are 90% in ten years, you can be assured that the risks are quite low and that you may be at greater risk for dying sooner if you jaywalk.

If the survival statistics for your diagnosis are around 50%, you are statistically in the flip-a-coin range if you don't do anything to improve your odds. If, however, the statistical survival numbers are low, such as 10% or less, this does not mean that you have to die. It does mean that one out of ten persons in a situation similar to yours survived and that you need to be the next one out of ten.

In fact, remissions occur regularly with patients whose situations are considered bleak. We are rarely able to determine how, but we know this happens. Whatever the survival statistics for your diagnosis, the strategy is to push yourself as hard as possible toward the survival side of the numbers, whether it's 90% or 10%.

It is wise, then, to use survival statistics as a tool of empowerment. Don't let the numbers bring you down. On the one hand, you don't want to ignore the seriousness of this information, but, on the other hand, you cannot allow it to depress your spirit or your quest for a positive final outcome. *Unexplained* remissions occur every day and there's no reason why the next one shouldn't be you.

Other Treatment Statistics

Some statistics describe what percentages of a group may have had a positive response from a particular treatment. This data, too, can provide in-

The truth about statistics is that they describe how groups of people respond, not how individuals respond.

valuable information for determining your treatment objectives.

Data that report treatment response describe cases where the cancer regressed when a particular treatment was used. Unless stated otherwise, it does not mean that there was a cure. If a certain diagnosis has a 70% response that means seven out of ten patients who fit the study criteria (i.e., diagnosis, stage, etc.) had tumor reduction or some other objective measure of regression with the treatment. These statistics do not address what happened at the conclusion of treatment.

Statistics and Complementary Cancer Therapies

Few cancer treatment studies take into account the supportive and preventive strategies available from natural medicine. The few research efforts that have investigated these areas have been mostly positive but not predictive of outcome. In other words, they show positive benefit in many cases but cannot be relied upon to provide statistical confidence that a particular outcome can be reached.

ESTABLISHING YOUR TREATMENT OBJECTIVES

Each human being and each treatment circumstance is different. Knowing what is best for you, what you wish for yourself, is the first step in the process of selecting your combined cancer therapies.

The therapy that might make sense for someone else may not meet your needs at all, even if you both have the same diagnosis. Issues such as quality of life, intensity of treatment, treatment timing, and even treatment choices can often be adjusted to fit your needs, condition, lifestyle, and beliefs.

Being hesitant about setting your objectives for treatment is common. This may be the result of a concern that you might change your mind later or you may just feel that thinking about treatments is upsetting.

I would still encourage you to give it a try. Nothing you do is set in stone. You can always change your mind later. Many of my patients—including those who initially resisted setting treatment objectives—have found that the objective-setting process and the results of it are both satisfying and supportive and that the process replaces anxiety with a sense of inner peace.

It would be helpful to keep written notes that you can refer back to later. Don't forget that your list can be changed at any time. Also keep in mind that it may take a few attempts before you arrive at the treatment objectives you feel most comfortable with. Since you are continually collecting data and expert advice, you can fine-tune your objectives as you gain additional information.

Treatment Objectives Include:

1. Maximum treatment, palliative treatment, or no treatment
2. Quality of life considerations
3. Special treatment objectives

Maximum Treatment, Palliation, or Neither?

Of course you want a cure, and, just for the record, you should make that your long-term goal. Going for the cure always has an attraction even when it means using the biggest and strongest conventional treatment available. But keep in mind that such a treatment can include greater risk and discomfort than some palliative treatments, which focus on reducing symptoms and attack the disease with fewer side effects. Such choices are available in every part of conventional oncology. Medical providers often make these decisions for their patients, but the purpose of this book is to involve you intelligently in that decision-making process.

Being hesitant about setting your objectives for treatment is common.

A more radical surgical procedure may offer the possibility of a better outcome but, at the same time, might affect your form or function. For almost every cancer diagnosis there are examples of such radical surgeries: mastectomy for breast cancer and total excision of an extensive brain tumor are just a few.

Less extensive variations of many surgical procedures are worth considering, however. One example would be a lumpectomy (with radiation) as opposed to mastectomy. Another example would be removing part of a brain tumor, leaving a person with better brain function than would removing it all. Such procedural choices can (but not always) produce significant differences in your quality of life. These are choices that need to be weighed carefully.

Each therapeutic choice involves additional decisions. Chemotherapy drug treatments, for example, can offer a variety of choices for the same diagnosis. In some cases, you can choose between high dose chemotherapy with significant side effects or lower dose programs with less toxicity.

Often, different drugs are available, ones with entirely different mechanisms of action in your body. There are differences in side effects during treatment, lingering effects after treatment, and, as you would have guessed, statistical differences in long-term survival.

Most patients choose therapy based on the first recommendation they receive, never realizing that other choices may be available. Patients who participate in the treatment-selection process, however, are much more likely to be satisfied with the results.

Three Key Questions to Help Determine the Best Treatment for You

1. What is the difference in survival rates among the maximum treatment, the less intense treatment, and no treatment at all?
2. What is the difference in risks and toxicity among maximum treatment, less intense treatment, and no treatment at all?
3. How much treatment can I endure?

As you learned earlier in this chapter, many conventional treatments are associated with research studies that statistically estimate patients' long-term survival rates. Perhaps of equal or greater importance are the differences in survival rates between treatments.

Patients who participate in the treatment-selection process are much more likely to be satisfied with the results.

For example, would you endure a much more toxic treatment for just a minimal statistical improvement in long-term survival? The answer probably depends on how toxic and how much improvement. If the maximum treatment offers a clear advantage over palliative treatment (one that is designed more to relieve symptoms than to cure) in long-term survival, this is obviously a positive. If the ten-year survival rate goes from 45% to 90%, your decision should be easy. However, if the improvement is modest, say 45% to 55%, you may want to consider more carefully if the difference is worth the increased toxicity of a stronger treatment. Your oncologist can provide you with the very latest statistics for your exact diagnosis since these figures change almost daily with new research studies.

As you review the statistical survival numbers don't forget to check the figures for no treatment at all. If treatment has just a small advantage over no treatment, you may want to explore the option of foregoing conventional treatment.

The differences in risk and toxicity are a necessary part of your decision as well. If the maximum treatment is not very toxic or the difference between treatment side effects is minimal, stronger treatment may be worth considering. More significant differences in toxicity, however, need to be weighed carefully against the potential benefits.

When you are comparing side effects, however, don't assume that refusing conventional treatment is without symptoms. The side effects of the untreated disease may be worse than those of some treatments, even when cure is not a probable outcome with the conventional therapy.

Your ability to tolerate treatment and potential toxicity plays an important role in your decision. If you are strong and in relatively good health, you will be much better able to endure maximum treatments than if you are having a lot of physical symptoms and problems. Your emotional, psychological, and spiritual status all affect your tolerance of treatment.

When a treatment is likely to overwhelm you, it can actually do you more harm than good, leaving you in worse condition than when you started. Such treatments will also reduce your opportunities to use supportive therapies later. On the one hand, if a conventional treatment offers specific benefits that outweigh the negatives and your only hesitation is that you don't want to do weeks or months of an unpleasant treatment, it sometimes helps to keep in mind that the time will pass whether you do it or not. So why not get it over with?

> Your emotional, psychological, and spiritual status all affect your tolerance of treatment.

Setting your objectives for intensity of treatment comes down to the answers to the three key questions on page 63. Put simply, if the potential benefits outweigh the potential risks and you are able to tolerate the treatment, it probably makes sense to go ahead with it.

The title of this section could have been *don't do the treatment just because it's there!* Medical specialists are increasingly recommending against treatments that don't have any real promise for improving status especially when those treatments have the potential to make things much worse. In the final analysis, you want to be certain that your treatment decision has been made correctly.

IMPORTANT QUESTIONS TO ASK YOUR PROVIDERS

Now that you have a better understanding of how to evaluate the different kinds of therapies, it's time to get the opinions of your health care providers. I can't emphasize strongly enough that selecting therapies should be done under the care and supervision of your conventional and alternative medical practitioners. Their opinions are the opinions of trained professionals, and the information they will share with you comes from years of experience with other patients like yourself.

Some important questions to ask your providers follow. In fact, it could be useful to provide a list of these questions to your providers prior to a visit with them, in order to provide them with the time to answer fully.

1. What treatments are available for me?
2. What specific improvement in survival is predicted for each?
3. What specific improvement in status (such as resolving pain) can I expect?
4. What are the side effects, toxicity, and recovery time for each?
5. How well do you think I will endure each of these treatments?
6. How do these treatments compare specifically with no treatment?

Be certain that your specialists know that you want specifics. If no data is available, they need to make that clear to you.

If few or no conventional treatment choices are available for you, your decision may be easy. If there are a number of close choices, it makes sense to write them down and review them. Always get a second opinion.

If a conventional treatment offers a real possibility for cure and you feel that you can accept the side effects, go for it. If you aren't impressed with the statistical outcome advantages of the strongest treatment program, go for the less toxic one. The stronger one may be available later if you need it.

If you want to do the strongest program but don't think you can endure it, you have several alternatives to consider. One useful strategy is to delay your decision for a short period of time while you build yourself up both nutritionally and emotionally. After a few days, weeks, or longer of getting yourself back in shape, you may be more able to move forward. The other alternative is to opt for the less toxic program. Depending on the specifics, the less toxic program may leave you more room to include nonconventional treatments.

If the only conventional treatments available are highly toxic and offer just the tiniest improvement in status, this may be the time to *just say no* rather than find yourself enduring a very difficult treatment that has literally no possibility to help. When circumstances are difficult and conventional medicine doesn't have anything to offer, it is not helpful to grasp at straws, looking to a treatment to be something it is not. At best, this is a very difficult decision. On the positive side, however, you can fill the space with supportive, nonconventional treatments.

TREATMENT AND QUALITY OF LIFE

Patients with the same diagnosis, in the same general condition, and with the same outcome often have a remarkably different quality of life during and after treatment. Some patients literally cruise through treatment. Others have a very difficult time. Here I will briefly explore how treatment objectives can affect a person's quality of life. (Chapter 11 discusses specific strategies for assessing and improving quality of life.) The issue of quality of life is tremendously important. For many, maintaining a good quality of life is the reason they became interested in nonconventional medicine in the first place.

Conventional treatment can affect quality of life in many positive and negative ways. In some cases, tumor shrinkage or removal can remarkably reduce or eliminate pain and improve other symptoms and complaints. These same treatments, however, can also cause pain and discomfort, nausea, vomiting, hair loss, fatigue, and other adverse reactions. Your specific response depends on the particular treatment(s), your diagnostics, and your general health.

Sometimes you have a choice of treatments that can provide the same end result but with altogether different side effects. Such choices are not always available, but when they are, you may do best by simply choosing the treatment protocol whose side effects would bother you the least.

If a real cure is available, you will likely be willing to endure reduced quality of life to get there. If conventional medicine's best offering is just a modest increase in survival status, however, you will want to look very hard at quality-of-life issues. A small statistical improvement may not be worth a more toxic treatment.

Be sure to keep an open mind and an open heart. Listen to your conventional as well as nonconventional medical providers, and remember that, in the end, the best treatment decisions are your decisions.

5

Understanding Your Conventional Therapy

Every challenge in life presents an opportunity. Selecting a course of treatment for cancer is no exception. This chapter will help you by providing the information you need to better understand your conventional medical treatment. Knowing about these conventional treatments will in turn help you to find the natural therapies that best complement your conventional care.

Having a good understanding of your conventional treatment will have other benefits as well. You'll gain the power to converse with your medical and radiation oncologists, surgeons, and the rest of your health care team. You'll be able to ask questions with confidence and to understand the answers you get. This knowledge will give you the understanding necessary to explore alternatives, exercising more control over your own life. And, of course, knowledge will enable you to understand the advice you will be given, but you'll still be able to make your own decisions. In your battle against cancer, knowledge and understanding will be two of the most powerful tools in your arsenal.

MAKING THE BEST USE OF THIS CHAPTER

If you and your physician have already decided on your conventional medical treatment, you can simply look it up in the pages that follow.

You'll find basic information about each treatment, how the treatment works, its potential side effects, and what to be aware of when combining it with natural treatments. For a more in-depth look at the side effects associated with chemotherapy and radiation therapy, see chapter 6. Once you've gained an understanding of your conventional medical treatment, you'll be ready to put together a treatment plan that makes optimum use of complementary cancer therapies. This we'll do in chapter 7.

THE PROOF BEHIND CONVENTIONAL CANCER TREATMENTS

"Scientifically proven" is a phrase we hear often. But when it comes to medicine, just what does it mean? Why are certain treatments "proved" to be effective and others not?

Most of the data concerning conventional cancer treatments is the result of scientific studies. Such studies are conducted carefully and analyzed thoroughly. Optimally, they involve large numbers of people over long periods of time. Researchers hope the information that comes from these studies will help them to determine how useful or how harmful a treatment might be. If a treatment is deemed effective, the resulting statistical data will then help physicians decide how beneficial it will be for each of their patients.

Not all conventional therapies have been scientifically studied, however. In fact, the Office of Technology Assessment for the U.S. Congress estimates that less than one-third of conventional medical practice has been proven effective with solid scientific studies. Conventional drugs and therapies that fall into the "not scientifically studied" category include some older medical treatments that are still used today, uses of FDA-approved medications that are "off label" (using a drug to treat a disease for which that drug is not FDA-approved), some surgical and radiation procedures, and newer drugs that are still being investigated.

Keep in mind that "not scientifically studied" doesn't mean that these treatments don't work but rather that no one has tested them scientifically. Some conventional treatments, for example, are the result of practical experience with individual patients rather than with a scientific study. For more information on how to understand the data about conventional cancer treatments, see page 56.

TYPES OF CONVENTIONAL TREATMENT

The most common conventional medical treatments for cancer are chemotherapy, radiation, and surgery. Within these categories are many individual therapies with widely varying results and side effects. Since conventional health care providers often combine these treatments, it's important that you have a good grasp of what treatments are available, how they work, and when they are considered appropriate.

Chemotherapy. Unlike many other diseases, cancer is not an illness that is treated by eliminating a foreign "invader" such as bacteria or a virus. Cancer is a disease process in which cells of the body undergo changes, causing them to multiply at a rapid and often uncontrolled rate. These cancerous cells become tumors that interfere with the body's normal functioning. Left unchecked, the results can be catastrophic.

While antibiotics attack and destroy invading viruses and bacteria, chemotherapy destroys these mutated human cells. And because cancer cells are so similar to human cells, the anticancer drugs often do damage to healthy tissue as well, causing a variety of side effects.

Radiation Therapy. Like chemotherapy, radiation also is used to destroy cancerous cells directly. This is most often accomplished by directing a beam of radiation at the tumor. One of the advantages of radiation therapy is that most of its effects occur in a small, discrete area where the cancer is located (as opposed to the effects of chemotherapy, which tend to reach many of the body's systems). Like chemotherapy, radiation can also damage healthy living cells, causing its own variety of side effects.

Surgery. Surgical removal of tumors is the oldest known treatment for cancer. The extent of surgery depends largely on the location, size, and type of cancer. Such surgical treatments can vary from a simple biopsy to procedures considerably more extensive.

Radiation therapies and chemotherapies are frequently used together. In many circumstances they are also combined with surgery.

Chemotherapy

Hardly a day goes by in my practice where a patient doesn't absolutely refuse chemotherapy. When I ask which chemotherapy they are refusing, they are often surprised that more than one even exists.

Seven common categories of chemotherapy agents and literally hundreds of different drugs and combinations are available. Each type of agent involves different actions in the body, different side effects, and a variety of predicted outcomes that range from outright cure to no effect at

Patients are often surprised that more than one type of chemotherapy even exists.

all. To assume that all types of chemotherapy are the same would be the equivalent of saying that a Piper Cub and a Boeing 747 are identical. It would be wise then to decide about chemotherapy only after you know which one is being suggested and what you can expect from it.

In discussing the varieties of chemotherapy, I will cover their therapeutic use as well as possible side effects that might result from each. Some of these side effects may be common and others quite rare. My aim is not to scare you but rather to give you a view of the larger picture. It is unlikely that you will experience all these effects, and it is important to know that almost all of them are reversible with the conclusion of treatment.

The Six Most Common Types of Chemotherapeutic Agents

- Alkylating agents
- Antitumor antibiotics
- Antimetabolites
- Biological agents
- Hormonal agents
- Plant-derived agents

Alkylating Agents

Alkylating agents attack cancer by creating substances known as *free radicals*, which are molecules capable of adding or removing an electron from human cells, thus damaging the cell. (Free radicals are discussed in more detail under "Radiation Therapy," page 84.) These highly reactive substances are especially damaging to tumor cells. Because the tumor cells are reproducing so rapidly and randomly, they are unable to repair the damage caused by free radicals before they are once again in the reproduction phase. So they simply expire.

Alkylating agents are routinely used to treat a wide variety of leukemias and lymphomas as well as solid tumors. Specific diseases treated include Hodgkin's disease; non-Hodgkin's lymphoma; acute and chronic leukemias; multiple myeloma; primary brain tumors; carcinomas of the breast, testes, bladder, ovaries, and cervix; head and neck cancers; and malignant melanomas.

Common Alkylating Agents

Generic Drug Name	*Trade or Other Common Names*
altretamine	Hexamethylmelamine
busulfan	Myleran
carboplatin	Paraplatin
carmustine	BCNU, BiCNU
chlorambucil	Leukeran
cisplatin	Platinol
cyclophosphamide	Cytoxan, Neosar, Endoxan
dacarbazine	DTIC
fotumestine	No other names
ifosfamide	Ifex
lomustine	CCNU, CeeNU
mechlorethamine	Mustargen
melphalan	Alkeran, L-PAM, L-Sarcolysin
procarbazine	Matulane, MIH
streptozocin	Zanosar
temozolide	No other names
thiotepa	No other names

SIDE EFFECTS OF ALKYLATING AGENTS

Alkylating agents have side effects that are associated primarily with the gastrointestinal system and with bone marrow suppression. Nausea and vomiting occur because of signals sent to the brain by the drug, not by anything going bad in the stomach.

The bone marrow suppression associated with alkylating agents is related to their ability to attack and destroy rapidly dividing cells. This action affects not only tumor cells, but also hair follicles, mucosal cells, and bone marrow, all of which are rapidly dividing cells. Both mouth sores and hair loss are common side effects of alkylating agents.

Because bone marrow cells manufacture the white blood cells of your immune system, the bone marrow suppression caused by chemotherapy means that you will be more vulnerable to infection. Your doctor's office will give you food and diet guidelines for microbial safety—in other words, you should avoid bacteria, molds, funguses, viruses, and other sources of infection.

The damage to the rapidly dividing cells of the bone marrow also results in a reduced number of red blood cells, producing anemia, which means that your blood's ability to carry oxygen is limited. Bone marrow suppression also reduces the number of platelets, which limits your ability to stop bleeding after being cut. These effects are usually reversible within a few weeks to a few months after treatment, depending on dosage and the patient's condition.

The alkylating drugs have a small chance of causing other cancers later on. In addition, they can also result in organ system toxicity, usually to the kidneys and/or liver, but in some cases to the nerves of the hands and feet, the ears (affecting the hearing), and the lungs. Most but not all of these toxicities are reversible as well.

THINGS TO BE WARY OF WHEN COMBINING ALKYLATING AGENTS WITH NATURAL TREATMENTS

Problems resulting from poor combinations usually occur in a variety of areas. For alkylating agents, these include absorption and gastrointestinal problems as well as stress and toxicity to various organs.

Absorption Considerations

With a few exceptions, alkylating agents are generally well-absorbed no matter how you take them—orally, intravenously, or by direct introduction into the body in the area of the tumor. However, you should avoid supplementary antioxidants while taking these chemotherapy agents since the antioxidants can reduce the effectiveness of the antitumor action. (A list of nonconventional treatments that have antioxidant activity are listed in appendix 3.)

Avoid using laxatives or therapies that might induce vomiting when taking oral alkylating agents, as these, too, can interfere with absorption.

High doses of amino acids, such as protein drinks, diet sodas, or individual amino acid preparations, should be avoided during the drug melphalan's absorption *protected zone*. **The protected zone is that time period and that part of your body where your conventional treatment does its work.** Amino acids can interfere with the body's ability to transport the drug from the digestive tract to the bloodstream. During intravenous administration of the drug carboplatin, avoid substances that contain aluminum, such as certain antacids, because aluminum can combine with the drug, thus reducing its effectiveness.

Gastrointestinal Problems

Since nausea and vomiting are common with these drugs, be certain that foods you eat during this period do not have a tendency to make things worse. Avoid raw fruits and vegetables, acid foods such as tomatoes, and rich foods such as cream sauces and dairy products. Even though dairy products may have an initial soothing effect, the proteins and sugars in them are difficult to digest and may eventually make you feel worse.

The drugs chlorambucil, thiotepa, and busulfan can cause serious diarrhea. This is the result of these drugs damaging the cells lining the intestines. Adhering to the simple diet mentioned above can help. You should avoid stimulants such as caffeine and ephedra. (A list of common foods and medicines that contain caffeine are listed in appendix 1.)

You may experience a loss of appetite resulting in weight loss if your treatment includes the drugs cyclophosphamide, thiotepa, dacarbazine, and procarbazine. If your weight is already low, this can be a serious problem. (See "Failure to Thrive" in chapter 11.)

Organ Stress and Toxicity

Since bone marrow toxicity is a direct result of these drugs, the use of immune stimulants may be possible in specific circumstances but should be avoided in general—they usually pose more potential risks than benefits. For instance, they may stimulate the wrong kind of (immune system) white blood cell production or detract from the immune system's ability to create the correct ones.

Mouth sores can occur with melphalan and procarbazine as a result of damage to the rapidly dividing cells of the mucosa and the lining of the digestive tract. Since the mouth sores represent a temporary breakdown in the *mucosal barrier*, which protects you from germs in your digestive tract, it is important to avoid any foods that are not verifiably germ-safe. Your oncologist's office will provide you with guidelines for a special diet and hygiene for your particular oncology treatment.

Alkylating agents tend to stress the kidneys and urinary tract. Non-conventional therapies, such as diuretics, that also do this should be avoided. (A list of nonconventional diuretics can be found in appendix 2.) Drinking large quantities of water is the best preventative for avoiding kidney toxicity from alkylators.

Some reversible liver stress may be experienced with busulfan, carmustine, chlorambucil, ifosfamide, lomustine, mechlorethamine, procarbazine, and streptozocin. Nonconventional therapies that add stress to the liver can increase the liver toxicity of these drugs, turning a mild side effect into a more serious one. (Nonconventional therapies that can stress the liver are listed in appendix 5.)

Nerve damage can result with altretamine, cisplatin, and carboplatin, usually as numbness to the hands and feet, but sometimes in the form of hearing damage. It is wise to avoid stimulants such as caffeine and ephedra, which can exacerbate these effects. Hair loss is most noticeable with cyclophosphamide and ifosfamide but is almost always reversible after treatment.

Pressors, certain foods and botanicals, including those that are aged, fermented, or spoiled, can precipitate a high blood pressure attack if used during the protected zone for procarbazine. (These pressors are listed in appendix 4.)

Antitumor Antibiotics

Antitumor antibiotics are a varied group of anticancer drugs that are so named because they are produced in a manner similar to conventional antibiotics. Like alkylating agents, most antitumor antibiotics create free radicals that attack rapidly dividing tumor cells. However, their actions, side effects, and usefulness are not as uniform as alkylating agents. They are used to treat a wide variety of cancers, including carcinomas of the breast, lung, stomach, and thyroid; lymphomas; certain leukemias; myelomas; and sarcomas.

Common Antitumor Antibiotics

Generic Drug Name	Trade or Other Common Names
bleomycin	Blenoxane
dactinomycin	Cosmegen
daunorubicin	Cerubidine
doxorubicin	Adriamycin, hydroxydaunorubicin
epirubicin	no other names
idarubicin	Idamycin
mitomycin C	Mutamycin
mitoxantrone	Novantrone
plicamycin	Mithracin

SIDE EFFECTS OF ANTITUMOR ANTIBIOTICS

The most common side effects with antitumor antibiotics are bone marrow suppression, nausea and vomiting, mouth sores, hair loss, and heart toxicity. A few exceptions are worth noting. Bleomycin does not usually result in bone marrow suppression, nausea and vomiting, or heart toxicity. Plicamycin usually doesn't cause mouth sores, hair loss, or heart toxicity, and dactinomycin does not typically cause heart toxicity.

THINGS TO BE WARY OF WHEN COMBINING ANTITUMOR ANTIBIOTICS WITH NATURAL TREATMENTS

Problems resulting from poor combinations with antitumor antibiotics include absorption and gastrointestinal problems as well as stress and toxicity to various organs.

Absorption

As with alkylating agents, the free radicals created by antitumor antibiotics can be adversely affected by antioxidant supplements. You should avoid antioxidant supplements within the protected zone for timing of these drugs. When reasonable estimates of this time are not available, the drug's terminal life can be estimated by an oncologist or an oncology pharmacist. (A list of nonconventional treatments that have antioxidant activity can be found in appendix 3.)

Gastrointestinal Problems

As in the case of the alkylating agents, the nausea and vomiting associated with these drugs is the result of signals generated by the drugs and sent to the brain, not the result of something happening in the stomach.

Organ Stress and Toxicity

Mitomycin C and plicamycin can be stressful to the kidneys and urinary tract. Such nonconventional therapies as diuretics are best avoided except in special circumstances. (A list of nonconventional diuretics can be found in appendix 2.) Drinking large amounts of water is the best preventive measure for avoiding kidney toxicity.

Dactinomycin and plicamycin can cause liver stress. Nonconventional therapies that add stress to the liver can increase the liver toxicity of these drugs, possibly creating more serious problems. (A list of alternative therapies that can stress the liver can be found in appendix 5.)

Cardiac toxicity is generally a result of damage to the heart and cardiovascular system, but it can also be caused by secondary actions, such as a fluid or metabolic imbalance brought on by the drug. Lung damage can occur with the use of bleomycin and mitomycin C. The mechanism of damage is not fully understood.

Antimetabolites

> Antimetabolites are anticancer drugs that interfere with the metabolism and reproduction of tumor cells.

Antimetabolites are anticancer drugs that interfere with the metabolism and reproduction of tumor cells. They restrict or otherwise disable cell-nucleus biochemicals, proteins, fats, and other critical components that the tumor cells require to sustain and reproduce themselves. These drugs seriously injure the tumor cells. They are often used with other chemotherapeutic agents that will destroy the tumor cells more readily once they have been weakened by the antimetabolite.

Antimetabolites are used in the treatment of a wide variety of cancers, including cancers of the digestive tract, liver, pancreas, head and neck, breast, ovaries, bone, and lung, as well as certain leukemias and lymphomas.

Common Antimetabolite Agents

Generic Drug Name	Trade or Other Common Names
asparaginase	ELSPAR, L-asparaginase
cladribine	2-CDA, 2-Chlorodeoxyadenosine, Leustatin
cytarabine	Cytosine arabinoside, ara-C, Cytosar-U
floxuridine	Fluorodeoxyuridine, 5-FUDR, FUDR
fludarabine phosphate	FLUDARA
fluorouracil	5-Fluorouracil, 5-FU
gemcitabine	Gemzar
hydroxyurea	Hydrea
leucovorin	no other names
mercaptopurine	6-mercaptopurine, 6-MP, Purinethol
methotrexate	MTX, Folex
pentostatin	NIPENT
thioguanine	6-thioguanine, 6-TG, Tabloid

SIDE EFFECTS OF ANTIMETABOLITES

While the specific actions of antimetabolites vary significantly, some can have far fewer side effects than other categories of chemotherapy drugs. The most common side effects are bone marrow suppression (except floxuridine, leucovorin, and asparaginase), mouth sores, hair loss, and diarrhea, all of which are normally reversible. These drugs also impair the ability of both men and women to reproduce, but this effect is usually more reversible than with other drug categories. Some of these drugs may cause nausea, vomiting, kidney toxicity, liver toxicity, allergic response, or nerve damage.

THINGS TO BE WARY OF WHEN COMBINING ANTIMETABOLITES WITH NATURAL TREATMENTS

Problems resulting from poor combinations usually occur in a variety of areas. For antimetabolic agents, these include absorption and gastrointestinal problems as well as stress and toxicity to various organs.

Absorption

You should avoid aspirin, anti-inflammatory herbs, and nonsteroidal anti-inflammatory drugs during the protected zone for this class of drugs, with the exception of leucovorin. Supplemental doses of B vitamins and folic acid should also be avoided. Amino acid supplements, including herbs high in the amino acid asparagine, should be avoided during the protected zone for asparaginase.

Gastrointestinal Problems

Nausea and vomiting can be a problem with cytarabine. The drugs 5-fluorouracil, methotrexate, and cytarabine can cause serious diarrhea, a result of damage to the intestinal lining; therefore, stimulants such as caffeine and ephedra are best avoided. (A list of common foods and medicines that contain caffeine can be found in appendix 1.)

Organ Stress and Toxicity

Pentostatin can be stressful to the kidneys and urinary tract. You should avoid alternative therapies that also stress these organs, including diuretics. (A list of nonconventional diuretics can be found in appendix 2.)

Floxuridine can cause liver stress, and nonconventional therapies that are stressful to the liver should be avoided. (A list of alternative therapies that can stress the liver can be found in appendix 5.)

Biological Agents

Biological agents are a variety of drugs that either are organisms on their own or mimic chemicals normally found in the human body. They include interleukins, interferons, bacteria, stimulating factors, hormone regulators, and vitamin A analogues. Biological agents have a wide range of actions and are currently the subject of a number of investigational studies.

Interleukins achieve their anticancer action by stimulating the activity of the immune system. More than twenty different interferons regulate cell proliferation and immune system reactions with a wide number of actions. Their anticancer action stems from their ability to slow down cell reproduction of both normal and tumor cells. Interferons are used in the treatment of specific types of leukemia, Kaposi's sarcoma, and a wide variety of infections.

Bacillus Calmette-Guerin (BCG) is one of the bacterial chemotherapy agents. It is a live bacterial strain that is administered directly to the site of certain urinary tract cancers. The immune system responds to the bacteria by attacking not only the bacteria, but also the local tumor cells.

Stimulating factors are modeled after the chemicals in the body that increase blood components, such as white blood cells and red blood cells. Stimulating factors have a positive effect on the immune system.

Hormone regulators have been used to control a variety of human growth factors, as well as to inhibit tumor growth. They have anticancer effects and reduce treatment side effects such as diarrhea. These drugs are still the subject of investigation.

Vitamin A analogues, known as *retinoids,* have demonstrated anticancer activity, but the way they work is not well understood. These agents are still the subject of investigation.

> Biological agents are a variety of drugs that either are organisms on their own or mimic chemicals normally found in the human body.

Common Biological Agents

Generic Drug Name	Class of Drug	Trade or Other Common Names
Bacillus Calmette-Guerin	bacteria	BCG, TICE, Thera-cys
epoetin	red blood cell stimulating factor	Erythropoietin, EPO, Epogen
filgrastim	red blood cell stimulating factor	G-CSF, Neupogen
IL-2	interleukin	Aldesleukin, Proleukin

Generic Drug Name	Class of Drug	Trade or Other Common Names
IL-3	interleukin	no other names
IL-4	interleukin	no other names
IL-10	interleukin	no other names
levamisole	immune system regulator	Ergamisol
octeotride	hormone regulator	Somatostatin analogue, Sandostatin
retinoids	vitamin A analogues	Isotretinoin, Tretinoin
sargramostim	white blood cell stimulating factor	GM-CSF, Leukine, Prokine

SIDE EFFECTS OF COMMON BIOLOGICAL AGENTS

Bone marrow suppression can occur with aldesleukin, bacillus Calmette-Guerin (although rarely), and levamisole. Anemia and thrombocytopenia (a decreased number of blood platelets), either of which can require transfusions, are commonly associated with the interleukins. Most biological agents can sometimes cause reduced thyroid function, which is not reversible and which may require long-term thyroid replacement therapy. Kidney, heart, and lung toxicity may also occur but are normally controlled and reversible.

Interferon alpha, the most common interferon in use, is fairly well tolerated. The most common side effects are flu-like symptoms, including fever, chills, muscle aches, headache, fatigue, and joint pain.

Side effects of bacillus Calmette-Guerin include bladder irritation, urinary urgency, burning with urination, and reduced bladder capacity. In addition, the symptoms one would normally expect from an infection, such as fever, chills, and fatigue, can also occur. These symptoms are not severe and usually resolve quickly.

Some white blood cell stimulators are rarely associated with toxic side effects, while others have dose-related side effects, including fluid build-up around the heart and lungs, edema of the hands and feet, headache, and flu-like symptoms. These symptoms commonly subside after treatment. Red blood cell stimulators tend to have few side effects; these include rare blood clots and increased blood pressure.

Biological agents usually have milder side effects than most other chemotherapy agents. They can include nausea, diarrhea, abdominal discomfort, headache, dizziness, depression and other emotional symptoms, hot flashes, fatigue, and blood-sugar metabolism problems.

The most common side effects of vitamin A retinoids are lip inflammation and eye dryness. Other less common side effects may include nosebleeds, rash, thinning hair, sensitivity to light, nausea, vomiting, and headache.

THINGS TO BE WARY OF WHEN COMBINING BIOLOGICAL AGENTS WITH NATURAL TREATMENTS

Problems resulting from poor combinations usually occur in a variety of areas. For biological agents, these include gastrointestinal problems and stress or toxicity to various organs.

Gastrointestinal Problems

Aldesleukin, bacillus Calmette-Guerin, sargramostim, and octeotride can cause serious diarrhea. It's helpful to avoid foods that are rich and high in acid content. Also avoid stimulants such as caffeine and ephedra. (Common foods and medicines that contain caffeine can be found in appendix 1.)

Organ Stress and Toxicity

Aldesleukin, bacillus Calmette-Guerin, sargramostim, and retinoids can be stressful to the kidneys and urinary tract. Natural diuretics and other nonconventional therapies that can stress the kidneys should be avoided. (See appendix 2 for a list of nonconventional diuretics.)

Both sargramostim and retinoids can stress the liver. (See appendix 5 for a list of natural treatments that should be avoided when taking these drugs.)

Hormonal Agents

Hormonal agents affect cancer cells by increasing or decreasing hormone activity in the body. This is done by regulating the actual levels of hormones as well as by interfering with the ability of some hormones to create a response in cells. Since the growth of some tumor cells is affected by the presence of natural hormones, hormone treatment interferes with that mechanism. Hormones are often used in conjunction with other chemotherapy agents.

Common Anticancer Hormonal Agents

Generic Drug Name	Class of Drug	Trade or Other Common Names
aminoglutethimide	antiadrenal	Cytadren
diethylstilbestrol	estrogen	DES
fluoxymesterol	steroid	Halotestin
flutamide	antitestosterone	Eulexin
goserelin acetate	antitestosterone, antiestrogen	Zoladex
ketoconazole	antitestosterone	Nizoral
leuprolide	antitestosterone	Lupron
megastrol acetate	progestin, antiestrogen	Megace
mifepristone	antiprogestin, antisteroid	no other names
tamoxifen	antiestrogen	Nolvadex

SIDE EFFECTS OF HORMONAL AGENTS

Hormonal agents have some common side effects, known together as *flare*. They include bone pain, redness around skin lesions, and increased blood calcium. Flare is considered by some as an indicator that the hormone treatment is having its desired antitumor effect.

Depression and other emotional symptoms can occur with diethylstilbestrol, fluoxymesterol, flutamide, goserelin acetate, leuprolide, and tamoxifen. Hot flashes can result from the hormonal action of flutamide, goserelin acetate, leuprolide, mifepristone, and tamoxifen. Individual hormonal agents have additional side effects consistent with their action in the body. Hormones are generally well tolerated when compared to other chemotherapy agents.

THINGS TO BE WARY OF WHEN COMBINING HORMONAL AGENTS WITH NATURAL TREATMENTS

Problems resulting from poor combinations usually occur in a variety of areas. For hormonal agents, these include gastrointestinal problems, antitumor actions, and stress or toxicity to various organs.

Gastrointestinal Problems

Nausea and vomiting can be a problem with diethylstilbestrol, fluoxymesterol, megastrol acetate, mifepristone, and tamoxifen. Avoid rich foods and foods with high acid content while taking these drugs.

Antitumor Actions

The use of plant-derived hormonal or hormone analogues, such as phytoestrogens or licorice root, can affect the action of conventional hormone agents in ways that have not been studied. Plant hormones can potentially increase the effects of some conventional hormone actions and reduce the effects of others. Before you use a hormone analogue, be certain that it does not interact in a negative way with other treatments or stimulate tumor growth.

Organ Stress and Toxicity

Diethylstilbestrol, fluoxymesterol, and ketoconazole can stress the liver. Nonconventional therapies that might be stressful to this organ should be avoided. (See appendix 5 for a list of nonconventional therapies that might be stressful to the liver.)

Plant-Derived Agents

Plant-derived agents have been in use for over 200 years and are the oldest form of chemotherapy. Their anticancer activity occurs when they interfere with the physical actions of the tumor cells as they attempt to divide and multiply. Different drugs interfere with different parts of the cell-division process. Some, like etoposide, also use free-radical generation to damage tumor cells.

Plant-derived agents are used in treating certain lung, breast, kidney, urinary tract, head and neck, testicular, and ovarian cancers, as well as specific lymphomas, leukemias, and sarcomas.

Common Plant-Derived Agents

Generic Name	Category	Trade or Other Common Names
docetaxel	diterpene	Taxotere
etoposide	podophyllotoxin	VePesid
irinotecan	camptothecan	no other names
paclitaxel	diterpene	Taxol
teniposide	podophyllotoxin	Vumon
topotecan	camptothecan	no other names

Generic Name	Category	Trade or Other Common Names
vinblastine	vinca alkaloid	Velban, Velsar
vincristine	vinca alkaloid	Oncovin, Vincasar PFS
vinorelbine	vinca alkaloid	Navelbine

SIDE EFFECTS OF PLANT-DERIVED AGENTS

With the exception of vincristine, bone marrow suppression is a common side effect among these agents. Hair loss and mouth sores occur from some of the agents, as does liver toxicity, but these are reversible. The vinca alkaloids, derived from the periwinkle plant, can cause nerve damage that is often but not always reversible. Diterpene-based drugs, from the bark of the Western yew tree, can cause significant allergic response, which is often treated prophylactically. The podophyllotoxins are derived from the May apple tree, and the camptothecan drugs are compounded from the Chinese tree *Camptotheca acuminata*. The camptothecan class of drugs can have significant toxicity, including severe diarrhea.

Nerve damage can also result with vincristine, as well as vinblastine, etoposide, paclitaxel, docetaxel, and vinorelbine.

THINGS TO BE WARY OF WHEN COMBINING PLANT-DERIVED AGENTS WITH NATURAL TREATMENTS

Problems resulting from poor combinations usually occur in a variety of areas. For plant-derived agents, these include absorption as well as stress and toxicity to various organs.

Absorption

Since some plant-derived chemotherapy drugs work by creating free radicals, you should avoid supplementary antioxidants during the protected zone for timing; the antioxidants can interfere with the antitumor effects of these drugs. (See appendix 3 for nonconventional treatments that have antioxidant activity.)

Organ Stress and Toxicity

Vinorelbine can stress the liver. Natural therapies that can add to this should be avoided. (See appendix 5 for nonconventional treatments that can be stressful to the liver.)

Chemotherapy Combinations

Most chemotherapy treatments include more than one chemotherapeutic agent. These drugs are combined to achieve a more complete tumor response. In combination, the dosage and timing of the individual drugs are often different from the dosages and timing that would be used if the drug was being employed by itself. This is done to optimize the actions of the individual drugs and to limit their combined toxic effects. As a result, combination drug protocols have different actions and side effects than might be predicted by simply combining their individual actions. Your medical specialist can help you understand the side effects and actions of your particular therapy.

Radiation Therapy

Radiation therapy has become increasingly useful in oncology. It is now recommended to 50% of cancer patients, and it is considered for most types of cancer. The advantage of radiation therapy is that most of its effects are restricted to the area where the tumor is located. In certain specialized circumstances, such as bone marrow transplant, radiation therapy may be administered to the whole body as total body irradiation (TBI) or radiation of specific systems, such as bone marrow irradiation (BMI).

Combination drug protocols have different actions and side effects than might be predicted by simply combining their individual actions.

Radiation therapy, also known as radiotherapy or ionizing radiation, is usually delivered either as an invisible stream of rays, known as an *external beam,* or by implanting near the tumor radioactive "seeds" (a process called *brachytherapy*), which release a slow, steady dose of radiation that eventually tapers off.

In the early days of radiation therapy, it was believed that the radiation rays simply hit the tumor cells and killed them. However, modern radiation physicists have shown that this is not the case. Radiation destroys tumor tissue by causing a series of events. Before we discuss how radiation therapy kills tumor cells, let me reassure those readers who successfully avoided biology class that it is not necessary to understand the next few paragraphs in order to understand the rest of this book.

All things in nature try to stay at equilibrium with their surroundings. Normally, the cells and atoms in our bodies have a neutral or balanced electrical charge—in other words, an equal number of negatively charged electrons and positively charged protons that balance each other. Radiation treatment has the effect of dislodging electrons from the atoms of local tissue wherever it is administered, causing them to lose an electron. Then those atoms are left with more positive charges than negative ones and become positively charged particles.

The advantage of radiation therapy is that most of its effects are restricted to the area where the tumor is located.

The electrons that were knocked free may join other atoms, adding their negative charge and creating negatively charged particles. These charged atoms are called *ions*, or *free radicals*. As these free radicals come into contact with local tissue, including tumor tissue, they either steal from or donate an electron to those cells, thus unbalancing them. Normal tissue cells often have time to repair the radiation damage before starting to reproduce, whereas tumor cells, which reproduce more rapidly and frenetically than normal cells, are usually unable to repair themselves before attempting to reproduce. In most cases, the radiation damage prevents those cells from reproducing and thus kills the tumor tissue. The free radicals quickly dissipate after treatment, but the destruction of tumor cells can continue for days and weeks after treatment.

Radiation therapy can destroy most or all of the tumor cells in the vicinity of the treatment. The imaging and administering technologies have advanced to the extent that external beam radiation can be aimed exactly and delivered in a precise dosage. It is now possible to accurately protect much more healthy tissue by using computerized delivery from multiple directions and by blocking tissue that should not be irradiated. This makes outcomes more predictable and reduces side effects. Radioactive implants have also enjoyed similar benefits from improved technology.

The effectiveness of radiation varies with the amount of each dose, how often the doses are administered, how they are aimed, nutritional factors, and other drugs and substances in use. A radiation oncologist will research and develop a treatment plan that will provide the optimum tumor-killing program for your specific type of tumor, its location, its size, and the many other factors that can affect treatment and outcome. A simulation is usually done before actual treatment, to align the computers and radiation beam exactly with your tumor. This helps the radiation technician minimize the treatment's effects on normal tissue.

Radiation can be a valuable addition to other conventional cancer treatments when used carefully. It can effectively destroy tumor tissue in a particular location for both palliation, such as pain relief, as well as cure. It has been used successfully to reduce the chances of a local cancer recurrence after surgery, as with a lumpectomy for breast cancer. Your specific results will depend on a wide range of factors that are particular to you. A radiation oncology specialist should explain these in detail before the start of your treatment.

THE SIDE EFFECTS OF RADIATION THERAPY

Radiation is not without side effects. Some damage is done to healthy tissue, and you may experience generalized symptoms such as fatigue, loss of appetite, nausea, vomiting, and emotional depression. In the area of application, minor superficial burning of the skin, the equivalent of a bad sunburn, can occur. If the tumor tissue is not located close to the surface, the radiation beam must travel through healthy tissue, such as muscle and/or organs in front of or behind the tumor. That healthy tissue will be affected by the radiation as well, but usually not to the extent of the tumor tissue damage. Side effects depend on the amount of radiation given and precisely where it is aimed. Radiation can also result in cell damage that can cause cancer many years later, but this risk is much less with today's modern technology.

The good news is that most, if not all, of these side effects are generally not severe and are usually reversible. The body's innate healing ability, along with modern nutritional technology, make the benefits of appropriate radiation technology far outweigh the risks.

Surgery

Surgical removal of tumors is the oldest medical form of treatment for cancer. In the early days of surgery, the lack of adequate anesthetics, poor control of bleeding, and minimal diagnostic technology resulted in hurried procedures and less-than-optimal results. Modern technology and techniques have considerably improved the safety and accuracy of surgical procedures, making them a worthwhile option under certain conditions.

Surgical procedures are now used for a number of reasons in cancer treatment, including:

- Diagnostic biopsy
- Diagnostic exploration
- Removal of the primary tumor
- Control of metastatic disease
- Control of related tumor problems

Diagnostic Biopsy

Diagnostic biopsy is the process of taking a small amount of tissue from the suspicious mass. The tissue sample is then sent to a pathologist, who analyzes the cells under a microscope and subjects them to a number of chemical tests. The pathologist's report tells you and your providers whether the sampled tissue is cancerous. If it is cancerous, the other tests can usually identify the kinds of cells, how fast the tumor will grow, specific characteristics such as tumor markers and hormone receptors, and, sometimes, which treatments will be most effective against it.

The procedure for a biopsy depends on the size, location, and presumed type of tumor. Biopsies are being done increasingly with the aid of diagnostic imaging technology, which allows the surgeon to electronically visualize the tumor and accurately guide the biopsy without having to make a large incision.

Biopsies done close to the surface and for well-defined tumors in accessible parts of the body are usually done by removing tissue with a device that looks like a hypodermic needle. Local anesthetic normally makes the procedure painless. After numbing the area, the needle is guided to the tumor, where a small piece of tissue is removed for analysis.

> The procedure for a biopsy depends on the size, location, and presumed type of tumor.

If the tumor is poorly defined or inaccessible, the surgeon may have to create a surgical opening to see the tumor in order to take an accurate biopsy. Such biopsies are done under general anesthetic, where the person is put to sleep during the procedure. The sample may be taken with a needle, a small sampling device, or a scalpel. Biopsies are real surgical procedures that include some risks associated with the anesthetic and a risk for bleeding. In most cases these risks are small.

Surgical biopsies have also generated some concern that the procedure could allow a new avenue for cells to escape from the tumor and spread. A number of studies investigating this question have not been able to identify this as a real risk for needle biopsy, although it may be a greater risk for certain other surgical biopsy procedures. Spread of the cancer, in many cases, may have more to do with the nature and the aggressiveness of the tumor cells than with the surgical procedure.

Surgical biopsy of a solid tumor is almost always a good idea if the patient can tolerate the procedure. It provides real data that can be of enormous help in selecting the right treatment. A competent surgeon can evaluate all of the risks for you.

Surgical biopsy of the lymph nodes can determine whether tumor tissue has spread. To biopsy a lymph node, it must first be removed, thus modifying the normal filtering and balancing function of the lymph system. In some cases, with removal of axillary (underarm) lymph nodes, swelling of the arm, known as *lymphedema,* can result. The good news is that new surgical procedures, such as *sentinel node biopsies,* in which only one or a few of the nodes are removed for diagnostics, are becoming available, thus bypassing much of the discomfort and side effects of older procedures.

Diagnostic Exploration

Diagnostic exploration is a procedure in which the surgeon makes an opening in the body in order to see what is going on inside. This is usually done when the diagnostic imaging and other techniques are unable locate or identify a tumor. Diagnostic exploration is almost always major surgery. Depending on the location and extent, the risks and discomfort can vary from mild to very serious. Diagnostic exploration should only be undertaken when less invasive methods have failed to identify or resolve the problem.

Removal of the Primary Tumor

Tumor removal is the most effective surgical procedure and is often a desirable option at this stage of cancer treatment technology. The objective is to remove the tumor as well as a margin of surrounding healthy tissue to ensure that all of the visible tumor is gone. The benefits of removing the primary tumor can include:

D iagnostic exploration should only be undertaken when less invasive methods have failed to identify or resolve the problem.

- Removing the primary source of cells that can cause spread.
- Stopping the local, immediate growth of the tumor and its effects on local tissue and organs.

In some cases, surgical removal of the primary tumor can be a cure. In other cases, it can result in a remission, slow the progress of the cancer, or help control side effects from the tumor.

Primary tumor removal may have better long-term results when accomplished in conjunction with other conventional treatments such as radiation or chemotherapy. Although the surgeon may do a good job of removing the tumor(s) along with a small safety zone of healthy tissue, known as a *clear margin,* small tumor cells (known as *micrometastases*) may still remain. We would hope that the immune system would dispense of these remaining cells, but often that does not happen, and these cells cause a local recurrence. Surgery in combination with other conventional treatments can, under certain conditions, remarkably reduce the chances of a recurrence from these leftover cells.

To avoid creating new problems, a good surgeon will try not to take any more healthy tissue than is necessary. If, after the procedure, the surgeon wants to go back and take more tissue because the margins from the surgery weren't adequate, don't be upset. This is fairly common and is not an indication that your surgeon did a poor job the first time around.

Control of Metastatic Disease

Metastatic disease means a secondary growth of cancer from the primary site. Control of metastases can sometimes be accomplished surgically. The decision is based on whether the benefits of the procedure outweigh the risks. Control of metastatic disease, by itself, does not result in cure but can remarkably improve quality of life and limit damage to healthy body systems. The potential risks, however, must be balanced against the potential benefits. These include not only the normal risks for surgery, such as those pertaining to the anesthesia, potential blood loss, trauma to the body, and discomfort, but also the possible worsening of the patient's overall ability to fight the disease.

It is usually a mistake to "chase" metastatic disease when the surgeries are frequent and the patient cannot tolerate them well.

In some circumstances, surgery can control metastatic disease for very long periods of time, but only when a person is strong enough to tolerate the procedure and there is a real, definable benefit. It is usually a mistake to "chase" metastatic disease when the surgeries are frequent and the patient cannot tolerate them well.

Control of Related Tumor Problems

Control of related tumor problems with surgery can also remarkably improve quality of life. If a tumor has damaged or interfered with a neighboring organ or tissue, surgical means are sometimes available to regain that function.

If a reasonable surgical solution exists in which potential benefits outweigh potential risks, it is almost always a good idea. In the case of a primary tumor that can be removed completely, it may be worth moving forward with minimum delay, especially if there is no identified spread of the disease. Eliminating the source of tumor cells puts you in a much better position to prevail.

Not all surgeons are created equally. Different levels of skill, training, and access to new procedures can produce remarkably different results. (See chapter 3 for more information.)

Miscellaneous Conventional Treatment Strategies

Several conventional medical strategies either use a combination of the three major types of conventional therapies or introduce something altogether different.

Bone Marrow and Peripheral Stem Cell Transplants

In certain circumstances, very high doses of some conventional treatments could eliminate most of the tumor tissue in the body, but because of their toxicity, these treatments would destroy the immune system beyond repair. Bone marrow transplants are procedures in which very high levels of chemotherapy and/or radiation are used to eradicate tumor cells. Afterward, the damaged bone marrow is replaced with either new bone marrow or immature blood cells known as stem cells.

Bone marrow consists of cells inside the bone that are the source of white blood cells, red blood cells, and platelets. The white blood cells make up the immune system and are our primary defense against infection and most diseases, including cancer. The red blood cells transport oxygen from our lungs to all the parts of our body that require it for existence. Platelets maintain the integrity of the arteries, veins, organs, and other blood-carrying tissue by stopping bleeding and blood loss. High doses of certain types of chemotherapy, radiation, and some other treatments can permanently damage the bone marrow cells. Different treatments may damage only specific components of the bone marrow.

The bone marrow used for the transplant may be your own cells, known as an *autologous* transplant, or the cells of someone else whose marrow is a close "match" to yours, known as an *allogeneic* transplant. In either case, the bone marrow from the donor is harvested and saved prior to the actual high-dose treatment. In a peripheral stem cell transplant, immature blood cells are taken from the circulating blood in a much simpler procedure.

The bone marrow procedure starts with *mobilization,* in which a drug is administered to increase the activity of the bone marrow and generate more marrow cells. The drugs used include some chemotherapy agents. A short time after mobilization, bone marrow is harvested for use later. *Harvesting* is a surgical procedure, usually accomplished under general anesthetic, in which a large needle is inserted into the center of the hip or other bone and the marrow is removed. This marrow is stored for use later. In some cases, the marrow is filtered or otherwise treated prior to being transplanted into the patient.

When it is certain that the marrow or stem cells are adequate for transplantation, the high-dose treatment begins. The high-dose treatment is normally chemotherapy but may also include total body irradiation (TBI) or bone marrow irradiation (BMI). At the completion of high-dose treatment, the bone marrow or stem cells are transplanted into the individual with what is, in effect, an intravenous (IV) infusion. It looks just like a typical IV bottle and line, except for the fact that this is more than just blood.

The infused marrow cells (or stem cells) magically find their way back to the bone where they settle in and begin generating new white blood cells, red blood cells, and platelets. This process, known as *engraftment*, begins immediately after the reinfusion, and blood cells from the new marrow, called *counts*, can be measured in blood cells within a few weeks. As the new marrow matures in its new home, the cells in circulation in the blood increase to normal levels and become more functional. It can take one year or more for the process to be complete, although the patient can usually begin a normal lifestyle in six months or less.

The high-dose chemotherapy and radiation cause the first side effects of bone marrow transplantation. These can include nausea, vomiting, fever, and inflammation of the parotid gland (like mumps). Mouth sores and complete hair loss occur approximately one week after the start of treatment.

Special Treatment Objectives

Don't be surprised if your medical specialist suggests a treatment for the sole reason that it helps another treatment work better. Combined therapies are finding increasing prominence in conventional medicine, along with some new and perhaps unfamiliar terminology.

Pre-surgical *debulking* is a process where the size of a tumor is reduced by radiation, chemotherapy, vaccine, or some combination of therapies. The objective for such treatments is to reduce the size of the tumor prior to removal. This allows less damage to surrounding healthy tissue and, in some cases, permits the removal of a complete tumor, which might not otherwise be possible. This is an example where a different treatment allows the surgical procedure to be more effective.

Chemotherapy can, in some cases, increase the tumor-killing capability of radiation therapy. For this reason, chemotherapy and radiation may be prescribed in very close time proximity or together.

Some of the drugs used in cancer treatment are in fact *rescues,* designed to undo the toxicity of a prior treatment in order for the first treatment to be administered at a higher dose. The rescue drugs may also have their own tumor-killing ability. The most dramatic rescue protocols are bone marrow transplantation and peripheral stem cell transplants, as previously described.

As you can see, a number of treatment options are available with conventional medicine. They are mostly interventions, designed to rid the body of tumor cells. Many of these treatments are worth a try because their gains can outweigh their risks. The true risk–benefit assessment is different for each person and must be evaluated individually. For more information about survival statistics and what they mean for you, see chapter 4.

I encourage you to at least carefully consider, with the assistance of a provider trained and familiar with these treatments, what conventional medicine has to offer. Use treatments that can significantly improve your status and avoid those that can worsen it. In this way, you will get the best that modern conventional medicine has to offer.

Don't be surprised if your medical specialist suggests a treatment for the sole reason that it helps another treatment work better.

The Side Effects of Conventional Treatments: How Alternative Medicines Can Help

Jenny was diagnosed with Hodgkin's disease on the twenty-fifth anniversary of her mother's diagnosis of breast cancer. She still remembers the day that her parents sat her down and explained how her mother would lose her hair and be unable to do housework for the next six months. Jenny would have to help out more around the house, but this would be a small price to pay to help with her mother's cure.

The technology and dosage schedules were very different twenty-five years ago. When Jenny's mom responded badly to the chemotherapy, her doctors insisted on continuing treatment. To make matters worse, her mom had a heart condition and suffered a heart attack four months into the treatment. Jenny swore that she would never put herself or her family through such an experience.

It was a busy Friday afternoon when Jenny's medical oncologist reached me. Jenny's Hodgkin's disease was most likely curable with chemotherapy, but Jenny was unwilling to use it. Without treatment, her prognosis was poor. The oncologist was very upset. She was unable to convince Jenny of the obvious benefits.

I had co-treated other patients with this oncologist, and she had seen these patients go through treatment with fewer side effects than had her general patient population. She also knew that I took meticulous care to avoid interfering with the effectiveness of her treatments.

Jenny arrived at my office late that afternoon with the demeanor of a prizefighter.

"Before we even start this conversation," she told me, "Let me tell you about my mother's experience with chemotherapy."

After telling me her mother's story, she wanted a guarantee that none of those symptoms will happen to her.

"My mother still talks about that awful experience," Jenny told me.

I spent the next hour explaining how we could use natural medicine to build her up and prepare her for treatment, to keep her healthy and strong throughout her chemotherapy and, after it was all done, start a cancer prevention plan. I also explained how, with some preparation, we could address the side effects of the drugs that were most likely to affect her, once again without interfering with their ability to cure.

Jenny decided to give it a try but warned that she would quit if the side effects got too bad. Her oncologist gave us three weeks to get ready. During that time we resolved some long-standing digestive problems and a few other health issues. We also took steps to protect her heart and cardiovascular system.

Natural medicine can provide significant help controlling the side effects of conventional cancer treatments.

Jenny completed her treatment without interruption. She lost her hair, but after her treatments it came back more manageable than before. Her other symptoms, such as mouth sores, were mild. Jenny stated that she felt guilty complaining about them since they were so much less than her expectations. It is now ten years later. Mother and daughter are doing just fine. Jenny's only other visits to the hospital since treatment were for the births of her two children.

For some, the prospect of chemotherapy, radiation, or surgery is as frightening as the cancer diagnosis. I have seen many patients reject all conventional treatment at the outset because they were concerned about side effects. There is no question that many conventional therapies can be toxic and difficult to tolerate.

The good news is that natural medicine can provide significant help in controlling the side effects of conventional cancer treatments. The proper combination of these treatments is a wonderful example of *complementary medicine*. While the conventional therapies are busy seeking and eliminating cancer cells, natural medicine treatments can limit the toxicity to healthy tissue, keeping you as strong and as healthy as possible.

THE SIDE EFFECTS OF CONVENTIONAL CANCER THERAPIES

Any discussion of side effects should begin by saying that it would be extremely unusual for one person to experience all the possible side effects associated with a particular conventional cancer treatment. It is important, though, to have an understanding of what effects these treatments can have. The possible side effects from all of the most common conventional treatments are combined and listed below for reference:

- Bone marrow suppression
- Nausea and vomiting
- Kidney and urinary tract toxicity
- Cardiac toxicity
- Allergic response
- Mouth sores
- Hair loss
- Numbness of the hands and feet
- Lung toxicity
- Liver toxicity

The World Health Organization (W.H.O.) uses the following statistical format to describe how common these side effects are:

Most patients means the particular side effect was experienced by 70 to 100% of participants who were part of valid studies using that treatment protocol.

More than half of patients means the particular side effect was experienced by 40 to 70% of persons who were part of valid studies using that treatment protocol.

Less than half of patients means that the particular side effect was experienced by 20 to 40% of the patients who were part of valid studies using that treatment protocol.

Not usual means that the particular side effect was experienced by less than 20% of the participants who were part of valid studies using that treatment protocol.

These descriptions are, of course, just statistics. Is there any way to know who will get which symptoms? No system can accurately predict your personal experiences with conventional cancer treatments. Your general health and physical condition will have some influence. The best strategy for preparing yourself for such cancer therapies as chemotherapy and radiation is to be as strong and as healthy as possible. Your medical specialist can provide you with insight as to how you will respond to chemotherapy.

A pre-existing condition can predispose you to problems. For example, lung toxicity may be common in less than half of those people receiving a particular treatment, but if you have a pre-existing lung disease, it is far more likely that your lungs will be affected by the added stress of that treatment. The best end result will be achieved when, given a choice, you select the conventional treatment that does not affect health issues that are already a problem. In addition, natural medicine can help you become less vulnerable to some side effects.

> The best strategy for preparing yourself for such cancer therapies as chemotherapy and radiation is to be as strong and as healthy as possible.

Bone Marrow Suppression

Bone marrow suppression is a direct result of treatment on the rapidly dividing cells of your body. While chemotherapy agents attack and destroy the rapidly reproducing cells of the tumor, they also destroy some other rapidly dividing cells in your body. These include bone marrow, the mucosal cells in the walls of your mouth and gastrointestinal tract, and hair follicles.

Bone marrow suppression means that the normal functioning of your bone marrow is reduced. Your bone marrow plays an important role in your health. It produces the white blood cells that fight infection, it makes red blood cells that transport oxygen to all areas of your body, and it creates platelets, which are cells that are vital to the clotting of blood. A decreased production of any of these cells will affect you.

You may already know that the reduction of red blood cells is known as *anemia*. This condition is likely to leave you feeling tired and listless. Your doctor may refer to your reduced number of white blood cells as *leukopenia,* and the reduction in platelets in your blood as *thrombocytopenia.* In some cases, bone marrow suppression requires direct medical intervention such as marrow-stimulating drugs or transfusion.

If you have bone marrow suppression at any level, you may be more vulnerable to infection. If bone marrow suppression is a possibility, it is wise to avoid avenues of infection, such as persons with colds or other contagious diseases, as well as foods that do not meet low-microbial hygiene requirements. Supplements other than a daily, clean-manufactured multiple vitamin and mineral capsule should be avoided during the period when the bone marrow is suppressed. This will be part of the calculation of the protected zone as described in chapter 1.

Bone marrow suppression usually requires medical monitoring in the form of periodic blood tests, at least until your response pattern is determined. For treatments in which bone marrow suppression is experienced by more than half or most patients, it is worthwhile to prioritize preventive strategies to reinforce the nutritional components that support marrow function, such as overall vitamin, mineral, and essential fatty acid nutrition. The use of immune stimulants such as certain herbs may be possible in specific circumstances, but they usually pose more potential risks than benefits and should generally be avoided. All treatments should be used outside the protected zone. For treatments in which bone marrow suppression is experienced by less than half of the patients, the same nonconventional treatments are still worthwhile but are not as critical.

ALTERNATIVE THERAPIES THAT MIGHT BE HELPFUL

- Overall vitamin, mineral, and essential fatty acid nutrition

ALTERNATIVE TREATMENTS TO AVOID

- Immune stimulants

Nausea and Vomiting

When nausea and vomiting occur with a particular treatment, it is wise to prioritize your preventive strategies. These symptoms usually occur because of signals generated and sent to the brain by the drugs, not because of something going bad in the stomach. Botanicals and other medications that are normally useful for an upset stomach or nausea may have some benefit, but that benefit is usually limited.

One useful strategy with drugs that cause nausea and vomiting is to be certain that the foods you eat during this period do not already have a tendency to cause these problems on their own and, as a result, make things worse. Don't wait until there is a problem to straighten out your diet. Start with simple, easily digested foods that you like. Avoid raw fruits and vegetables, highly acidic foods such as tomatoes, and rich foods such as cream sauces and dairy products. Even though dairy foods initially may have a soothing effect, the proteins and sugars they contain are difficult to digest and may eventually make you feel worse. Supplementation with B-complex vitamins at a safe time outside the protected zone can help replace some of the nutrients lost from disrupted absorption.

Nausea and vomiting can occur for reasons other than drug side effects. Foods that are difficult to digest, an unusual eating schedule, and stress can all contribute to these problems. If you are experiencing nausea or vomiting, whether or not they're a direct result of chemotherapy, try to eat at normal times and concentrate on foods that don't bother you, even if they are not the best foods in terms of cancer prevention. Try to avoid eating when you're stressed or in a hurry and avoid noisy, chaotic eating places.

Alternative Therapies That Might Be Helpful

- Licorice root
- Marshmallow root

Note: Care must be taken to be certain that the protected zone is being respected.

Alternative Treatments to Avoid

- High doses of oral vitamin C
- Cleansing herbs such as beet
- Excessive juicing

Kidney and Urinary Tract Toxicity

Preventive strategies should be used with all treatments that are stressful to the kidneys and urinary tract, even when this side effect is not a major one. A history of kidney disease, bladder infections, or urinary tract problems make prevention even more important.

Nonconventional therapies that can also stress the kidneys, such as diuretics, are best avoided except in special circumstances. A list of nonconventional diuretics can be found in appendix 2.

Large quantities of water are the best preventive measure for avoiding kidney toxicity from chemotherapy protocols. This is because of water's simple diluting effect. Good mineral nutrition and essential fatty acids, taken outside the protected zone, can help strengthen and prevent kidney damage.

If, before chemotherapy, you are experiencing urinary urgency, burning with urination, or having to get up more than once at night to urinate, mention this to your medical specialist. Resolving these problems prior to conventional treatment can avoid problems later. The appropriate non-conventional treatments may take care of the problem as long as there is time before the protected zone.

ALTERNATIVE THERAPIES THAT MIGHT BE HELPFUL

- Omega-3 DHA fatty acids
- Marshmallow root

ALTERNATIVE TREATMENTS TO AVOID

- Diuretic herbs (they may initially help but can cause later dehydration)

Cardiac Toxicity

If you are being treated with a therapy that causes cardiac toxicity in most or more than half of those using it, you should be alert for any signs or symptoms of this problem. The first sign of cardiac toxicity is normally elevated heart enzymes, which can been seen in blood tests. By the time you can feel the effects of cardiac toxicity—such as the symptoms of heart failure—the damage has been done.

Cardiac toxicity should also be discussed with your health care providers if you have a history of heart, cardiovascular, or lung conditions or impairments, even if cardiac toxicity is unusual for this treatment.

This side effect is generally the result of damage to the heart and cardiovascular system but can also be caused by secondary actions such as fluid, metabolic, or other imbalances brought on by the drug. The damage can usually be reduced by antioxidant tissue stores, such as found in coenzyme Q10. The dilemma, however, is that these antioxidants, if administered during the protected zone, can interfere with the actions of most of the drugs that cause cardiac toxicity.

The recommended plan is to use a broad combination of antioxidants, including coenzyme Q10 and vitamin E, taking them before and after—*not during*—the protected zone of treatment.

ALTERNATIVE THERAPIES THAT MIGHT BE HELPFUL

- Antioxidants, before or after the protected zone of treatment
- Coenzyme Q10, before or after the protected zone
- Vitamin E, before or after the protected zone

ALTERNATIVE TREATMENTS TO AVOID

- Heart-stimulating herbs such as cactus, fox glove, lily-of-the-valley

Allergic Response

Certain drugs and combinations of drugs can cause an allergic response. Conventional medicine has remarkably reduced and suppressed this occurrence by pre-treatment with antihistamines and other drugs, but it can still occur.

If you tend to be allergic, have known or suspected allergies to particular drugs or foods, or have a history of asthma, it would be wise to be vigilant for signs of allergic response. Ask your conventional provider to tell you what symptoms to be wary of. Also, if you have noticed that you wheeze after eating certain foods or after exercise, feel bad after eating certain foods or being around animals or other allergens, be alert for a possible allergic reaction.

Certain drugs and combinations of drugs can cause an allergic response.

There are no accepted tests for predicting an allergic response to chemotherapy, but if you tend to be allergic, you can do a few things to minimize the possibility. If you have experienced any previous allergic symptoms or are concerned that you might respond badly, you should alert both your conventional and nonconventional providers. If you have time before starting conventional treatment, work with your providers to avoid allergic foods and situations and, where possible, treat the allergies. This preparation is best done with your provider and not alone, since you want to be certain that you are not in the process of withdrawing from an allergy and thus vulnerable when you start chemotherapy.

- Pay attention to and treat allergies prior to treatment if possible

ALTERNATIVE TREATMENTS TO AVOID

- Avoid introducing new herbal treatments prior to starting conventional treatment

Mouth Sores

Mouth sores occur as a result of damage to the rapidly dividing cells of the mucosa, the lining of the digestive tract. Good general nutrition *prior* to the treatment has anecdotally helped with but not eliminated mouth sores. Saline, a mild mixture of salt and water, can be very helpful. It is not only soothing, but also helps control inflammation. Water without chlorine and without carbonation seems to work best.

Since the mouth sores represent a temporary breakdown in the *mucosal barrier* that protects you from the germs in your digestive tract, it is important to avoid any foods or other substances that are not verifiably germ-safe. Your oncologist's office will give you guidelines for low-microbial diet hygiene for your particular oncology treatment. A folate mouthwash may also help healing. As always, take care with the protected zone for treatment.

ALTERNATIVE THERAPIES THAT MIGHT BE HELPFUL

- Mild saline mouthwash
- Folate mouthwash
- Low-microbial diet hygiene

ALTERNATIVE TREATMENTS TO AVOID

- High doses of oral vitamin C

Hair Loss

Hair loss is almost always reversible after treatment. Adequate B-vitamin and mineral nutrition outside the protected zone, both before and after treatment, can potentially shorten the period somewhat, but not eliminate it.

In Europe and Asia, hair loss has been avoided by using ice packs on the scalp during treatment, which reduces blood flow and thus drug saturation to the chilled area. However, this process also introduces the risk of the drug missing some tumor cells. Until this procedure is well studied and fine-tuned, the risks of not allowing the chemotherapy to do its job far outweigh the potential benefits, and it is therefore not recommended.

> Hair loss is almost always reversible after treatment.

If hair loss usually occurs with a treatment you are going to receive, shop for a wig beforehand. Have some fun and try to make this an adventure. I have had literally hundreds of patients tell me that their significant other found them very physically appealing when they lost their hair, and some brag that their sex lives hadn't been as good in years. If there is a silver lining in the chemotherapy cloud, you should take advantage of it.

ALTERNATIVE THERAPIES THAT MIGHT BE HELPFUL

- B-vitamin nutrition before treatment, taking care to avoid the protected zone
- Adequate B-vitamin and mineral nutrition outside the protected zone

ALTERNATIVE TREATMENTS TO AVOID

- Ice packs

Numbness of the Hands and Feet

When nerve damage results from chemotherapy, it is usually in the form of numbness to the hands and feet. This is known as *peripheral neuropathy*. The best defense against it is to use adequate nervous system nutrition, including a broad scope of vitamins and minerals, essential fatty acids, and a variety of antioxidants outside the protected zone for these drugs, both before and after treatment. Exercise and movement are very useful for maintaining nerve function and may help nerve regeneration. You should avoid stimulants such as caffeine and ephedra; they could make you feel worse.

ALTERNATIVE THERAPIES THAT MIGHT BE HELPFUL

- Adequate nutrition: a broad scope of vitamins, minerals, and fatty acids

- Antioxidants outside the protected zone of treatment
- Exercise

ALTERNATIVE TREATMENTS TO AVOID

- Stimulants such as caffeine and ephedra

Lung Toxicity

Lung damage can occur with a number of chemotherapy regimes. If your treatment has caused lung toxicity in more than half of the people using it or if you have a history of lung disease, heart disease, or cardiovascular disease, or if you have experienced shortness of breath or wheezing, you should advise your conventional and nonconventional providers.

The mechanisms of damage are not well understood, but improved tissue stores of antioxidants may reduce some of the damage. The dilemma, as with cardiac toxicity, is that antioxidant nutrition may not be a good risk during treatment. Using a combination of antioxidants outside the protected zone is recommended, to be certain that tissue stores in the lung are not low. Avoid stressing the lungs around the time of treatment, since this can worsen the effects.

If you use oxygen just part of the time, it may be helpful not to use it any more than necessary during treatment if there are agents in your protocol that use free radical mechanisms for destroying tumor tissue. Theoretically, the extra oxygen can increase the local oxidative damage to the lungs.

ALTERNATIVE THERAPIES THAT MIGHT BE HELPFUL

- Antioxidants outside the protected zone of treatment

ALTERNATIVE TREATMENTS TO AVOID

- Any herb or natural treatment that could cause an allergic response

Liver Toxicity

If the drug treatment you are using has caused liver toxicity in more than half of the people taking it—or if you have a history of liver disease; have ever been jaundiced (yellow tinting of your skin); regularly take over-the-counter pain relievers, such as Tylenol; have ever used alcohol more than occasionally; or have used recreational drugs or needles—you should advise your conventional and nonconventional providers.

Antioxidants, including *Silybum marianum,* used outside the protected zone, can be helpful preventive strategies. Nonconventional therapies that add stress to the liver can increase the liver toxicity of these drugs, turning a mild side effect into a more serious one. Nonconventional therapies that can stress the liver are listed in appendix 5. In addition, avoid other liver-stressing substances such as alcohol, over-the-counter pain relievers, and other drugs (prescription or recreational) that cause liver stress.

ALTERNATIVE THERAPIES THAT MIGHT BE HELPFUL

- Antioxidants outside the protected zone
- *Silybum marianum*

ALTERNATIVE TREATMENTS TO AVOID

- Excess vitamin A
- Excess synthetic (not natural) vitamin K (a.k.a. menadione)
- Herbs. Many herbs are processed by, and therefore increase the stress on, the liver. This includes most herbs. Only the most common herbs that can be toxic to the liver are listed here:

  Allium sativum (a.k.a. garlic), in large doses
  Cheledonium (a.k.a. tetterwort, celandine)
  Citrullus (a.k.a. watermelon)
  Hydrastis (a.k.a. goldenseal)
  Larrea (a.k.a. chaparral)
  Senecio (a.k.a. ragwort, life root)

- Any herbal product in alcohol

Your Personal Plan for Combining Conventional and Nonconventional Care

We are now to the point where we can develop a combined therapy program designed just for you. This plan will provide you with every possible advantage for a positive long-term outcome. It will reflect all of the factors that make you and your circumstances unique.

In this chapter I discuss cancers by type. From adrenal cancers to tumors of the thyroid, I'll provide you with an overview of both conventional and alternative treatments. For ease of navigation, the cancers in this chapter are arranged alphabetically.

For specific nonconventional treatments, see chapter 8, *The ABCs of Alternative Therapies.*

DEVELOPING YOUR OWN PLAN
FOR COMBINED THERAPIES

Your combination plan should consider all of the following factors:

- Your diagnostic information
- Your conventional oncology treatment

- Your previous oncology treatments
- Other concurrent health problems
- Your personal and family health history
- Your personal needs and objectives

Diagnostic Information

This important information includes the type of cancer you have, its location, and its stage. Of course, different types of cancers necessitate different treatments. The diagnosis of breast cancer would obviously require a different plan than would colon or lung cancer. While many basic strategies are similar, the specifics of each diagnosis must be addressed with approaches that emphasize the potential positives and the treatment's anticipated effects.

Stage, lymph node and metastasis status, pathology, tumor markers, genetic testing, and other diagnostic data are all indicators of the aggressiveness of the tumor, how far it has spread, and how it can be expected to respond to conventional therapy. In some cases, we can also infer from such diagnostic information how well the cancer will respond to nonconventional treatments.

Staging is an important concept to understand because it is a way to classify tumors with respect to how far they have progressed and to their potential for responding to treatment.

The TNM system of staging was developed by the American Joint Committee on Cancer (AJCC) to describe the history and extent of the tumor. The T represents the primary tumor. The size and sometimes other characteristics of the primary tumor are considered. The N represents regional (i.e., close to the primary tumor) lymph nodes and takes into account the number and sometimes location of nodes showing signs of tumor cell invasion, if any. This is a measure of tumor spread in the vicinity of the primary tumor. The M reflects distant tumor metastases if they exist. In some cases, staging includes tumor grade and patient age. In the future, data such as tumor markers and other parameters may be added to provide a more complete picture.

Lymph node and metastasis status tell us whether or not the cancer has spread from its primary site. All this information together will help determine treatment and probable response.

Staging indicates how far tumors have progressed and their potential for responding to treatment.

Your Conventional Oncology Treatment

The nature of your conventional oncology treatment will determine which nonconventional treatments are appropriate and when they can be used. Avoiding undesirable interactions between conventional and nonconventional therapies is a primary objective. The principle of noninterference is all-important. It is absolutely vital that your alternative medicines not detract from or interfere with your conventional cancer treatments. The protected zone is that time period and that part of your body where your conventional treatment does its work. Protecting this zone is the very essence of the principle of noninterference. See chapter 5 for more information about how to avoid interfering with the absorption and antitumor actions of your conventional cancer treatment.

Previous Oncology Treatments

Any oncology treatments you've already received should be taken into consideration as well. Some of these therapies have long-term effects, including side effects, which can change the priorities for your current nonconventional treatment.

Concurrent Health Problems

These are any health problems that currently affect you, whether or not they are associated with your cancer. A complete review of your total health status is an important part of your plan. You will tolerate treatment and recover much more efficiently if your body is not dealing with other problems that stress your healing power.

Personal and Family Health History

Your personal and family health histories are also important factors, providing useful clues about how you got to this point in your personal health and how certain long-standing problems can be resolved. These histories can also highlight risk factors that should be avoided in the future, thus reducing your chances for a recurrence.

Your family health history also can provide important insights into patterns that can be genetic or the result of family habits and behavior. It can be a clue for seeking additional testing to more completely understand your health and can underscore health issues that can be addressed in your nonconventional treatment plan.

Personal Needs and Objectives

Your personal needs and objectives need to be an integral part of your treatment plan. Patients frequently do not pay enough attention to this important guiding tool, and as a result, their quality of care invariably suffers.

ADRENAL CANCER

Almost all the systems of the body are influenced by the actions of the adrenal glands. Interference with their normal function can result in a wide variety of problems.

Considering Your Diagnosis

Adrenal cortical carcinoma is described by the TNM staging system that takes into account:

- Tumor size
- Local spread
- Local lymph node involvement
- Metastatic spread to other parts of the body

Stage I
Stage I is a tumor less than 5 cm, without local lymph node involvement, and without spread to other sites.

Stage II
Stage II is a tumor greater than 5 cm, without local lymph node involvement, and without spread to distant metastatic sites.

Stage III
Stage III is either a tumor less than 5 cm, with local lymph node involvement, or a tumor greater than 5 cm, without local lymph node involvement. In either case, there is no spread to distant metastatic sites.

Stage IV
Stage IV is any time there are distant metastases or if the primary tumor has grown beyond the adrenal gland.

Conventional Treatment Strategies for Adrenal Cancer

Adrenal tumors, also known as adrenal cortical tumors, are usually treated with conventional surgery if they are early stage (stage I or stage

II). If the tumor has advanced, however, chemotherapy will be added. Radiation is only used locally for disease that has spread to the bone.

Surgery

Surgical treatment involves removal of the tumor and the affected adrenal gland, often removing adjacent structures as well, such as parts of the vena cava (a large vein) and the diaphragm. Surgery is also used to control metastatic disease.

Chemotherapy

Chemotherapy may be useful with more advanced disease. The most common chemotherapy treatment is the combination of the agent mitotane, a pesticide derivative, and the alkylating agent cisplatin.

A Guide to Using Alternative Medicines in Treating Adrenal Cancer

Many of the adrenal cancer chemotherapy regimens are vulnerable to interference, especially from high-level antioxidants. Antimetabolite drugs are not commonly used as a treatment for adrenal tumors, but if they are, specific nutrient supplements can interfere with them in some instances, especially if they are at high levels. And of course, always be certain that nonconventional treatments are administered outside the protected zone.

With the support of your trained nonconventional provider, use natural treatments to help deal with the side effects most common with both surgery and chemotherapy, the most likely treatments for adrenal cancers. When the conventional treatment plan can result in immune system suppression, be certain that any supplements you may be taking are screened for microbial safety. You may have to stop taking supplements when your white blood cell count is low, which happens as a result of immune system suppression.

Supplemental nutrition should be based on your actual physiological needs. Avoid high doses of supplements during conventional treatment. Follow the preventive diet, lifestyle, and environmental strategies suggested in chapter 10. These may have some curative effect and at the minimum will reduce risk factors, as well as help your immune system to function properly.

BILIARY CANCERS (*see* Liver, Gall bladder, and Biliary Cancers)

BLADDER CANCER (*see* Genitourinary Cancers)

Breast cancer can affect either women or men, although malignant tumors of the male breast are rare. Breast cancer in women has become a national tragedy in Western culture. One out of eight women will experience breast cancer in her lifetime.

Considering Your Breast Cancer Diagnosis

Breast cancer is described by the TNM staging system, which takes into account:

- The cell type of tumor
- The size of the tumor
- The tumor location with respect to the muscles that form the chest wall
- Whether local lymph nodes are involved
- Tumor metastatic spread to other parts of the body

Stage 0

Stage 0 is carcinoma in situ, or Paget's disease of the nipple with no tumor. This is a very slow-growing condition that rarely spreads. It is usually treated conventionally by surgery (lumpectomy), followed by radiation or mastectomy.

Stage I

Stage I is a breast tumor whose greatest dimension is no greater than 2 cm, with no lymph node involvement or metastases. There are no distant metastases and the tumor does not extend back to the chest wall.

Stage IIA

Stage IIA describes two separate conditions. It can be the same as stage 0 or stage I, with the addition of involvement of local axillary (underarm) lymph node(s). Stage IIA can also be a tumor between 2 cm and 5 cm, with no lymph node involvement. In either case, there are no distant metastases and the tumor does not extend back to the chest wall.

Stage IIB

Stage IIB also describes two separate conditions. It can be either a tumor between 2 cm and 5 cm, with axillary (underarm) lymph node involvement, or a tumor greater than 5 cm without lymph node involvement. In either case, there are no distant metastases and the tumor does not extend back to the chest wall.

Stage IIIA

Stage IIIA can be any tumor up to 5 cm, with axillary (underarm) lymph node involvement, which can include lymph nodes fixed to each other. There are no distant metastases and the tumor does not extend back to the chest wall.

Stage IIIB

Stage IIIB can be a tumor of any size that extends to the chest wall or skin, causes skin swelling or skin ulceration, or is an inflammatory carcinoma with involvement of the axillary (underarm) lymph nodes. It can also be any tumor where the internal mammary lymph nodes are involved. In either case, there are no distant metastases.

Stage IV

Stage IV describes any tumor where there is spread to a distant metastatic site.

The staging system for breast cancer was devised primarily to aid in the selection of conventional therapies and to assess long-term survival. It has some value when selecting nonconventional treatments but also some limitations. In general, one can assume that lower-stage tumors will be more amenable to nonconventional treatment whereas higher-stage ones are more advanced and thus less likely to respond to more gentle, nonconventional treatments.

The smaller the tumor, the greater the chance it will respond to nonconventional treatment.

The size of the tumor has a significant effect on the place of nonconventional therapy in the combination plan. The smaller the tumor, the greater the chance it will respond to nonconventional treatment. The larger the tumor, the more important it is to use interventions that will quickly limit its further growth and spread. Tumors less than 2 cm are more likely to benefit from nonconventional therapies than larger tumors are, based on their behavior in studies with and without conventional therapies.

The grade of the tumor has a significant impact on the short-term usefulness of nonconventional therapies. Grade is not a part of the TNM staging system. Low-grade tumors are essentially slower growing and less aggressive. As a result, they usually do not develop as quickly and are therefore more likely to respond to nonconventional therapy. Higher-grade tumors may be beyond the reach of alternative treatments and the body's immune system and may respond more favorably to conventional intervention.

The aggressiveness of the tumor, as well as its short- and long-term behavior, are increasingly better predicted with a variety of new tests, such as one identifying tumor markers. Tumor markers are substances in the blood that serve as indicators of the genetic and other individual characteristics of the tumor. As with tumor grade, when tumor markers predict behavior that is less aggressive or more responsive to conventional treatment, it is more likely that the cancer will respond to nonconventional therapy as well. Lymph node involvement signals the tumor's spread beyond its primary site. The lymph nodes act as filters, screening tumor cells out of lymph channels before they can travel to other parts of the body. In the past, most or all lymph nodes were removed for staging. In some cases today, however, a new technology known as sentinel node biopsy allows a surgeon to remove just one or a few lymph nodes to determine the extent of disease. If there is no axillary (underarm) lymph node involvement, there is a better chance that tumor cells are confined to the local area.

Nonconventional therapies have a much better chance of affecting the tumor when there is no axillary node involvement. If there is lymph node involvement, the more nodes involved, the greater the likelihood that a more aggressive treatment will be necessary to eliminate tumor growth.

Spread to a location other than the original tumor site, known as a distant metastasis, makes nonconventional treatment more difficult and raises the importance of conventional methods, at least for the short term.

Locally advanced, aggressive breast cancer, such as inflammatory breast cancer, so named because of the local inflammation and skin changes that accompany it, should be considered very aggressive even if there is no evidence of lymph node or metastatic spread.

Conventional Treatment Strategies for Breast Cancer

The diagnostic and conventional-treatment options for breast cancer are increasing at a rapid rate. As a result, the treatment recommendations for early, low-grade tumors are often very different from those for more advanced diagnoses.

Treatments for breast cancer usually include a combination of therapies. This could mean one or more of either surgery, radiation, chemotherapy, peripheral stem cell transplant, and vaccines. Early-stage tumors can often be treated successfully with a lumpectomy (the removal of the tumor only) and radiation. To significantly improve the outcome for more advanced breast cancer, chemotherapy and more extensive surgery, such as a mastectomy, are also used. Additional therapies, such as peripheral stem cell transplants, are effective under certain conditions. Vaccines are currently being investigated and tested.

Surgery

Surgical interventions are designed to remove tumor tissue. This has the advantage of removing the cancer cells that can provide a source for spread, but it involves the side effects and risks inherent with any surgical procedure. Surgery is usually undertaken in combination with other treatment methods.

A lumpectomy removes only the breast tumor and a small amount of surrounding tissue. It is a useful procedure for certain breast tumors when clear margins can be realized, which means that the tumor can be removed with a small margin of tissue that has no visible cancer. A lumpectomy is a relatively safe procedure when done by a competent surgeon. In most cases, a lumpectomy has the advantage of providing positive outcomes equivalent to mastectomy but with less trauma and a much better cosmetic result. Historically, the greatest drawback to the lumpectomy has been the risk of local recurrence. The addition of local radiation therapy, however, has remarkably reduced that risk.

The diagnostic and conventional-treatment options for breast cancer are increasing at a rapid rate.

A mastectomy, the removal of most or all breast tissue, is done when the size and characteristics of the tumor indicate that a lumpectomy will not provide the best outcome. For most women considering a mastectomy, a modified radical mastectomy, which does not remove the muscles of the chest wall, has been shown to be equally as effective as the more aggressive radical mastectomy.

Other surgical procedures include ovarian ablation and treatment of metastatic disease. Ovarian ablation, also known as ablative oophorectomy, essentially deactivates the ovaries, thus reducing the amount of estrogen in the body. Surgical treatment for removal of metastatic disease is recommended when the benefits of the surgery outweigh the risks and trauma of the procedure. These procedures should be considered carefully before being undertaken.

Radiation Therapy

Radiation therapy in the treatment of breast cancer has two possible objectives: the prevention of a local recurrence and the control of local metastatic tissue.

If breast cancer recurs, it is often in the area of the surgical incision. This is likely the result of small tumor cells that could not be seen by even the most careful surgeon or the microscope. This recurrence can happen with either a lumpectomy or a mastectomy. Radiation can destroy many of these local cells and thus reduce the chances of a local recurrence. The scientific studies for this use of radiation are very persuasive.

When dealing with metastatic tissue, it is often possible to improve quality of life, reduce pain, and shrink the tumor with localized radiation. Every case is different and you'll want to be certain that the potential gains are greater than the risks.

Chemotherapy

Chemotherapy is usually applied in a combination of drugs, and often in combination with surgery and/or radiation, to simultaneously attack the rapidly dividing cells by a number of different mechanisms. An increasing number of chemotherapy choices are available.

The most common drugs used by themselves are the alkylating agent cyclophosphamide (Cytoxan), the antitumor antibiotic doxorubicin (Adriamycin), and the plant-derived drug paclitaxel (Taxol). The following are combinations of chemotherapy agents that are used to treat breast cancer.

CA

CA is the abbreviation for Cytoxan and Adriamycin when they are used together. The combination is usually administered weekly or every three weeks. Side effects include bone marrow suppression, mouth sores, and hair loss occurring in more than half (40 to 70%) of those treated. Nausea, vomiting, and heart toxicity occur in less than half (20 to 40%) of the patients receiving treatment with CA.

CA Plus Taxol

CA plus Taxol has been shown to produce better long-term outcomes than CA alone for certain categories of patients. A number of variations in protocols exist, but basically the CA is administered for six weeks, followed by Taxol for six weeks. Radiation may be included in the middle of the protocol. Side effects for CA are as previously mentioned. Side effects for Taxol commonly include bone marrow suppression, hair loss, and, less frequently, numbness of the hands and feet.

CAF

CAF is the abbreviation for Cytoxan, Adriamycin, and 5-fluorouracil (a.k.a. 5-FU) when used together. The Cytoxan is commonly administered in a daily oral dose, whereas the Adriamycin and 5-FU are given intravenously once per week. Bone marrow suppression and mouth sores occur in more than half (40 to 70%) of those patients being treated, whereas nausea and vomiting, heart toxicity, and hair loss occur in less than half (20 to 40%).

CMF

CMF is the abbreviation for the Cytoxan, the antimetabolite methotrexate, and the antimetabolite 5-fluorouracil. The timing of the administration can vary, but usually the Cytoxan is given by pill daily and the methotrexate and 5-FU are given by IV once per week. The treatment period is normally three to six months. The side effects of CMF are normally milder than for CA or Taxol. Bone marrow suppression occurs in more than half (40 to 70%) of those treated. Nausea and vomiting, heart toxicity, mouth sores, and hair loss occur in less than half (20 to 40%).

DC1

DC1 denotes the plant-derived docetaxel and the alkylating agent cisplatin administered every twenty-one days. More than half of the patients experience bone marrow suppression and hair loss, whereas less than half (20 to 40%) experience hand and foot numbness and allergic response to the drugs.

DC2

DC2 is the combination of the plant-derived docetaxel and the alkylating agent cyclophosphamide administered intravenously once every three weeks. Most (70 to 100%) patients experience bone marrow suppression, more than half (40 to 70%) experience hair loss, while less than half (20 to 40%) experience an allergic response to the drugs.

DD

DD is the combination of the plant-derived docetaxel and the antitumor antibiotic doxorubicin administered intravenously once every three weeks. Most (70 to 100%) patients experience bone marrow suppression, more than half (40 to 70%) experience hair loss, while less than half (20 to 40%) experience mouth sores, an allergic response to the drug, and numbness of the hands and feet.

DF
DF is the plant-derived docetaxel and the antimetabolite 5-FU administered intravenously. The docetaxel is given on day 1 while the 5-FU is administered on days 1 through 5. This schedule is repeated every twenty-one days. Most (70 to 100%) patients experience bone marrow suppression, more than half (40 to 70%) experience hair loss, while less than half (20 to 40%) experience digestive system problems and an allergic response to the drugs.

DV
DV is the combination of the plant-derived drugs docetaxel and vinorelbine. Both drugs are administered intravenously on day 1 and the vinorelbine is repeated on day 5. This schedule is repeated every twenty-one days. Most (70 to 100%) patients experience bone marrow suppression, more than half (40 to 70%) experience mouth sores and hair loss, and less than half (20 to 40%) experience digestive tract problems, numbness of the hands and feet, and an allergic response to the drugs.

Mitomycin C Plus Vinblastine
The antitumor antibiotic mitomycin C can be combined with the plant-derived vinblastine. It is normally used when other chemotherapy agents have not worked. Administration is IV for both drugs, with the mitomycin C administered every four weeks and the vinblastine every two weeks. The most common side effects are fevers, nausea and vomiting, loss of appetite, and bone marrow suppression. Side effects for this protocol can vary greatly depending on patient condition and the individual drug dosages used. Ask your medical specialist to estimate how you will respond based on your specific circumstances.

PD1 and PD2
PD1 and PD2 both combine the plant-derived paclitaxel with the antitumor antibiotic doxorubicin but at different dosages. Drugs are administered on the same day once every three weeks. More than half (40 to 70%) of the patients taking PD1 experience hair loss and bone marrow suppression, whereas less than half (20 to 40%) have mouth sores. More

than half (40 to 70%) of the patients taking PD2 experience hair loss, bone marrow suppression, and heart toxicity, whereas less than half (20 to 40%) have mouth sores.

PFF1 and PFF2

PFF1 and PFF2 both combine the plant-derived paclitaxel with the antimetabolites 5-FU and leucovorin, although with different schedules and dosages. With PFF1, the Taxol is administered every three weeks and the other drugs are administered weekly. With PFF2, all the drugs are administered over a three-day period and repeated again in four weeks. More than half (40 to 70%) of the patients experience hair loss and less than half (20 to 40%) experience bone marrow suppression with both programs. Less than half (20 to 40%) of the patients taking PFF1 experience numbness of hands and feet, whereas this symptom is rare with patients taking PFF2.

TAC

TAC denotes the combination of the plant-derived docetaxel, the antitumor antibiotic doxorubicin, and the alkylating agent cyclophosphamide administered once every three weeks. Bone marrow suppression occurs in nearly all patients, hair loss is experienced by more than half (40 to 70%), and nausea and vomiting are experienced by less than half (20 to 40%).

VD

VD is the combination of the plant-derived vinorelbine and the antitumor antibiotic doxorubicin administered intravenously. The vinorelbine is given on days 1 and 8, while the doxorubicin is given on day 1. The schedule is repeated every three weeks. More than half (40 to 70%) of the patients experience bone marrow suppression and hair loss.

VF

VF is the combination of the plant-derived vinorelbine and the antimetabolite 5-FU administered intravenously. The vinorelbine is given on days 1 and 5, while the 5-FU is administered on days 1 through 5. The schedule is repeated every twenty-one days. Most (70 to 100%) patients experience bone marrow suppression, more than half (40 to 70%) experience mouth sores and hair loss, while less than half (20 to 40%) experience nausea and vomiting.

The role of nonconventional therapy in the overall treatment plan for breast cancer should be decided with the advice of a skilled medical specialist. If the tumor is slow-growing, small, lacking aggressive characteristics, and has not spread, you might begin with nonconventional therapies only. This decision will depend on whether there is time enough before the tumor can advance and become less treatable should the alternative treatment not work.

The progress of the tumor should be carefully monitored so that you will know whether the nonconventional therapy is working. For example, while monitoring progress, ductal carcinoma in situ may be slow enough and well defined enough to use only nonconventional therapy for months or longer. If the tumor is shrinking and resolving, conventional care (other than regular monitoring) may not be needed.

Other situations, such as potentially precancerous breast calcifications, can be trickier. Even though these calcifications may be benign (noncancerous) for long periods of time, if they begin to convert to breast cancer, they may actually get smaller rather than larger, making it very difficult to know if they are responding to treatment or advancing. Every situation is unique, and in such cases it is important to get an informed clinical judgment from a medical specialist who is able determine how well the tumor situation can be monitored.

If you and your medical specialist agree that there is time and monitoring capability to use nonconventional treatments alone, a strict monitoring program must be set up so that you know where you are. If the tumor regresses, which would be great news, be certain that you keep up the nonconventional program and the monitoring over the long term. Don't go back to unhealthful behaviors and habits that may have precipitated the cancer in the first place.

If, on the other hand, the tumor needs to be dealt with immediately, then you and your providers can develop a conventional plan that will provide intervention. It is hoped that this will still leave you plenty of time to use nonconventional strategies to prevent a recurrence.

Lymphedema is a possible side effect of the surgical removal of axillary (underarm) lymph nodes. This accumulation of fluid in the arm can be very troublesome. Regular exercise, starting as soon as possible after surgery, helps limit this side effect. In addition, if you are overweight or in poor physical condition, losing weight and increasing your muscle mass will help. Even though you may not much feel like it, exercise and stretching during conventional therapy can improve your condition greatly.

With the support of a trained nonconventional provider, select nonconventional therapies from chapter 5 that most closely match your symptoms and best address the side effects of your conventional therapy.

Many of the breast cancer chemotherapy and radiation regimes are vulnerable to interference, especially from high-level antioxidants. The antimetabolite drugs can, in some cases, be interfered with by specific nutrients, especially if they are supplemented at high levels.

When the conventional treatment plan results in immune-system suppression, be certain that the supplements you are using have been screened for microbial safety. Often, you should stop taking supplements when your white blood cell counts are low (which happens as a result of immune-system suppression from treatment), but keep in mind that, under certain conditions, white blood counts may be high and the immune system may still not be fully functional.

Follow the recommendations for phytoestrogens in the next chapter.

It is always worthwhile to introduce preventive strategies, which become even more important at the conclusion of conventional treatment. Follow the diet, lifestyle, and environmental strategies suggested in chapter 10. These may have some curative effect and at the minimum will reduce risk factors, as well as help your immune system to function properly. Supplemental nutrition should be based on your actual physiological needs. Avoid very high doses of any supplements during conventional treatment. Always be certain that nonconventional treatments are administered outside the protected zone.

> Always be certain that nonconventional treatments are administered outside the protected zone.

CARCINOID TUMORS

Carcinoid tumors secrete hormones. In some cases, they may not be noticed because the location of the tumor allows the body to deactivate them prior to having any effect. When the carcinoid tumor is located on the liver or a vulnerable part of the digestive system or some other rare site, the secreted hormones can create the carcinoid syndrome, which can include hot flashes (not associated with menopause), diarrhea, breathing difficulty, and heart problems. These symptoms can be treated with chemotherapy.

Considering Your Diagnosis

There is no commonly used staging system for carcinoid tumors.

Conventional Treatment Strategies for Carcinoid Tumors

Carcinoid tumors are generally slow-growing and are treated primarily with surgery. Carcinoid syndrome symptoms can be treated with chemotherapeutic agents.

Surgery

Surgery involves removal of the tumor and repairing any local problems caused by the spread of the tumor.

Chemotherapy

Chemotherapy generally provides symptomatic relief. The most common protocol is the combination of the biological agents octeotride and interferon alpha.

A Guide to Using Alternative Medicines in Treating Carcinoid Tumors

With the support of a trained nonconventional provider, select nonconventional therapies that most closely address your symptoms. Supplemental nutrition should be based on your actual physiological needs. Avoid very high doses of any supplements during conventional treatment.

When the conventional treatment plan results in immune system suppression, be certain that the supplements you use are screened for microbial safety. You may have to stop taking supplements when your white blood cell counts are low (which happens as a result of immune system suppression from treatment), but keep in mind that, under certain conditions, white blood counts may be high and the immune system may still not be fully functional.

It is recommended that serotonin-affecting drugs and nutritional supplements, such as certain antidepressants, the amino acid tryptophan, and 5-HTP, be avoided, especially if there is a danger of carcinoid syndrome. In addition, avoid stimulants such as coffee, tea, chocolate, and other caffeine-containing substances, as well as stimulating herbs such as ephedra.

Follow the diet, lifestyle, and environmental strategies described in chapter 10. These may have some curative effect and at the minimum will reduce risk factors, as well as help the immune system to function properly.

Always be certain that nonconventional treatments are administered outside the protected zone.

CERVICAL CANCER (*see* Gynecological Cancers)

COLON AND RECTAL CANCER

The incidence of colorectal cancers is high in the Western world but remains quite low in such places as Japan and the sub-Saharan areas of Africa. Studies suggest that major risk factors for colorectal cancers include the high-fat and low-fiber diets common in Western cultures.

Considering Your Diagnosis

Colon and rectal cancer is described by a number of staging systems, the most common being the TNM and Dukes'.

Studies suggest that major risk factors for colorectal cancers include the high-fat and low-fiber diets common in Western cultures.

Stage 0

Stage 0 TNM does not have an equivalent Dukes' stage. This stage describes carcinoma in situ, which is very slow-growing and usually has not spread. There is no local lymph node involvement and no distant metastatic spread.

**Stage A Dukes' or
Stage I TNM**

Stage A Dukes' and stage I TNM is a tumor limited to the inner layer of the colon or rectal wall. There is no local lymph node involvement and no distant metastatic spread.

Stage B1 Dukes'

Stage B1 Dukes' is still stage I TNM, a tumor limited to the inner layer and the middle muscular layer of the colon or rectal wall. There is no local lymph node involvement and no distant metastatic spread.

Stage B2 Dukes' or Stage II TNM

Stage B2 Dukes' or stage II TNM is a tumor that has grown into all three layers of the colon or rectal wall. There is no local lymph node involvement and no distant metastatic spread.

Stage B3 Dukes'

Stage B3 Dukes' is still stage II TNM, a tumor that has grown into all three layers of the colon or rectal wall and also invaded surrounding structures or organs. There is no local lymph node involvement and no distant metastatic spread.

Stage C Dukes' or Stage III TNM

Stage C Dukes' or stage III TNM is any tumor that includes local lymph node involvement and no distant metastatic spread.

Stage D Dukes'

Stage D Dukes' is still stage III TNM, any tumor that includes local lymph node involvement and distant metastatic spread.

Conventional Treatment Strategies for Colon and Rectal Cancer

Surgery is the principal treatment for colon and rectal cancer and can be very effective in cases where the tumor is found early and has not spread. Radiation and chemotherapy are also used in the treatment of colorectal cancers, with a number of possible objectives, including the reduction of the tumor to an operable size, eradication of the tumor, and control of metastatic disease.

Still under investigation are a number of early-stage vaccine trials.

Surgery

Surgical interventions depend on the extent and location of the tumor. In cases where it is localized and accessible, a skilled surgeon can often remove the tumor with no noticeable long-term effects and complete cure.

With more advanced tumors, surgery is often combined with other treatments. In some cases, larger sections of the bowel are removed and with others an ostomy (Greek word for *opening*), also known as a colostomy, is created where the bowel exits into an appliance in the side rather than the anus. Some colostomies can be reversed later and reconnected normally. Depending on the exact procedure, the colostomy may require special dietary and hygiene considerations. The newer colostomy appliances are much easier to use and less conspicuous. Most colostomy users lead essentially normal lives.

Radiation Treatments

Radiation can be used locally to reduce the size of the tumor, to eliminate it completely, or to prevent a recurrence in the area of a surgical removal. Radiation damage to surrounding structures is sometimes a concern, as well as irritation to the bowel during and shortly after the procedure.

Chemotherapy

Chemotherapy strategies include both single-drug and combination strategies. The most common single agent is the antimetabolite 5-fluorouracil (5-FU), usually administered with a continuous infusion IV pump.

Most of the combination-drug regimes include 5-FU plus either the antimetabolite leucovorin, the biological agent levamisol, the biological agent interferon alpha two, the plant-derived irinotecan, or the antitumor antibiotic mitomycin C. Most of these treatments and combinations have fewer side effects than other chemotherapy protocols. The drug camptothecan (Irinotecan) has also been used for colorectal cancers.

A Guide to Using Alternative Medicines in Treating Colorectal Cancers

Colon and rectal cancers are often treatable surgically. It is important to resolve concurrent digestion and bowel problems to the extent possible prior to surgery, to reduce inflammation and improve healing. Conditions such as irritable bowel syndrome, long-standing constipation, or diarrhea should be dealt with to assure the best surgical result.

With the support of a trained nonconventional provider, select nonconventional therapies from chapter 8 that most closely match your symptoms and best address the side effects of your conventional therapy.

Radiation and some lesser used chemotherapy treatments for colon and rectal cancer are vulnerable to interference, especially from high-level antioxidants. The antimetabolite drugs can, in some cases, be interfered with by specific nutrients, especially if they are supplemented at high levels.

When the conventional treatment plan results in immune system suppression, be certain that the supplements you are using have been screened for microbial safety. You may have to stop taking supplements when your white blood cell counts are low (which happens as a result of immune-system suppression from treatment), but keep in mind that, under certain conditions, white blood counts may be high and the immune system may still not be fully functional.

Follow the diet, lifestyle, and environmental strategies described in chapter 10. These may have some curative effect and at the minimum will reduce risk factors, as well as help the immune system to function properly. Supplemental nutrition should be based on your actual physiological needs. Avoid very high doses of any supplements during conventional treatment.

Always be certain that nonconventional treatments are administered outside the protected zone.

ENDOMETRIAL CANCER (*see* Gynecological Cancers)

ESOPHAGEAL CANCER

The esophagus is a muscular tube that connects the throat to the stomach. Located just behind the heart and the air passage (trachea) to the lungs, it is very close to the centerline of the body but wanders slightly to the left of center in places. The esophagus is soft and flattens out when there is no food in it. The wall of the esophagus is generally described as having three layers, the inner mucosa, the middle muscle layer that propels food toward the stomach, and the outer adventitia.

Considering Your Diagnosis

Esophageal cancer is described by a TNM staging system that takes into account:

- Tumor location within the wall of the esophagus
- Whether local lymph nodes are involved
- Spread beyond the esophagus

Stage I
Stage I is a tumor limited to the inner layer of the esophageal wall, without local lymph node involvement, and without distant metastatic spread.

Stage IIA
Stage IIA is a tumor that has grown through the esophageal wall, still without local lymph node involvement, and without distant metastatic spread.

Stage IIB
Stage IIB is a tumor that has grown no farther than from the inner surface to the muscle layer, with local lymph node involvement, but without distant metastatic spread.

Stage III

Stage III is either a tumor that has grown through the esophageal wall, with local lymph node involvement but without distant metastatic spread, or any tumor that has spread to the structures immediately surrounding the esophagus, regardless of local lymph node involvement but without distant metastatic spread.

Stage IV

Stage IV is any tumor, regardless of lymph node status, where there is distant metastatic spread.

Conventional Treatment Strategies for Esophageal Cancer

Treatments include surgery, radiation, and chemotherapy, often in combination. Early stage tumors are often treated with surgery only. More advanced tumors may also include chemotherapy and radiation.

Surgery

Surgical interventions include removal of the tumor and control of metastases. Surgery is the mainstay of conventional treatment for esophageal cancer. Tumor removal can include removal of part or all of the esophagus. Depending on the position of the tumor, part of the stomach may also be involved.

Radiation Therapy

Radiation therapy is used alone or with chemotherapy for advanced tumors and those that cannot be removed surgically. Depending on the location of the tumor, side effects, in addition to the general side effects for radiation, can include difficulty in swallowing as well as some damage to surrounding structures, such as the lungs and heart.

Chemotherapy

Chemotherapy regimes for esophageal cancer include a number of combination therapies that are useful for palliation (relieving discomforts but not curing) and little else. A number of drugs are currently being investigated that may hold more promise than those currently in use, but results so far have not been encouraging.

The alkylating agent cisplatin combined with the antimetabolite 5-fluorouracil are the most common chemotherapy treatments. They are often combined with local radiation therapy.

A Guide to Using Alternative Medicines in Treating Esophageal Cancer

Surgical intervention, when appropriate, should not be delayed in order to try nonconventional therapy on its own. Early tumors are surgically treatable and can have good results but, if left, can grow unpredictably.

Prior to surgery and/or radiation, it is important to use the preventive strategies described in chapter 10; these will help limit the poor digestive actions that can force stomach contents into the esophagus and add irritation during conventional treatment. The use of herbs following surgery and radiation should be delayed until healing is far enough along that there is no longer risk for local infection, contamination, or irritation.

Depending on the size and location of the tumor, some difficulty in swallowing may be experienced with stage IIA, III, and IV tumors, which will be more uncomfortable during treatment. It is especially important to eat solid foods rather than liquids, but the foods should be soft enough to pass the tumor location without causing a backup of food.

Follow the diet, lifestyle, and environmental strategies described in chapter 10. These may have some curative effect and at the minimum will reduce risk factors, as well as help the immune system to function properly.

With the support of a trained nonconventional provider, select the nonconventional therapies from chapter 8 that best address the side effects you are experiencing. Supplemental nutrition should be based on your actual physiological needs. Avoid very high doses of any alternative medicines during conventional treatment.

The chemotherapy and radiation regimes for esophageal cancer are vulnerable to interference, especially from high-level antioxidants. When the conventional treatment plan can result in immune-system suppression, be certain that the supplements you use are screened for microbial safety. Often, you should stop taking supplements when your white blood cell counts are low (which happens as a result of immune-system suppression from treatment), but keep in mind that, under certain conditions, white blood counts may be high and the immune system may still not be fully functional. The antimetabolite drugs can, in some cases, be interfered with by specific nutrients, especially if they are supplemented at high levels.

Take special care with the use of digestive enzymes and antacids. If not carefully dosed and administered, digestive enzymes can irritate the tumor. Antacids may have a short calming effect on digestion but can interrupt the proper digestion of food, causing more discomfort later.

Always be certain that nonconventional treatments are administered outside the protected zone.

GALLBLADDER CANCER (*see* Liver, Gallbladder, and Biliary Cancer)

GENITOURINARY CANCERS

Genitourinary cancers include renal cell carcinoma of the kidney, transitional cell carcinoma of the urinary bladder, and, for men, cancer of the prostate and testes.

Considering Your Diagnosis

Genitourinary cancers are described by a number of staging criteria that take into account:

- Tumor cell type
- Local tumor spread
- Local lymph node involvement
- Tumor metastatic spread to other parts of the body

Conventional Treatment Strategies for Genitourinary Cancers

Renal cell carcinoma is primarily treated by surgical removal of the tumor. Radiation and chemotherapy are generally used when the tumor has spread beyond the kidney. Transitional cell carcinoma of the bladder is usually treated with a combination of surgery and chemotherapy.

Prostate cancer can be treated with surgery, radiation, and chemotherapy, but in many cases when the tumor is slow-growing, conventional therapies are not indicated.

Testicular cancer is treated with surgery, chemotherapy, and, rarely, radiation.

Surgery

Surgery is designed to remove the primary tumor. With renal cell carcinoma, part or all of the kidney may be removed. Fortunately, we have two kidneys. Surgery of the bladder can result in loss of part of the bladder. Prostate surgery almost always involves loss of the prostate tissue, but recent improvements in surgical technique spare the nerves that create erection. Testicular surgery often involves the removal of one or both testicles.

Radiation Therapy

Radiation therapy is not a primary tool in the treatment of genitourinary cancers, but it has found a growing use under special conditions such as palliation of metastatic sites.

Chemotherapy

Chemotherapy involves a wide range of agents. For renal cell carcinoma, chemotherapy is only used when the tumor has spread beyond the kidney. The most common drugs are the biological modifiers interferon alpha and interleukin-2. Transitional cell carcinoma is treated with single agent BCG (bacillus Calmette-Guerin), as well as with some drug combinations. Prostate cancer has been treated primarily with hormones and hormone-opposing drugs. Testicular cancer has responded well to a number of chemotherapy regimens.

PEE and BEP

PEE and BEP both represent the alkylating agent cisplatin (Platinol), the plant-derived drug etoposide, and the antitumor antibiotic bleomycin. With PEE the cisplatin and etoposide are administered by IV on days 1 through 5. The bleomycin is administered by IV on days 1 and 8. The cycle is repeated every fourteen days. The BEP schedule is slightly different. Most (70 to 100%) patients receiving treatment experience lung toxicity, numbness of hands and feet, kidney toxicity, mouth sores, and bone marrow suppression; and more than half (40 to 70%) treated experience mouth sores, hair loss, and allergic response to the drugs.

VAB-6

VAB-6, used in the treatment of testicular cancer, denotes the plant-derived drug vinblastine, the alkylating agent cyclophosphamide (Cytoxan), the antitumor antibiotics bleomycin and dactinomycin, and the alkylating agent cisplatin. The vinblastine, cyclophosphamide, dactinomycin, and bleomycin are administered on day 1 of the cycle. Bleomycin is also administered in a continuous infusion from days 1 through 3. The cisplatin is administered on day 4. The cycle is then repeated in four weeks. More than half (40 to 70%) of the patients treated experience bone marrow suppression, kidney toxicity, allergic response to the drugs, hair loss, numbness of hands and feet, and lung toxicity, while less than half (20 to 40%) experience liver toxicity and mouth sores.

M-VAC

This protocol is for the treatment of transitional cell carcinoma of the urinary bladder. M-VAC is the acronym for the combination of the antimetabolite methotrexate, the plant-derived drug vinblastine, the antitumor antibiotic Adriamycin (doxorubicin), and the alkylating agent cisplatin. The methotrexate is administered on days 1, 15, and 22. The vinblastine is administered on days 2, 15, and 22. The doxorubicin and cisplatin are administered on day 2. The cycle is then repeated in three weeks. Most (70 to 100%) patients receiving it experience bone marrow suppression; more than half (40 to 70%) experience mouth sores, kidney toxicity, and hair loss; while less than half (20 to 40%) experience cardiac toxicity, allergic response to the drugs, and numbness of hands and feet.

A Guide to Using Alternative Medicines in Treating Genitourinary Cancers

With the support of a trained nonconventional provider, select nonconventional therapies from chapter 5 that most closely match your symptoms and best address the side effects you are experiencing from your conventional therapies. When the conventional treatment plan results in immune system suppression, be certain that the supplements you are using have been screened for microbial safety. You may have to stop taking supplements when your white blood cell counts are low (which happens as a result of immune system suppression from treatment). But keep in mind that under certain conditions, white blood counts may be high and the immune system may still not be fully functional.

Many of the genitourinary cancer chemotherapy and radiation regimes are vulnerable to interference, especially from high-level antioxidants. Specific nutrients, especially if they are supplemented at high levels, can in some cases interfere with the antimetabolite drugs.

Follow the diet, lifestyle, and environmental strategies described in chapter 10. These may have some curative effect and at the minimum will reduce risk factors, as well as help the immune system to function properly. Supplemental nutrition should be based on your actual physiological needs. Avoid very high doses of any supplement during conventional treatment.

Always be certain that nonconventional treatments are administered outside the protected zone.

GLIOMAS

Gliomas are tumors of the central nervous system, primarily brain tumors. They include astrocytomas and glioblastomas.

Considering Your Diagnosis

No staging system exists for gliomas, but there is a grading system that takes into account the aggressiveness of the tumor. Grades begin with the least aggressive, grade I, and extend to the most aggressive, grade IV. These tumors are made up of specific kinds of nervous system cells known as astrocytes. The least aggressive tumors are known as astrocytomas. More aggressive tumors are known as anaplastic astrocytomas which means astrocytomas whose borders have invaded surrounding tissue. Glioblastoma multiforme is the most aggressive form of astrocytoma with the most invasion of surrounding tissue.

Grades I and II are astrocytomas.
Grade III is an anaplastic astrocytoma.
Grade IV is a glioblastoma multiforme.

Conventional Treatment Strategies for Gliomas

Gliomas are generally treated with surgery, radiation, and chemotherapy.

Surgery
Surgical treatment is for the purpose of removing some or all of the tumor mass. The extent of surgery is almost always governed by the size and location of the tumor. Brain function and quality of life issues greatly affect surgical decisions. When the tumor has been interfering with surrounding brain tissue, removal of its bulk can restore form and function to a remarkable degree.

Radiation Treatment
Radiation is commonly used for the treatment of brain tumors. If surgery is an option, radiation also may be used to destroy any remaining tumor and to help prevent a recurrence. When surgery is not an option, radiation may be used for local control of the tumor since it can often destroy tumor tissue with less damage to surrounding brain tissue.

Chemotherapy
A number of chemotherapy agents are used for the treatment of gliomas. Since the brain is separated from the blood in the rest of the body by the-

Combining Conventional and Nonconventional Care

blood-brain barrier, these agents must be capable of crossing that barrier. In addition, their action must be capable of damaging tumor tissue without doing extensive harm to the rest of the brain.

Many combination therapies are in use, both FDA-approved and experimental, which are specific to the particular circumstances of the person and the tumor. The following are the most common.

BCNU Plus Cisplatin

The alkylating agents carmustine (BCNU) and cisplatin are combined for use in certain cases following surgery. Common side effects for this glioma treatment include bone marrow suppression, nausea and vomiting, reversible liver toxicity, lung toxicity, kidney toxicity, numbness of hands and feet, and hearing deficit that is often reversible. Side effects for this protocol can vary greatly depending on patient condition and the individual drug dosages used. Ask your medical specialist to estimate how you will respond based on your specific circumstances.

Carmustine, Streptozocin, and Mercaptopurine

The alkylating agents carmustine and streptozocin are combined with mercaptopurine (6-MP) for the treatment of a wide variety of gliomas. Common side effects for this glioma treatment include bone marrow suppression, nausea, vomiting, diarrhea, reversible liver toxicity, lung toxicity, and kidney toxicity. Side effects for this protocol can vary greatly depending on patient condition and the individual drug dosages used. Ask your medical specialist to estimate how you will respond based on your specific circumstances.

Gene Therapy

The unique gene therapy combination of the enzyme herpes simplex thymidine kinase and the antiviral ganciclovir has been used for treatment of glioma. Side effects for this category of glioma protocols are generally mild but can vary greatly depending on patient condition and the individual drug dosages and timing used. Ask your medical specialist to estimate how you will respond based on your specific circumstances.

A Guide to Alternative Medicines in Treating Gliomas

With the support of a trained nonconventional provider, select nonconventional therapies from chapter 8 that most closely match your symptoms and best address the side effects of your conventional therapies. Many of the glioma chemotherapy and radiation regimes are vulnerable to interference, especially from high level antioxidants. Specific nutrients, especially if they are supplemented at high levels, can in some cases interfere with the antimetabolite drugs.

When the conventional treatment plan results in immune system suppression, be certain that the supplements you are using have been screened for microbial safety. You may have to stop taking supplements when your white blood cell counts are low (which happens as a result of immune system suppression from treatment), but keep in mind that, under certain conditions, white blood counts may be high and the immune system may still not be fully functional.

Follow the diet, lifestyle, and environmental strategies described in chapter 10. These may have some curative effect but at the minimum will reduce risk factors, as well as help the immune system to function properly. Supplemental nutrition should be based on your actual physiological needs. Avoid very high doses of any supplements during conventional treatment.

Always be certain that nonconventional treatments are administered outside the protected zone.

GYNECOLOGICAL CANCERS

These cancers pertain to the female organs of reproduction and include ovarian cancer and cancers of the cervix and endometrium.

Considering Your Diagnosis

Gynecological cancers are described by a number of staging criteria that take into account:

- Tumor cell type
- Local tumor spread
- Local lymph node involvement
- Tumor metastatic spread to other parts of the body

Conventional Treatment Strategies for Gynecological Cancers

The most common cancers of the female reproductive system include ovarian, cervical, and uterine. Early-stage ovarian cancer is treated by surgical removal of the ovaries, with good long-term results. If the tumor is more advanced, treatment protocols will include more extensive surgery and chemotherapy.

Cancer of the uterine cervix is almost always treated surgically. If detected early, the tumor can be removed locally. If it is more advanced, more radical surgery such as hysterectomy may be necessary, along with radiation and chemotherapy.

Cancer of the endometrium, the inner lining of the uterus, is almost always treated surgically by hysterectomy. In some cases, chemotherapy and radiation are also recommended.

The most common cancers of the female reproductive system include ovarian, cervical, and uterine.

Surgery

Surgical interventions are used to remove the tumor and surrounding structures. When gynecological tumors are caught early enough, local surgery may be the only recommended treatment. If the tumor is more advanced or has spread, surgery is still recommended to remove all or as much tumor as possible.

Radiation Therapy

Radiation therapy is used for local control, usually after surgery, for certain uterine and endometrial tumors.

Chemotherapy

Chemotherapy agents include a wide variety of drugs and combinations. The single-agent drugs that have been most successful are the alkylating agents cisplatin, carboplatin, melphalan, hexamethylmelamine (altretamine), thiotepa, ifosfamide, and chlorambucil; the plant-derived drugs topotecan, Taxol, and vincristine; the antitumor antibiotic doxorubicin; and the antimetabolites 5-fluorouracil and methotrexate.

Carboplatin Plus Taxol

The combination therapy of carboplatin plus Taxol is used for the treatment of advanced ovarian carcinoma. Common side effects for this ovarian cancer treatment include bone marrow suppression, hair loss, nausea and vomiting, numbness of hands and feet, diarrhea, mouth sores, heart toxicity, kidney toxicity, and hearing toxicity. A rare side effect is allergic response. Side effects for this protocol can vary greatly depending on patient condition and the individual drug dosages used. Ask your medical specialist to estimate how you will respond based on your specific circumstances.

Cisplatin Plus Taxol

Cisplatin plus Taxol is also used in combination for the treatment of advanced ovarian carcinoma. Common side effects for this ovarian cancer treatment include bone marrow suppression, hair loss, nausea and vomiting, numbness of hands and feet, diarrhea, mouth sores, heart and kidney toxicity, hearing toxicity, and rare allergic response. Side effects for this protocol can vary greatly depending on patient condition and the individual drug dosages used. Ask your medical specialist to estimate how you will respond based on your specific circumstances.

Megace

The hormone megastrol acetate (Megace) is commonly used for the treatment of endometrial cancer. Common side effects include weight gain, nausea, fluid retention, breakthrough bleeding, shortness of breath, hair loss, and blood sugar metabolism difficulties.

Cis-retinoic Acid Plus Interferon Alpha

The biological agents cis-retinoic acid and interferon alpha are combined for the treatment of advanced cervical cancer. Common side effects include flu-like symptoms (such as fever, chills, body aches, and headache), skin itching and irritation, dry mouth, nausea, vomiting, eye irritation, and fatigue.

CA

CA is the abbreviation for Cytoxan and Adriamycin when they are used together. They are usually administered weekly or every three weeks. Common side effects include bone marrow suppression, mouth sores, and hair loss occurring in more than half (40 to 70%) of the patients. Nausea, vomiting, and heart toxicity occur in less than half (20 to 40%) of all patients.

A Guide to Alternative Medicines in Treating Gynecological Cancers

With the support of a trained nonconventional provider, select nonconventional therapies from chapter 5 that most closely match your symptoms and best address the side effects of your conventional therapy.

Many of the gynecological cancer chemotherapy and radiation regimes are vulnerable to interference, especially from high-level antioxidants. The antimetabolite drugs can, in some cases, be interfered with by specific nutrients, especially if they are supplemented at high levels. With gynecological tumors, it is important to account for any hormone activity that might be included with the nonconventional therapies.

When the conventional treatment plan results in immune system suppression, be certain that the supplements you are using have been screened for microbial safety. You may have to stop taking supplements when your white blood cell counts are low (which happens as a result of immune system suppression from treatment), but keep in mind that, under certain conditions, white blood counts may be high and the immune system may still not be fully functional.

> Many of the gynecological cancer regimes are vulnerable to interference, especially from high-level antioxidants.

Follow the diet, lifestyle, and environmental strategies described in chapter 10. These may have some curative effect and at the minimum will reduce risk factors, as well as help the immune system to function properly. Supplemental nutrition should be based on your actual physiological needs. Avoid very high doses of any supplements during conventional treatment.

Always be certain that nonconventional treatments are administered outside the protected zone.

HEAD AND NECK CANCERS

Head and neck cancers can include tumors of the nose, throat, salivary glands, voice box, and surrounding structures.

Considering Your Diagnosis

Head and neck cancers are described by a TNM staging system that takes into account:

- Tumor size
- Local lymph node involvement
- Spread to local structures
- Tumor metastatic spread to other parts of the body

Stages I and II

Stages I and II are small local tumors without local lymph node involvement and without distant metastatic spread.

Stage III

Stage III is a tumor that has spread to local structures, with just one local lymph node involved, and without distant metastatic spread.

Stage IV

Stage IV is a tumor that has spread to local structures, with multiple local lymph nodes involved, and with distant metastatic spread.

Conventional Treatment Strategies for Head and Neck Cancers

Many similarities exist in the conventional treatments for head and neck cancers. Localized head and neck tumors are normally treated with surgery and/or radiation. The results and long-term outcomes can be very good in early-stage cases. With advanced and metastatic disease, chemotherapy is usually added.

Surgery

Surgery is used to remove the tumor whenever possible. The head and neck area is among the most challenging surgically because of the many nerves, blood vessels, and critical structures so close together. Even if the tumor can be removed completely, radiation therapy might also be suggested.

In some cases surgery is used simply to debulk the tumor, that is, reduce the size of it rather than remove it entirely, especially if it is located in a place that interferes with function. Such surgical interventions are often useful. The addition of chemotherapy may offer a statistical improvement in long-term outcome in instances where the tumor has been either completely or partially removed.

Radiation Therapy

Radiation therapy can be used to destroy a tumor that cannot be removed by surgery, to reduce the size of a tumor to make it surgically removable, and to prevent recurrence by destroying any tumor cells that might remain after surgery . Radiation, depending on exactly where it is applied, can result in dry mouth and difficulty in swallowing that can last for some time.

Chemotherapy

Chemotherapy is used primarily to treat metastatic and recurrent tumors, but new drugs are being tested that may be useful in earlier treatment.

Combining Conventional and Nonconventional Care

CF

CF, the combination of the alkylating agent cisplatin with the antimetabolite 5-fluorouracil (5-FU), is the most common chemotherapy regime. The usual administration is cisplatin by IV on day 1 and 5-FU continuously infused from days 1 to 5. The cycle is then repeated in three to four weeks. More than half (40 to 70%) of the patients experience kidney toxicity, nausea, and vomiting; less than half (20 to 40%) experience bone marrow suppression, mouth sores, and numbness of hands and feet.

PFL

PFL is the combination of the alkylating agent cisplatin (Platinol), the antimetabolite 5-fluorouracil (5-FU), and the antimetabolite leucovorin. The administration is cisplatin by IV on day 1, 5-FU by IV on days 1 through 5, and the leucovorin orally (sometimes mixed with 5-FU) on days 1 through 5. Most (70 to 100%) patients experience mouth sores; more than half (40 to 70%) experience bone marrow suppression and kidney toxicity; and less than half (20 to 40%) experience nausea, vomiting, and numbness of hands and feet.

Cisplatin, 5-FU, and Hydroxyurea

The other common chemotherapy treatment for head and neck cancer is the combination of the alkylating agent cisplatin, the antimetabolite 5-fluorouracil (5-FU), and the antimetabolite hydroxyurea. This combination is normally administered along with radiation. The cisplatin is given by IV on day 1, the 5-FU by continuous IV infusion on days 1 through 5, and the hydroxyurea orally on days 1 through 5. The process is repeated every three to four weeks, but the cisplatin is given only every other cycle. Common side effects include nausea and vomiting, diarrhea, numbness of hands and feet, kidney toxicity, hearing toxicity, liver toxicity, mouth sores, loss of appetite, headache, and fatigue. Side effects for this protocol can vary greatly depending on patient condition and the individual drug dosages used. Ask your medical specialist to estimate how you will respond based on your specific circumstances.

A Guide to Alternative Medicines in Treating Head and Neck Cancers

If a good conventional treatment is available for your particular circumstances, do not delay treatment in order to try a nonconventional therapy unless you and your medical specialist are certain that you have time. In some cases, conventional therapies have a limited window of opportunity during which they can provide a predictable good outcome. Wait too long and the opportunity could be lost or reduced in value. It is also vital you not risk the rapid growth or spread of the cancer. The progress of the tumor should be carefully monitored if conventional treatment is delayed, to be certain things do not get out of hand. Use a folate mouthwash for several weeks prior to treatment.

With the support of a trained nonconventional provider, select nonconventional therapies from chapter 5 that best address the symptoms of your cancer and the side effects of your conventional therapy.

Many of the head and neck cancer chemotherapy and radiation regimes are vulnerable to interference, especially from high-level antioxidants. The antimetabolite drugs can, in some cases, be interfered with by specific nutrients, especially if they are supplemented at high levels.

Always be certain that all nonconventional treatments are administered outside the protected zone.

When the conventional treatment plan results in immune system suppression, be certain that the supplements you are using have been screened for microbial safety. You may have to stop taking supplements when your white blood cell counts are low (which happens as a result of immune system suppression from treatment), but keep in mind that, under certain conditions, white blood counts may be high and the immune system may still not be fully functional.

Follow the diet, lifestyle, and environmental strategies described in chapter 10. These may have some curative effect and at the minimum will reduce risk factors, as well as help the immune system to function properly. They are especially important for healing following surgery or radiation. Supplemental nutrition should be based on your actual physiological needs. Avoid very high doses of any supplement during conventional treatment.

Always be certain that all nonconventional treatments are administered outside the protected zone.

HODGKIN'S DISEASE

Hodgkin's disease, also known as lymphoreticuloma, is the most common cancer of the lymphatic system. In its early stages the disease is characterized by local, painless swelling of one or more lymph nodes and sometimes by swelling of the spleen, liver, or other organs. Other symptoms may include fever, weight loss, and weakness.

Hodgkin's disease can be confirmed only by microscopic examination of affected tissue, usually from a lymph node. The cause of the disease remains unknown, but numerous infectious agents, including bacteria, protozoa, and viruses, have been suggested.

Considering Your Diagnosis

Hodgkin's disease is staged by a system that takes into account:

- Lymph node involvement
- Lymph system organ involvement
- Tumor spread outside the lymph nodes and organs

Stage I

Stage I is the involvement of a single lymph node region, such as the spleen or thymus.

Stage II

Stage II is the involvement of two or more lymph node regions on the same side of the diaphragm (the structure that separates the chest cavity from the abdominal or stomach cavity).

Stage III

Stage III is the involvement of lymph structures on both sides of the diaphragm.

Stage IV

Stage IV is extensive or bulky disease outside the lymph node regions.

Conventional Treatment Strategies for Hodgkin's Disease

Hodgkin's disease is generally treated with chemotherapy and radiation. Surgery is only employed under rare circumstances. Radiation therapy might be used alone and in combination with chemotherapy. Hodgkin's tumors are often very responsive to radiation.

Two principal chemotherapy protocols, ABVD and MOPP, are commonly used singly or together. ABVD combines the antitumor antibiotics Adriamycin (doxorubicin) and bleomycin with the plant-derived vinblastine and the alkylator dacarbazine. The drugs are administered every two weeks. Most (70 to 100%) patients treated experience bone marrow suppression; more than half (40 to 70%) experience nausea and vomiting, hair loss, and lung toxicity; and less than half (20 to 40%) experience cardiac toxicity, allergic response to the drugs, mouth sores, and numbness of hands and feet.

MOPP combines the alkylating agents mechlorethamine and procarbazine with the plant-derived vincristine (Oncovin) and the steroid hormone prednisone. The mechlorethamine and vincristine are administered on days 1 and 8. The procarbazine and prednisone are administered daily on days 1 through 14. The cycle is then repeated in twenty-eight days. More than half (40 to 70%) of the patients experience bone marrow suppression and numbness of hands and feet, while less than half (20 to 40%) experience nausea, vomiting, and hair loss. Infertility following treatment can be a problem with MOPP but is usually not a result of ABVD.

A Guide to Alternative Medicines in Treating Hodgkin's Disease

Conventional medicine often produces excellent outcomes with Hodgkin's disease. In most cases it is not wise to delay conventional treatment in order to try nonconventional protocols.

With the support of a trained nonconventional provider. select nonconventional therapies from chapter 5 that best address your symptoms and the side effects of your conventional therapy.

> Conventional medicine often produces excellent outcomes with Hodgkin's disease.

Many of the Hodgkin's disease chemotherapy and radiation regimes are vulnerable to interference, especially from high-level antioxidants. The antimetabolite drugs can, in some cases, be interfered with by specific nutrients, especially if they are supplemented at high levels.

When the conventional treatment plan results in immune system suppression, be certain that the supplements you are using have been screened for microbial safety. You may have to stop taking supplements when your white blood cell counts are low (which happens as a result of immune system suppression from treatment), but keep in mind that, under certain conditions, white blood counts may be high and the immune system may still not be fully functional.

Follow the diet, lifestyle, and environmental strategies described in chapter 10. These may have some curative effect and at the minimum will reduce risk factors, as well as help the immune system to function properly. Supplemental nutrition should be based on your actual physiological needs. Avoid very high doses of anything during conventional treatment.

Always be certain that nonconventional treatments are administered outside the protected zone.

LEUKEMIA

Leukemia is a cancer of the bone marrow that can also affect the lymph nodes and spleen.

The first symptoms of leukemia are usually fatigue and weakness. In acute leukemia, these symptoms are often severe and the disease progresses rapidly. Early chronic leukemia can be so insidious that it might not be detected until more advanced symptoms such as enlargement of the lymph nodes and spleen occur.

Considering Your Diagnosis

Leukemias are not described by a staging system but are instead named for their individual cell types and their aggressiveness. Leukemias in general describe the rapid growth of specific types of white blood cells that, in effect, crowd out other important blood cells, such as other white blood cells (there is more than one kind of white blood cell), red blood cells, and platelets. AML refers to acute myeloid leukemia, ALL is shorthand for acute lymphoblastic leukemia, CML is chronic myeloid leukemia, and CLL is chronic lymphocytic leukemia. A fifth leukemia, which is chronic, is hairy cell leukemia. Acute leukemias are faster growing than chronic leukemias.

Conventional Treatment Strategies for Leukemia

Conventional treatment for leukemia is aimed at reducing the numbers of the excess blood cells by selectively killing them with chemotherapy. Destroying the progenitor cells that produce them is also important.

In some cases, specific radiation protocols are combined with chemotherapy. In addition, bone marrow and peripheral stem cell transplants are used to provide more lasting effects. A great number of protocols are in use, both approved and experimental. The antimetabolite cytarabine (cytosine arabinoside or ara-C) is used alone or in combination with the antitumor antibiotic daunorubicin for the treatment of AML. In some cases, the cytarabine is combined with other antitumor antibiotics, including Idarubicin or mitoxantrone.

The alkylating agent mitoxantrone is combined with the plant-derived drug etoposide for the treatment of AML in relapse. The chemotherapeutic treatment of ALL usually involves the use of a wide variety of drugs, arranged in different combinations for different phases of treatment. The treatment protocols are often very long-running, for a year or more, and are sometimes combined with radiation.

The drugs that are used, normally in a variety of combinations, include the alkylating agent cyclophosphamide; the antitumor antibiotics daunorubicin and doxorubicin; the antimetabolites L-asparaginase, cytarabine, 6-mercaptopurine, methotrexate, thioguanine, and leucovorin; the plant-derived agents vincristine and etoposide; the biological agent interferon alpha; as well as some steroid hormones.

The antimetabolite hydroxyurea and the biological interferon alpha are used for the treatment of CML. The alkylating agent chlorambucil is used alone or in combination with a steroid hormone for the treatment of CLL in certain cases. The antimetabolites cladribine and fludarabine phosphate, as well as interferon alpha, are also used singly for the treatment of CLL. The antimetabolites cladribine and pentostatin, as well as interferon alpha, are used in the treatment of hairy cell leukemia.

Side effects for the various leukemia treatment protocols above can vary greatly depending on patient condition and the individual drug dosages and timing used. Ask your medical specialist to estimate how you will respond based on your specific circumstances.

A Guide to Alternative Medicines in Treating Leukemia

With the support of a trained nonconventional provider, select nonconventional therapies from chapter 5 that best address your symptoms and the side effects of your conventional therapy.

Many of the leukemia chemotherapy and radiation regimes are vulnerable to interference, especially from high-level antioxidants. The antimetabolite drugs can, in some cases, be interfered with by specific nutrients, especially if they are supplemented at high levels. When the conventional treatment plan results in immune system suppression, be certain that the supplements you are using have been screened for microbial safety. You may have to stop taking supplements when your white blood cell counts are low (which happens as a result of immune system suppression from treatment), but keep in mind that, under certain conditions, white blood counts may be high and the immune system may still not be fully functional.

Follow the diet, lifestyle, and environmental strategies described in chapter 10. These may have some curative effect and at the minimum will reduce risk factors, as well as help the immune system to function properly. Supplemental nutrition should be based on your actual physiological needs. Avoid very high doses of any supplement during conventional treatment.

Always be certain that nonconventional treatments are administered outside the protected zone.

LIVER, GALLBLADDER, AND BILIARY CANCER

The liver secretes bile into the gallbladder, where it is stored. Bile has a number of functions, including acting as an enzyme for the digestion of fats as well as a vehicle for removing toxins from the body after they have been processed by the liver. The gallbladder stores the bile until it is needed—until you eat a meal with fats. At that time, the gallbladder constricts, pushing the bile out through the biliary ducts to the small intestine.

Considering Your Diagnosis

Liver cancer and biliary/gallbladder cancer each have a TNM staging system.

The staging system for liver cancer takes into account:

- Tumor size
- Number of tumors
- Local lymph node involvement
- Metastatic spread to other parts of the body

Stage I
Stage I is a tumor less than 2 cm that has not involved liver blood vessels. There is no local lymph node involvement and there is no distant metastatic spread.

Stage II
Stage II is either a tumor less than 2 cm that has involved liver blood vessels or a tumor greater than 2 cm that has not involved liver blood vessels. There is no local lymph node involvement and no distant metastatic spread.

Stage III
Stage III is either a tumor greater than 2 cm that has involved liver blood vessels or multiple tumors in only one lobe of the liver. These may have local lymph node involvement, but there is no distant metastatic spread.

Stage IV

Stage IV is a tumor involving more than one lobe of the liver or distant metastatic spread.

The TNM staging system for biliary and gallbladder cancer takes into account:

- Tumor location
- Tumor growth in the wall of the gallbladder
- Local spread of the tumor
- Regional lymph node involvement
- Metastatic spread to other parts of the body

Stage I

Stage I is a tumor that involves only the inside and middle layer of the gallbladder wall. There is no local node involvement and no metastatic spread to other parts of the body.

Stage II

Stage II is either a tumor that has grown through the wall of the gall-bladder or a biliary tumor that has involved adjacent structures. There is no local node involvement and no metastatic spread to other parts of the body.

Stage III

Stage III is either a tumor that has grown through the wall of the gallbladder and has involved an adjacent organ, including the liver, or a biliary tumor that has involved adjacent structures. There may be local node involvement but no metastatic spread to other parts of the body.

Stage IV

Stage IV is either a tumor that has grown through the wall of the gallbladder and has involved an adjacent organ, including the liver, or a biliary tumor that has involved surrounding muscle layers. There may be local node involvement and/or metastatic spread to other parts of the body.

Conventional Treatment Strategies
for Liver, Gallbladder, and Biliary Cancers

Localized tumors, including hepatoma cholangiocarcinoma, are treated surgically by removal of the tumor when possible. When surgery is not an option or when there is metastatic disease, then chemotherapy is used, with the objective of either palliation or reducing the tumor to an operable size. Radiation and organ transplantation are options but are used less often. New vaccines are in early trials.

Surgery

Surgical procedures are normally used when all or a substantial amount of tumor can be removed. Removal of parts of the liver, all of the gallbladder, and parts of the biliary system can be accomplished with controllable long-term effects. Many different procedures exist for specific circumstances.

Chemotherapy

Chemotherapy regimes center around the antimetabolites 5-fluorouracil (5-FU), floxuridine (FUDR), and leucovorin for both primary tumors and metastases to the liver. The side effects of these treatments are generally milder than those of other chemotherapeutic agents. Interferon alpha has also been used to treat liver cancers.

A Guide to Alternative Medicines in Treating Liver, Gallbladder, and Biliary Cancers

With the support of a trained nonconventional provider, select nonconventional therapies from chapter 5 that best address your symptoms and the side effects of your conventional therapy. Many of the liver, gallbladder, and biliary cancer chemotherapy and radiation regimes are vulnerable to interference, especially from high-level antioxidants. The antimetabolite drugs can, in some cases, be interfered with by specific nutrients, especially if they are supplemented at high levels.

When the conventional treatment plan results in immune system suppression, be certain that the supplements you are using have been screened for microbial safety. You may have to stop taking supplements when your white blood cell counts are low (which happens as a result of immune system suppression from treatment), but keep in mind that, under certain conditions, white blood counts may be high and the immune system may still not be fully functional.

Follow the diet, lifestyle, and environmental strategies described in chapter 10. These may have some curative effect and at the minimum will reduce risk factors, as well as help the immune system to function properly. Avoid all liver-stressing drugs, including alcohol. Supplemental nutrition should be based on your actual physiological needs. Avoid very high doses of any supplement during conventional treatment.

In the early stages of lung cancer, there are often no symptoms. As the disease progresses, symptoms may include coughing, shortness of breath, chest pain, and coughing up blood. Loss of appetite, weakness, and weight loss often accompany the disease. Cigarette smoking is a major cause of lung cancer. Other factors that put patients at risk for lung cancer are exposure to asbestos, radon gas, and other environmental toxins.

There are two basic kinds of lung cancer. Small-cell carcinoma accounts for about 25% of all lung cancer cases. Non–small-cell carcinomas include squamous-cell carcinomas, large-cell carcinomas, and adenocarcinomas.

Considering Your Diagnosis

Lung cancer is described by a TNM staging system that takes into account:

- Tumor size
- Tumor local spread
- Local lymph node involvement
- Tumor metastatic spread to other parts of the body

Stage I
Stage I is a tumor that has not spread out of the lung space, without local lymph node involvement, and without distant metastatic spread.

Stage II
Stage II is a tumor that has not spread out of the lung space, with local lymph node involvement, but without distant metastatic spread.

Stage III
Stage III is either a tumor that has not spread out of the lung space, with advanced local lymph node involvement but without distant metastatic spread, or a tumor that has grown out of the lung space, with possible local lymph node involvement, but without distant metastatic spread.

Stage IV
Stage IV is a tumor that has spread to a distant metastatic site.

The staging system does not account for the different cell types of lung cancer.

Conventional Treatment Strategies for Lung Cancer

Lung cancer can be treated with surgery and/or radiation and/or chemotherapy, depending on the type of cancer and its extent. Surgery can be successful in early stages. Radiation and chemotherapy may be added with small-cell or more advanced tumors. Tumor response and outcomes are particular to the many combinations of circumstances possible.

Surgery

Surgical treatment can provide significant benefits when all of the tumor can be removed. Surgical removal of a large portion of the tumor also can be useful. When there is significant metastasis, however, care must be exercised to be certain that the potential benefits of surgery are not outweighed by the risks and trauma associated with the procedure.

Radiation Therapy

Radiation therapy can be used to destroy a tumor that cannot be removed by surgery, to reduce the size of a tumor to make it surgically removable, or to destroy any tumor cells that might be left after surgery to prevent a recurrence. Radiation can also be used to control metastatic disease, reduce pain, and improve function. Depending on the exact location of the treatment, radiation can result in difficulty in swallowing and heart damage, but most symptoms resolve after treatment.

Chemotherapy

Chemotherapy regimes include the single use of the plant-derived Taxol (paclitaxel), the antimetabolite gemcitabine, as well as etoposide. In addition, a number of combination therapies are used but these are primarily for non–small-cell lung cancer.

Taxol Plus Carboplatin

Taxol plus the alkylating agent carboplatin are used together, usually administered at the same time, once every three weeks by IV. Common side effects for this lung cancer treatment include bone marrow suppression, numbness of hands and feet, nausea, vomiting, diarrhea, mouth sores, heart toxicity, and kidney toxicity. Side effects for this protocol can vary greatly depending on patient condition and the individual drug dosages used. Ask your medical specialist to estimate how you will respond based on your specific circumstances. The side effects for Taxol plus carboplatin are generally milder than with Taxol plus cisplatin.

Taxol Plus Cisplatin

This treatment is normally for non–small-cell lung cancer. Taxol is used in combination with the alkylating agent cisplatin, administered together by IV once every three weeks. Common side effects for this lung cancer treatment include bone marrow suppression, numbness of hands and feet, nausea, vomiting, diarrhea, mouth sores, heart toxicity, and kidney toxicity. Side effects for this protocol can vary greatly depending on patient condition and the individual drug dosages used. Ask your medical specialist to estimate how you will respond based on your specific circumstances.

Navelbine Plus Cisplatin

This treatment is normally for non–small-cell lung cancer. The plant-derived vinorelbine (Navelbine) may be combined with cisplatin. The vinorelbine is administered by IV once per week and the cisplatin on days 1 and 29. The cycle is then repeated every six weeks. Common side effects for this lung cancer treatment include bone marrow suppression. Numbness of hands and feet, nausea, vomiting, hair loss, and fatigue are generally mild to moderate. Side effects for this protocol can vary greatly depending on patient condition and the individual drug dosages used. Ask your medical specialist to estimate how you will respond based on your specific circumstances.

PJ

PJ is the combination of the plant-derived paclitaxel and the alkylating agent carboplatin, both administered intravenously every twenty-one days. Most (70 to 100%) patients experience bone marrow suppression and numbness of hands and feet.

CAE

CAE is the combination of cyclophosphamide, Adriamycin, and etoposide administered intravenously. The cyclophosphamide and Adriamycin are administered on day 1, the etoposide is administered on days 1 through 5, and the cycle is repeated in twenty-one days. It is often applied for six cycles, followed by radiation. More than half (40 to 70%) of the patients receiving it experience bone marrow suppression and hair loss, while less than half (20 to 40%) of patients experience mouth sores, nausea and vomiting, heart toxicity, and numbness of hands and feet.

CAV

CAV is the combination of the alkylating agent cyclophosphamide (Cytoxan), the antitumor antibiotic doxorubicin (Adriamycin), and the plant-derived vincristine. All three drugs are administered by IV once every twenty-one days. CAV is used to treat both small-cell and non–small-cell lung cancers. More than half (40 to 70%) of the patients receiving it experience bone marrow suppression, hair loss, nausea, and vomiting; while less than half (20 to 40%) experience cardiac toxicity, urinary tract toxicity, mouth sores, and numbness of hands and feet.

CEV
CEV is the combination of the alkylating agent carboplatin, the antitumor antibiotic epirubicin, and the plant-derived etoposide, all administered intravenously. The carboplatin and epirubicin are administered on day 1, the etoposide is administered on days 1 through 3, and the cycle is then repeated in four weeks. Most (70 to 100%) patients experience bone marrow suppression; more than half (40 to 70%) experience nausea, vomiting, and hair loss; and less than half (20 to 40%) experience mouth sores and cardiac toxicity. This treatment is usually accompanied by radiation.

CG1 and CG2
CG1 and CG2 are combinations of the alkylating agent cisplatin and the antitumor antibiotic gemcitabine, administered intravenously weekly in different orders. More than half (40 to 70%) of the patients taking CG1 experience bone marrow suppression and mouth sores, while the mouth sores symptoms are less with CG2. The ability of these protocols to destroy tumor cells is similar.

MVP
MVP is shorthand for the antitumor antibiotic mitomycin C, the plant-derived vinblastine, and the alkylating agent cisplatin (Platinol). They are administered once every twenty-one days and are used for both small-cell and non–small-cell lung cancers. Common side effects include numbness of hands and feet, bone marrow suppression, nausea, vomiting, and diarrhea. Mouth sores and hair loss are less common. Side effects for this protocol can vary greatly depending on patient condition and the individual drug dosages used. Ask your medical specialist to estimate how you will respond based on your specific circumstances.

PE
PE is the abbreviation for cisplatin (Platinol) and the plant-derived etoposide. The cisplatin is administered by IV on day 1 and the etoposide by IV on days 1, 2, and 3. The cycle is repeated every twenty-one days. PE is used to treat both small-cell and non–small-cell lung cancers. More than

half (40 to 70%) of the patients receiving it experience hair loss and bone marrow suppression, while less than half (20 to 40%) experience nausea and vomiting.

A Guide to Alternative Medicines in Treating Lung Cancer

Lung cancer may respond to moderate doses of cis-beta carotene. At dosages less than 30,000 IU per day, this supplement may be helpful. Conflicting studies exist on this subject, but the moderate dosage level of the natural cis- form of this provitamin should avoid the potential negative effects while providing any available potential benefit. Other antioxidants may also be helpful.

With the support of a trained nonconventional provider, select nonconventional therapies from chapter 5 that most closely match your symptoms and address the side effects of your conventional therapy.

> Lung cancer may respond to moderate doses of cis-beta carotene.

Many of the lung cancer chemotherapy and radiation regimes are vulnerable to interference, especially from high-level antioxidants. The antimetabolite drugs can, in some cases, be interfered with by specific nutrients, especially if they are supplemented at high levels. When the conventional treatment plan results in immune system suppression, be certain that the supplements you are using have been screened for microbial safety. You may have to stop taking supplements when your white blood cell counts are low (which happens as a result of immune system suppression from treatment), but keep in mind that, under certain conditions, white blood counts may be high and the immune system may still not be fully functional.

Follow the diet, lifestyle, and environmental strategies described in chapter 10. These may have some curative effect and at the minimum will reduce risk factors, as well as help your immune system to function properly. Even if you have a lung cancer that is not the result of tobacco smoke, it is still useful to avoid tobacco and other airborne carcinogens. Supplemental nutrition should be based on your actual physiological needs. Avoid very high doses of anything during conventional treatment.

Always be certain that nonconventional treatments are administered outside the protected zone.

MYELOMA

A myeloma is a malignant tumor originating in the bone marrow. Usually occurring in people of at least middle age, myelomas usually affect flat bones such as the vertebrae, skull, pelvis, and shoulder blades. Signs and symptoms include anemia, weakness, pain, kidney insufficiency, pathological bone fractures, and a tendency toward hemorrhaging.

Considering Your Diagnosis

The staging system for myeloma is complex and does not have direct applicability here.

Generally, however, the staging system takes into account:

- Blood analysis
- X-ray
- Urine tests

Conventional Treatment Strategies for Myeloma

The conventional treatment for myeloma is centered around chemotherapy agents.

Chemotherapy Drugs

MP

MP is the most common protocol, using the alkylating agent melphalan along with the steroid hormone prednisone. Both drugs are administered daily on days 1 though 4 and the cycle is then repeated in four weeks. This treatment is often continued for years. Common side effects for this myeloma treatment include bone marrow suppression with increased risk for infection, infertility, weight gain, and mental status dysfunction, especially in elderly. Long-term risks can include infertility and loss of periods in women, and leukemia. Side effects for this protocol can vary greatly depending on patient condition and the individual drug dosages used. Ask your medical specialist to estimate how you will respond based on your specific circumstances.

VAD

VAD is usually used with patients in relapse or preparing for a bone marrow transplant and includes the plant-derived vincristine, the antitumor antibiotic Adriamycin (doxorubicin), and the steroid hormone dexamethasone (Decadron). The three drugs are given daily on days 1 through 4. The Decadron is repeated on days 9 through 12 and 17 through 20. Common side effects for this myeloma treatment include bone marrow suppression, nausea, vomiting, heart toxicity, numbness of hands and feet, hair loss, osteoporosis, mental status dysfunction, especially in the elderly, high blood pressure, and weight gain. Side effects for this protocol can vary greatly depending on patient condition and the individual drug dosages used. Ask your medical specialist to estimate how you will respond based on your specific circumstances.

VBMCP

VBMCP is short for the plant-derived vincristine, along with the alkylating agents BCNU (carmustine), melphalan, and cyclophosphamide, and the steroid hormone prednisone. The vincristine, BCNU, and cyclophosphamide are administered on day 1 of the cycle. The melphalan is administered daily on days 1 through 4. The prednisone is administered daily from days 1 through 15, with a lower dose the last seven days. Common side effects for this myeloma treatment include bone marrow suppression, nausea, vomiting, liver and kidney toxicity, numbness of hands and feet, hair loss, and lung toxicity. Long-term risks can include impotence in men, infertility and loss of periods in women, and leukemia. Side effects for this protocol can vary greatly depending on patient condition and the individual drug dosages used. Ask your medical specialist to estimate how you will respond based on your specific circumstances.

VBMCP Plus Interferon

VBMCP is also administered with the biological agent interferon alpha. In this protocol, the VBMCP plan is followed except that the interferon alpha is substituted in place of the last seven days of prednisone. Common side effects include flu-like symptoms (such as fever, chills, body aches, and headache), bone marrow suppression, nausea, vomiting, liver and kidney toxicity, numbness of hands and feet, hair loss, and lung toxicity. Long-term risks can include impotence in men, infertility and loss of periods in women, and leukemia. Side effects for this protocol can vary greatly depending on patient condition and the individual drug dosages used. Ask your medical specialist to estimate how you will respond based on your specific circumstances.

VMCP/VBAP Plus ABCM

VMCP/VBAP plus ABCM utilizes the alkylating agents cyclophosphamide, melphalan, and BCNU in combination with the plant-derived vincristine, the antitumor antibiotic doxorubicin, and the steroid hormone prednisone. The vincristine is administered on days 1 and 22 of the cycle. The melphalan, cyclophosphamide, and prednisone are given daily on days 1 through 4, and the prednisone is given again daily on days 22 through 25. The BCNU and doxorubicin are given once in the cycle on day 22. (There are variations to this schedule.) The entire cycle is then repeated. Common side effects include bone marrow suppression with increased risk for infection, nausea, vomiting, constipation, liver toxicity and kidney toxicity, numbness of hands and feet, hair loss, and lung toxicity. Long-term risks can include impotence in men, infertility and loss of periods in women, and leukemia. Side effects for this protocol can vary greatly depending on patient condition and the individual drug dosages used. Ask your medical specialist to estimate how you will respond based on your specific circumstances.

A Guide to Alternative Medicine in Treating Myeloma

With the support of a trained nonconventional provider, select nonconventional therapies from chapter 5 that most closely match your symptoms and best address the side effects of your conventional therapy.

Many of the myeloma chemotherapies are vulnerable to interference, especially from high level antioxidants. The antimetabolite drugs can, in some cases, be interfered with by specific nutrients, especially if they are supplemented at high levels.

When the conventional treatment plan results in immune system suppression, be certain that the supplements you are using have been screened for microbial safety. You may have to stop taking supplements when your white blood cell counts are low (which happens as a result of immune system suppression from treatment), but keep in mind that, under certain conditions, white blood counts may be high and the immune system may still not be fully functional.

Follow the diet, lifestyle, and environmental strategies as described in chapter 10. These may have some curative effect and at the minimum will reduce risk factors, as well as help the immune system to function properly. Supplemental nutrition should be based on your actual physiological needs. Avoid very high doses of supplements during conventional treatment.

Always be certain that nonconventional treatments are administered outside the protected zone.

NON-HODGKIN'S LYMPHOMA

The causes of this disease, which involves a group of malignant tumors of lymphoid tissue, are unknown. It is 50% more frequent in men than in women, and patients who have received immunosuppressive therapies are more likely to develop non-Hodgkin's lymphoma.

Considering Your Diagnosis

Lymphomas are generally described by grade—namely, low-grade, intermediate-grade, and high-grade lymphomas. The grading system for lymphoma is complex and does not have direct applicability here. Generally, however, staging protocols for lymphoma take into account:

- Patient history
- Blood analysis
- X-ray and other imaging diagnostics
- Cell analysis

Conventional Treatment Strategies for Non-Hodgkin's Lymphoma

Non-Hodgkin's lymphoma is generally treated in conventional medicine with chemotherapy and radiation. Surgery is rarely used. Bone marrow transplant is used increasingly for this diagnosis as well.

Radiation Therapy

Radiation therapy is used for both local control and as total body irradiation (TBI). Treatment is usually administered daily for a period of one to two months.

Chemotherapy

Chemotherapy is applied in drug combination protocols.

CHOP

CHOP denotes the alkylating agent cyclophosphamide, the antitumor antibiotic hydroxydaunorubicin (doxorubicin), the plant-derived vincristine, and the steroid hormone prednisone. The cyclophosphamide, hydroxydaunorubicin, and vincristine are administered on day 1 of the cycle; the prednisone is administered on days 1 through 5. The cycle is repeated every three to four weeks. More than half (40 to 70%) of the patients treated experience bone marrow suppression, hair loss, and numbness of hands and feet, while less than half (20 to 40%) experience nausea, vomiting, and cardiac toxicity.

Combining Conventional and Nonconventional Care

CVP

CVP is the acronym for the alkylating agent cyclophosphamide, the plant-derived vincristine, and the steroid hormone prednisone. The cyclophosphamide and prednisone are administered daily on days 1 through 5, whereas the vincristine is given only on day 1. The cycle is then repeated in four weeks. Less than half (20 to 40%) of the patients receiving it experience bone marrow suppression, nausea and vomiting, hair loss, and numbness of hands and feet.

Pro-mACE-CytaBOM

Pro-mACE-CytaBOM represents the steroid hormone prednisone, the antitumor antibiotic doxorubicin, the alkylating agent cyclophosphamide, the plant-derived drug etoposide, the antimetabolite cytarabine, the antitumor antibiotic bleomycin, the plant-derived drug vincristine, and the antimetabolites methotrexate and leucovorin. The prednisone is administered daily for fourteen days. The doxorubicin, cyclophosphamide, and etoposide are administered on day 1. The cytarabine, bleomycin, vincristine, and methotrexate are given on day 8, and the leucovorin is given on days 9 and 10. More than half (40 to 70%) of the patients receiving it experience bone marrow suppression, nausea and vomiting, mouth sores, hair loss, numbness of hands and feet, and lung toxicity, while less than half (20 to 40%) experience cardiac toxicity, allergic response to the drugs, and liver toxicity.

DHAP

DHAP, which is normally used when one of the previous protocols does not work, includes the alkylating agent cisplatin, the antimetabolite cytarabine, and the steroid hormone dexamethasone (Decadron). Common side effects include profound bone marrow suppression with risk for infection, kidney toxicity, and hearing problems. Side effects for this protocol can vary greatly depending on patient condition and the individual drug dosages used. Ask your medical specialist to estimate how you will respond based on your specific circumstances.

The Vanderbilt Regime

The Vanderbilt regime, commonly used for specific high-grade lymphomas, includes the alkylating agent cyclophosphamide, the plant-derived drugs etoposide and vincristine, the antitumor antibiotic bleomycin, the antimetabolites methotrexate and leucovorin, and the steroid hormone prednisone. The drugs are administered in a complex fifty-day schedule, which is repeated. Common side effects include bone marrow suppression, nausea, vomiting, diarrhea, mouth sores, digestive discomfort, osteoporosis, depression, lung toxicity, hair loss, thinning and darkening of skin and nails, infertility, and numbness of hands and feet. Side effects for this protocol can vary greatly depending on patient condition and the individual drug dosages used. Ask your medical specialist to estimate how you will respond based on your specific circumstances.

A Guide to Alternative Medicines in Treating Non-Hodgkin's Lymphoma

With the support of a trained nonconventional provider, select nonconventional therapies from chapter 5 that most closely match your symptoms and best address the side effects of your conventional therapies.

Many of the non-Hodgkin's lymphoma chemotherapy and radiation regimes are vulnerable to interference, especially from high-level antioxidants. Specific nutrients, especially if they are supplemented at high levels, can in some cases interfere with the antimetabolite drugs.

When the conventional treatment plan results in immune system suppression, be certain that the supplements you are using have been screened for microbial safety. You may have to stop taking supplements when your white blood cell counts are low (which happens as a result of immune system suppression from treatment), but keep in mind that, under certain conditions, white blood counts may be high and the immune system may still not be fully functional.

Follow the diet, lifestyle, and environmental strategies as described in chapter 10. These may have some curative effect and at the minimum will reduce risk factors, as well as help the immune system to function properly. Supplemental nutrition should be based on your actual physiological needs. Avoid very high doses of any supplement during conventional treatment.

Always be certain that nonconventional treatments are administered outside the protected zone.

OVARIAN CANCER (*see* Gynecological Cancers)

PANCREATIC CANCER

The pancreas has many functions in the body, which include adding certain digestive enzymes to the duodenum (the first section of the small intestine following the stomach) and secreting insulin and glucagon, both of which play an important role in controlling blood sugar.

Considering Your Diagnosis

Pancreatic cancer is described by a TNM staging system that takes into account:

- Local extent of the tumor beyond the pancreas
- Local lymph involvement
- Tumor metastatic spread to other parts of the body

Stage I

Stage I is a tumor that has not spread beyond the pancreas or has spread locally to the duodenum, the bile duct (which connects the pancreas to the duodenum for the purpose of delivering digestive enzymes), or the stomach but that is still surgically removable, with no local lymph node involvement, and without distant metastatic spread.

Stage II

Stage II is a tumor that has spread locally to the duodenum, the bile duct, or the stomach and is not surgically removable, with no local lymph node involvement, and without distant metastatic spread.

Stage III

Stage III is a tumor that has spread locally to the duodenum, the bile duct, or the stomach and is not surgically removable, with local lymph node involvement, but without distant metastatic spread.

Stage IV

Stage IV is a tumor that has spread locally to the duodenum, the bile duct, or the stomach and is not surgically removable, with possible local lymph node involvement, and with distant metastatic spread.

Conventional Treatment Strategies for Pancreatic Cancer

Pancreatic cancer is treated conventionally with surgery, chemotherapy, and radiation. If possible, the tumor is removed surgically. Surgery is then followed by a course of both radiation and chemotherapy. The extent, exact location, and particular type of pancreatic cancer will affect the choice of conventional treatment.

Surgery

The most common surgical intervention is the Whipple procedure, a complex operation that involves removal of the lower part of the stomach, a section of the small intestine, and part of the pancreas. New variations on this surgery have reduced its side effects, but various digestive and diabetic side effects still exist, depending on the specifics. In some cases, parts or all of the tumor can be removed without utilizing the more radical Whipple.

Radiation Therapy

Radiation therapy, when useful, is normally used in combination with chemotherapy. Side effects, in addition to the normal systemic effects of radiation, can include further aggravation of digestive symptoms.

Chemotherapy

Chemotherapy regimes depend on the type of tumor and are mostly palliative. Adenocarcinoma is usually treated with the antimetabolite 5-fluorouracil (5-FU), either during or following radiation. The side effects for this treatment are normally mild.

Islet cell (pancreatic) carcinoma is treated with a combination of the alkylating agent streptozocin and the antitumor antibiotic doxorubicin (Adriamycin).

A new antimetabolite, gemcitabine (Gemzar), and a new plant-derived drug, camptothecan (Irinotecan), have also been used to treat pancreatic tumors.

A Guide to Alternative Medicines in Treating Pancreatic Cancer

Before and after surgery it is useful to take digestive enzyme supplements to make up for what the pancreas, stomach, and other organs may not be able to supply. In addition, intestinal digestion and issues such as constipation and diarrhea should be addressed to assure proper bowel function, including the absorption of necessary nutrients and proper elimination of toxins. The enzyme plan should be developed by a licensed provider experienced with your particular circumstances, with pancreatic cancer, and with the details of your conventional treatment.

With the support of a trained nonconventional provider, select nonconventional therapies from chapter 5 that most closely match your symptoms and best address the side effects of your conventional therapy.

Some lesser-used pancreatic cancer chemotherapy and radiation regimes are vulnerable to interference, especially from high-level antioxidants. The antimetabolite drugs can, in some cases, be interfered with by specific nutrients, especially if they are supplemented at high levels.

When the conventional treatment plan results in immune system suppression, be certain that the supplements you are using have been screened for microbial safety. You may have to stop taking supplements when your white blood cell counts are low (which happens as a result of immune system suppression from treatment), but keep in mind that, under certain conditions, white blood counts may be high and the immune system may still not be fully functional.

Follow the diet, lifestyle, and environmental strategies described in chapter 10. These may have some curative effect and at the minimum will reduce risk factors, as well as help the immune system to function properly. Supplemental nutrition should be based on your actual physiological needs. Avoid very high doses of supplements during conventional treatment.

Always be certain that nonconventional treatments are administered outside the protected zone.

SARCOMAS

Sarcomas include a wide variety of tumors that originate in bone; soft tissue, including joints, muscle, tendons, skin, and veins; and vascular structures, including arteries, veins, and lymph ducts. The most common type is the osteosarcoma, a malignancy of immature bone tissue. Sarcomas are relatively rare in adults but are one of the most common malignancies in children.

Considering Your Diagnosis

Sarcomas are staged by a scheme that takes into account:

- Tumor grade (how fast it grows)
- Local lymph node involvement
- Distant metastases

Stage 1
Stage 1 is a low-grade tumor without local lymph node involvement and without spread to a distant metastatic site.

Stage 2
Stage 2 is an intermediate-grade tumor, without local lymph node involvement, and without spread to a distant metastatic site.

Stage 3

Stage 3 is a high-grade tumor, without local lymph node involvement, and without spread to a distant metastatic site.

Stage 4A

Stage 4A is any tumor with local lymph node involvement and without spread to a distant metastatic site.

Stage 4B

Stage 4B is any tumor with spread to a distant metastatic site.

Conventional Treatment Strategies for Sarcomas

Surgery, radiation, and chemotherapy are used, often in combination, to treat sarcomas.

Surgery

Surgical interventions are designed to remove the tumor and also spare a limb, often a prime objective considering where these tumors arise. Surgery is often combined with preoperative and postoperative radiation and/or chemotherapy, depending on the particular circumstances.

Radiation Therapy

Radiation therapy is used to control tumor size and to prevent local recurrence. It is administered both prior to and following surgery.

Chemotherapy

Chemotherapy is used often with sarcomas. Numerous experimental protocols are under study, some of them very complex and lasting for years. The most common protocols are:

MAID

MAID is the acronym for the antioxidant Mesna, the antitumor antibiotic Adriamycin (doxorubicin), and the alkylating agents ifosfamide and dacarbazine (DTIC). This combination is used for soft-tissue sarcomas. The drugs can be administered in a continuous IV infusion. Common side effects include bone marrow suppression, nausea, vomiting, heart toxicity, kidney and urinary tract toxicity, and confusion. Side effects for this treatment protocol can vary greatly depending on patient condition and the individual drug dosages used. Ask your medical specialist to estimate how you will respond based on your specific circumstances.

MABCDP

MABCDP represents the combination of the antimetabolite methotrexate, the antitumor antibiotics Adriamycin (doxorubicin) and bleomycin, the alkylating agent cyclophosphamide (Cytoxan), the antitumor antibiotic dactinomycin, and the alkylating agent cisplatin (Platinol). This protocol is used for the treatment of osteosarcoma. Common side effects include bone marrow suppression with risk for infection, nausea, vomiting, heart toxicity, kidney and urinary tract toxicity, liver toxicity, lung toxicity, osteoporosis, mouth sores, and allergic responses. Side effects for this protocol can vary greatly depending on patient condition and the individual drug dosages used. Ask your medical specialist to estimate how you will respond based on your specific circumstances.

VACD

VACD is the combination of the plant-derived drug vincristine, the antitumor antibiotic Adriamycin (doxorubicin), the alkylating agent cyclophosphamide, and the antitumor antibiotic dactinomycin. This protocol is for the treatment of rhabdomyosarcoma and Ewing's sarcoma. It is known to be more effective with children than with adults. Side effects for this sarcoma treatment protocol can vary greatly depending on patient condition and the individual drug dosages used. Ask your medical specialist to estimate how you will respond based on your specific circumstances.

IE

IE is the alkylating agent ifosfamide and the antioxidant Mesna. It is primarily used for the treatment of recurrences of sarcomas. Common side effects for this sarcoma treatment include bone marrow suppression, nausea, vomiting, diarrhea, confusion, fatigue, cough, shortness of breath, hair loss, and liver toxicity. Renal and urinary tract toxicity is significantly reduced with Mesna. Side effects for this protocol can vary greatly depending on patient condition and the individual drug dosages used. Ask your medical specialist to estimate how you will respond based on your specific circumstances.

VACD Plus IE

VACD plus IE combines the VACD and IE protocols mentioned above. This combination is used primarily to treat Ewing's sarcoma. Side effects for this Ewing's sarcoma treatment protocol can vary greatly depending on patient condition and the individual drug dosages used. Ask your medical specialist to estimate how you will respond based on your specific circumstances.

With the support of a trained nonconventional provider, select nonconventional therapies from chapter 5 that most closely match your symptoms and best address the side effects of your conventional therapy.

Many of the sarcoma chemotherapy and radiation regimes are vulnerable to interference, especially from high-level antioxidants. Specific nutrients, especially if they are supplemented at high levels, can in some cases interfere with the antimetabolite drugs.

When the conventional treatment plan results in immune system suppression, be certain that the supplements you are using have been screened for microbial safety. You may have to stop taking supplements when your white blood cell counts are low (which happens as a result of immune system suppression from treatment), but keep in mind that, under certain conditions, white blood counts may be high and the immune system may still not be fully functional.

Follow the diet, lifestyle, and environmental strategies described in chapter 10. These may have some curative effect and at the minimum will reduce risk factors, as well as help the immune system to function properly. Supplemental nutrition should be based on your actual physiological needs. Avoid very high doses of any supplement during conventional treatment.

Always be certain that nonconventional treatments are administered outside the protected zone.

SKIN CANCER

Skin cancer is one of the most common malignancies to affect people. A skin tumor arises on the surface of the body and usually appears as a small ulcer, pimple, or mole. They may appear singly or in groups and can invade blood vessels, lymph glands, and connecting ducts. There are two types of skin tumors: epidermal and dermal.

Considering Your Diagnosis

Most types of skin cancer, such as squamous cell and basal cell carcinoma, are generally not staged. Melanoma, a less common but more dangerous type of skin cancer, is described by a TNM staging system that takes into account:

- Tumor size
- Tumor local spread

- Local lymph node involvement
- Metastatic spread to other parts of the body

Stage IA
Stage IA is a tumor that is no larger than 0.75 mm, without local lymph node involvement, without spread to local skin tissue, and without distant metastatic spread.

Stage IB
Stage IB is a tumor that is greater than 0.75 mm but no larger than 1.5 mm, without local lymph node involvement, without spread to local skin tissue, and without distant metastatic spread.

Stage IIA
Stage IIA is a tumor that is greater than 1.5 mm but no larger than 4.0 mm, without local lymph node involvement, without spread to local skin tissue, and without distant metastatic spread.

Stage IIB
Stage IIB is a tumor that is greater than 4.0 mm or has small, separate tumor masses within 2 cm of the primary tumor, without local lymph node involvement, and without distant metastatic spread.

Skin cancer is one of the most common malignancies.

Stage III
Stage III is a tumor with limited local lymph node involvement or less than five in-transit metastases, without local lymph node involvement.

Stage IV
Stage IV is a tumor with advanced local metastases or with distant metastases.

Conventional Treatment Strategies for Skin Cancer

Squamous cell and basal cell carcinoma of the skin are the most common kinds of skin tumor. These are treated primarily by local surgical removal and are largely curable. They are rarely treated with chemotherapy.

Melanoma is much less common but much more dangerous. Localized melanoma is treated surgically, with good outcomes if there has not been spread. With spread, chemotherapy options are also used.

Surgery

Surgical intervention involves removal of the tumor with cryosurgery (very cold, freezing the tumor), laser surgery, or conventional surgery. With melanoma, a traditional surgical removal is made with wide margins.

Radiation Therapy

Radiation is not used as a primary treatment. It is not indicated for squamous and basal cell carcinoma, and melanoma is considered to be radiation-resistant. Radiation is used, however, for the control of brain metastases.

Chemotherapy

Chemotherapy is most frequently used with advanced melanoma. Several drugs and combinations have been used. In addition, a number of vaccines are currently being tested. The alkylating agent dacarbazine (DTIC) has been given alone and in combination with other drugs, including the biological agent interferon alpha-2, the alkylating agent cisplatin, the plant-derived vinblastine, and the hormonal drug tamoxifen, for the treatment of melanoma (except melanoma of the eye). Chemotherapy agents are less effective than surgery and other interventions and are therefore not used extensively.

Interferon alpha-2 has been used to treat advanced melanoma that has not spread. A number of administration protocols run from four weeks to two years. The alkylating agent melphalan is sometimes heated and administered directly into the artery of the affected area after surgical removal of the melanoma. This is most often done with the arm or leg when the melanomas cannot be otherwise controlled.

The antimetabolite 5-fluorouracil (5-FU) has been used as a topical (surface) treatment for a number of nonmelanomas, including multiple basal cell carcinomas.

A Guide to Alternative Medicines in Treating Skin Cancer

Surgical treatment should not be delayed for the purpose of trying nonconventional treatments, especially for stages I and II melanoma, which can often be cured when caught early.

With the support of a trained nonconventional provider, select nonconventional therapies from chapter 5 that most closely match your symptoms and best address the side effects of your conventional therapy.

Many of the skin cancer chemotherapy and radiation regimes are vulnerable to interference, especially from high-level antioxidants. Specific nutrients, especially if they are supplemented at high levels, can interfere with the antimetabolite drugs.

Immune-suppressive treatments are not usually used with skin cancer, but when the conventional treatment plan results in immune-system suppression, be certain that the supplements you are using have been screened for microbial safety. You may have to stop taking supplements when your white blood cell counts are low (which happens as a result of immune system suppression from treatment) but keep in mind that, under certain conditions, white blood counts may be high and the immune system may still not be fully functional.

Follow the diet, lifestyle, and environmental strategies described in chapter 10. These may have some curative effect and at the minimum will reduce risk factors, as well as help the immune system to function properly. Supplemental nutrition should be based on your actual physiological needs. Localized melanoma is treated surgically while more advanced tumors are usually treated first with chemotherapy. Chemotherapy after surgery may be useful in some instances.

UTERINE CANCER (*see* Gynecological Cancers)

The ABCs of Alternative Therapies

This chapter describes the nonconventional therapies available for treating cancer. The first thing we'll do once again, however, is to focus on your objectives: For instance, are you fighting an active tumor or are you in remission? Once you become clear about your treatment goals, you're ready to learn about how natural medicines work and the general categories of treatment. Then we'll review the current nonconventional therapies suggested for treating cancer, including their treatment objectives, the evidence for how they work (if there is any), their side effects, and whether they may be appropriate for use.

This is an opportunity to look over the many recent and ancient, promoted and forgotten, regal and common methods used for the treatment of cancer. You can browse this chapter to discover the many herbs, nutrients, and procedures that are available. Remember that most are relatively inexpensive and safe, when used appropriately.

Many of these treatments come without the scientific backing we would all like to see, but if a treatment catches your eye or tugs at your heart, and the potential gains outweigh the risks, it might be worth a try. Since you can't possibly do all of the treatments listed here, use this chapter to sort out those that suit you best.

Remember, it is extremely important that you consult chapter 7 and your nonconventional provider to ensure that your nonconventional treatments do not have unpleasant interactions with your conventional therapies.

BE CLEAR ABOUT YOUR OBJECTIVES

If you're dealing with an active tumor, you need to address strategies that can help you achieve a cure. This means not only helping to directly or indirectly destroy tumor cells but also supporting the body or organ system(s) involved.

During remission, however, your objective is to prevent a recurrence. Preventive strategies are similar to marching toward a cure, but their application will be different. You will concentrate more on developing your innate ability to resist the cancer, as opposed to removing it. During remission, you'll make dietary, lifestyle, and other changes that can have long-term, positive effects. Nonconventional therapies also can be used to improve your quality of life in a number of interesting ways. (See chapter 11 for a more complete discussion of quality-of-life issues.)

Often, you can focus on more than one objective at a time. When doing this, be certain that you aren't inadvertently combining nonconventional therapies that interact in a negative manner, cancel each other's actions, or multiply those actions in a way that results in a negative effect.

It has been suggested in the media and elsewhere that natural therapies are inherently safe and foolproof, but this is not always true. Many natural treatments are powerful medicines with the ability to significantly affect your body, to interact with other medicines and procedures, and to cause side effects. Used properly, however, natural medicine opens up a whole world of opportunities for cancer survival. Remember, the emphasis is on *used properly*.

It's also important to know that most natural therapies have not been scientifically studied. Remember, though, that "not scientifically studied" doesn't mean that these therapies don't work, merely that they have not been tested scientifically, and as a result, their use is based on less than stringent evidence.

A cancer diagnosis may make you, your family, and your friends vulnerable to believing that which may not be completely true. In fact, you may get downright angry with anyone who suggests that you're trusting

It has been suggested in the media that natural therapies are inherently safe and foolproof, but this is not always true.

The ABCs of Alternative Therapies

the wrong people. Listen to your heart, but guide yourself with as much good evidence as possible. The information about scientific evidence in chapter 7 and the decision-making process from chapter 2 should help you wend your way through the wild claims and the hype of the marketplace so that you can get the very best treatment.

HOW NATURAL MEDICINES WORK

Nonconventional therapies can play a positive role in the treatment and prevention of cancer in a number of specific ways:

- Supporting the immune system
- Stimulating the immune system
- Attacking tumor cells
- Reducing the total workload of the immune system (antioxidants)
- Relieving the side effects of the tumor
- Minimizing the side effects of conventional therapies
- Dealing with health problems that are not a result of cancer or cancer treatments

Supporting the Immune System

The immune system is your main defense against invading pathogens, such as bacteria and viruses. This system identifies and attacks such invaders, keeping you safe from illness and infection.

The immune system consists of white blood cells and the systems that produce and regulate them. Much like the other systems of your body, your immune system functions more effectively when it receives all of the nutrients and body inputs necessary for optimum performance. Strategies to support the immune system do not make it operate at a superhuman level but instead supply what is necessary for it to function, some of which is lacking in our modern diet and environment. Cancer has reached epidemic proportions in modern times, and this phenomenon is undoubtedly the result of the changes in our world.

If the nutritional and other needs of your immune system have not been met over the years, your immune system may not be able to perform as well as possible.

Immune system support is accomplished with vitamins, minerals, and other important nutrients, as well as by improving physiological and psychological balance. It is important to understand the difference between supporting the immune system and stimulating it, which I'll discuss next.

Stimulating Your Immune System

When you are healthy, your immune system maintains a steady baseline level of the various kinds of white blood cells. When the immune system detects either an infection, the presence of abnormal cells, or some other challenge, it rapidly increases the number and activity of white blood cells in order to deal with this emergency.

What's more, each kind of white blood cell is specialized to deal with a different kind of problem. Some eliminate viruses, some destroy bacteria, and others attack defective cells such as precancerous cells. The immune system normally has the ability to sense the need for and to increase only the particular type of white blood cells that are needed.

In nonconventional medicine, methods exist for creating or amplifying such an alert, thus increasing the number of white blood cells and, in some cases, even increasing the particular types of white blood cells that your body needs. These methods employ various nutrients, botanicals, and a number of physical and psychological protocols.

Stimulating bone marrow or immune system activity does not necessarily lead to an improved response against cancer, however. In fact, using stimulating substances such as herbs may actually *reduce* your body's abil-

U sing stimulating sub-stances such as herbs may actually *reduce* your body's ability to eliminate cancer cells.

ity to eliminate cancer cells by activating the wrong cells or by giving incorrect signals to the immune system's target, the tumor cells. More human studies on anticancer activity are needed to demonstrate which immune stimulators help the disease-fighting process and which may interfere with it.

Natural immune-stimulating substances should not be used to counter the effects of immune-suppressing drugs without professional guidance. The immune-stimulating activity may act on different white blood cells than those that were suppressed by the immune-suppressing drug. Another risk is that the immune-stimulating action may further stress the bone marrow and result in worse rather than better performance.

Attacking Tumor Cells

A number of methods in nonconventional medicine directly attack tumor cells, either by damaging the cells and causing them to expire, by creating a hostile environment for the cells, or by interfering with their ability to reproduce. These methods for attacking tumor cells include the use of enzymes, herbs, diet, and certain physical therapies.

The ABCs of Alternative Therapies

Reducing the Total Workload of the
Immune System (Antioxidants)

The immune system goes on day after day with its business of protecting you from infection and neutralizing unwanted invaders. In nonconventional medicine, we reduce this workload as much as possible by using preventive strategies to maximize the immune system's ability to fight cancer.

Such preventive strategies include avoiding risk factors that might cause illness as well as using the "damage-control" effects of substances known as antioxidants. These substances play an important role in your body because they can protect you from substances known as free radicals. Free radicals are highly reactive, which means that they are able to bond with other substances in your body. The result can cause damage to the cells of your body, in ways that can predispose you to cancer. Antioxidants also help in cell-repair mechanisms.

Antioxidants are found in a wide variety of foods, vitamins, minerals, botanicals, and other substances.

Nonconventional methods for controlling tumor effects include nutrition, botanicals, diet, lifestyle, physical therapies, and psychological strategies.

Relieving the Side Effects of the Tumor

Cancer can create many problems that affect you, such as interfering with the normal function of body systems, secreting unusual hormones, and creating discomfort or pain. Nonconventional treatments can often be used to help control these unwanted effects.

The nonconventional methods for controlling tumor effects include nutrition, botanicals, diet, lifestyle, physical therapies, and psychological strategies.

Minimizing the Side Effects of Conventional Therapies

Many cancer treatments bring with them undesirable side effects, some of which include significant health risks. Nonconventional strategies can help control these effects without interfering with the antitumor action of the cancer treatment.

Such nonconventional treatments include botanical medicines, clinical nutrition, diet, lifestyle, physical therapies, and psychological strategies. Keep in mind that nonconventional therapies can interfere with conventional cancer treatments. Chapter 6 addresses these interactions, so reading it should be an essential part of your strategy for minimizing the side effects of your cancer therapies.

Dealing with Health Problems That Are Not a Result of Cancer or Cancer Treatments

People who have cancer may also be coping with other physical or psychological problems not directly related to the tumor or treatment. In some cases, the cancer treatment may even interfere with the treatments for these other situations. If this is your situation, you may discover that ailments you've been able to live with in the past have become more difficult to deal with now that you're also coping with cancer.

Nonconventional medicine can help reduce the stress of other health issues and may be used at times when conventional treatments are unavailable or inappropriate. Once again, during conventional treatment, it is important to consider the principles of noninterference, covered in chapter 1. It's vital that you don't interfere with the tumor-destroying ability of your conventional cancer treatments.

THE TYPES OF NONCONVENTIONAL TREATMENTS

- Botanical medicines include all herbs and plant-derived substances
- Nutritionals include all vitamins, minerals, and substances from which the vitamin or mineral constituents are most important
- Enzymes include all physiological enzymes, regardless of source
- Hormones include substances with hormonelike activity in humans
- Combinations and miscellaneous substances
- Proprietary treatments
- Procedures include treatments that are done to an individual
- Strategies include plans for adjusting diet, lifestyle, or behavior

Botanical Medicines

Botanical medicines include all herbs and plant-derived substances. These medicines have been used to treat human illness since the beginning of recorded time. Herbs and other plants contain a wide variety of physiological ingredients known as *alkaloids*, which have medicated literally every human malady. Many modern drugs are imitations of the chemicals in plants.

Describing and understanding the medicinal use of botanicals is such a large field that it has its own name, *pharmacognosy*. For many years pharmacognosy was a required study for every pharmacist. That training all but disappeared over the last few decades but is now undergoing renewed interest.

Unlike most drugs, one plant can have dozens of active ingredients and many different actions in humans. For this reason, it is wise to know all of an herb's activities before taking it. Otherwise, you could resolve one problem only to make something else worse.

Botanicals, as a whole, are less toxic than drugs, but many do have side effects and some of these are serious. Such side effects are almost always dosage-related, which makes it all the more important to adhere to an appropriate dose schedule. In addition, some interact with other herbs and treatments.

Interestingly, most botanicals have some antioxidant activity and as a result show some cancer-prevention effect. Most of these antioxidant levels and effects have not been well studied.

Consult chapter 7 and seek the services of a licensed, competent non-conventional provider to tailor a botanical program that "fits you to a tee" and to ensure that you don't use these botanicals in a way that will worsen your outcome.

This chapter lists not only the botanicals generally used to treat cancer but also those others commonly used to treat certain side effects. If you find an herb you like whose actions are not studied well enough to determine its anticancer activity, you may still want to try it if the toxicity risks are not an issue. In the future, real benefits may be discovered from using many of the substances on this list. The best result occurs when you are certain you are doing no harm.

The Botanicals Listed in This Chapter

aloe	goldenseal
angelica	green tea
astragalus	laetrile
barberry	marijuana (indian hemp)
beet root	marshmallow root
bromelain	milk thistle
burdock	mistletoe
chaparral	mushrooms
chlorella	noni
cottonseed oil	Oregon grape
echinacea	Pau d'Arco
garlic	red clover

The Botanicals Listed in This Chapter, *continued*

rosemary	tolpa torf preparation
saw palmetto	turmeric
Siberian ginseng	Venus's-flytrap
tetterwort	wheatgrass

Nutritionals

Vitamins, minerals, and other nutrients exist everywhere in foods and plants. They generally do not occur alone in nature but instead are found in combinations. In some cases, these naturally occurring combinations have advantages over the use of single nutrients, even in high doses. These nutrients are required for literally every normal and emergency function of the body. While there is often debate about dosages and the best sources for these nutrients, the scientific community rarely disagrees about their importance.

Nutritionals Listed in This Chapter
Vitamins

beta-carotene	vitamin C
B vitamins in genera	vitamin D
vitamin A	vitamin E
vitamin B_6	vitamin K, as K_1 or K_3

Minerals, Oils, and Other Nutritionals

arginine	germanium
calcium	inositol
chromium	iodine
coenzyme Q10	molybdenum
copper	selenium
essential fatty acids	tellurium
flavonoids	zinc

Enzymes

For nearly a decade, enzyme manipulation through diet and supplementation has been part of nonconventional medicine for the treatment of cancer, heart disease, infection, and a wide variety of other ailments. There has never been a standard or definitive human testing of these methods to determine if they really work, but anecdotal evidence is abundant. Enzymes are used in a number of ways in nonconventional medicine.

Enzyme Treatments Listed in This Chapter
enzyme balancing
pancreatic enzyme

Hormones

Hormones are substances secreted by certain glands, then conveyed to another part of the body where they affect physiological activity, such as metabolism or growth. Phytoestrogens are plant substances that appear to have effects that are similar to the human hormone, estrogen.

Hormone Treatments Listed in This Chapter
DHEA
melatonin
phytoestrogens

Combinations and Miscellaneous Substances

These natural substances either are combinations of various substances or simply don't fit into the other categories.

Combinations and Miscellaneous Substances Listed in This Chapter
alkylglycerols
aspirin
essiac tea
Hoxsey formula
kampo
shark cartilage

Proprietary Treatments

Literally hundreds of proprietary cancer treatments are marketed directly to the public. These include individual substances, combinations of substances, procedures, and just about everything in between. Unfortunately, very little verifiable data exists about most of them.

Some of the more popular proprietary treatments are listed here with a brief description. The majority of these treatments include individual strategies described elsewhere in this chapter. However, no conclusive human studies suggest that they cure cancer. This doesn't mean that these treatments have no value, but if they do, there is no reliable information about their actual effectiveness or safety. Some are currently the subject of human studies and will soon produce new evidence. These descriptions are not meant to be an endorsement or a criticism, but rather an overview of the claims being made.

If you have an interest in any of these treatments, you should get the most recent information from the source and compare it against the known benefits of the therapies in this chapter. Don't let the lure of medical claims and testimonials, combined with the mystery of no supporting human data, lead you to a strategy that may prove a waste of time and money. Without strict research methods, statements such as "80% of participants were alive after five years" are meaningless as well as deceptive. Use the strategies from this book, as well as the support of a knowledgeable provider, to evaluate potential usefulness and safety before starting. New proprietary treatments are being offered almost daily. Apply the same standards of credibility, safety, and data to any new treatment you are considering.

Proprietary Treatments Listed in This Chapter

American Biologics	Immuno-augmentive therapy
Antineoplastin Therapy	Issels' Whole Body Therapy
Cancell	Kelley Nutritional Metabolic
Carnivora	Therapy
Clark	Live cell therapy
Coley's Toxins	Livingston therapy
Colloidal silver	PC-SPES
Evers therapy	Poly MVA
Gerson therapy	Revici therapy
Gonzalez program	714X therapy

Procedures

These regimens cover nearly everything from acupuncture and homeopathy to massage and simple exercise.

Procedures Listed in This Chapter

acupuncture and Oriental medicine
colonic therapy
exercise
homeopathy
hydrotherapy

The ABCs of Alternative Therapies

hyperthermia
manipulation
massage
oxygen treatments
polarity therapy
qigong
therapeutic touch

Strategies

Not quite procedures, these strategies are more like techniques and lifestyle changes that are designed to bring about certain health benefits.

Strategies Listed in This Chapter

acid/alkaline cleansing diet
grape cure
macrobiotic diet

A GUIDE TO NONCONVENTIONAL THERAPIES FOR THE TREATMENT OF CANCER

The nonconventional therapies discussed in this chapter are arranged alphabetically. This list will allow you to look up whatever therapy interests you so that you will be able to learn its general effects, what category of treatment it belongs to, and its overall objectives. Some nonconventional treatment protocols have been the subject of a great deal of media attention, as well as underground claims. We will review these as well, considering which are credible and which are not.

Don't let the lure of medical claims and testimonials lead you to a strategy that may prove a waste of time and money.

A Word of Warning

Serious risks can be involved in both natural and conventional therapies and in combining the two. It is wise to plan your alternative choices with both your conventional provider and a knowledgeable alternative medicine provider. If something needs to be added or subtracted for safety or effectiveness, it will be prudent to find that out *before* you begin treatment. Your conventional medical specialist should also know the details of your nonconventional plan. By using all the members of your health care team, you will ensure for yourself the best possible care.

ACID/ALKALINE CLEANSING DIET

CATEGORY: STRATEGY

This diet is purported to improve the body's chemistry by balancing the acid and alkaline foods in the diet. Creating a more alkaline environment is believed to improve resistance to cancer.

The diet consists of avoiding acid-creating foods such as cow's milk, caffeine, alcohol, tobacco, beef, pork, fried foods, sugar, refined or processed foods, artificial foods, or foods containing additives, preservatives, or colors.

Regardless of the validity of the theory, these diet strategies have other scientific benefits that make them worthwhile. These principles are also incorporated in other programs such as macrobiotics. If this diet interests you, consult with a licensed provider to be certain that you are getting adequate nutrition.

ACUPUNCTURE AND ORIENTAL MEDICINE

CATEGORY: PROCEDURE

Acupuncture is the use of needles, electrical voltage, or pressure to stimulate "meridians of energy flow" in the body. This Oriental system uses organ names such as "liver" and "kidney" in their diagnostics and treatment, but these terms are not identical to the organ definitions of Western medicine. The theory is that the needle application will affect the organ system in the proper manner, such as by stimulating, sedating, or strengthening.

Oriental (or Chinese) herbs are used within the Oriental system of diagnosis, with logic and applications that often differ significantly from Western thinking.

Some practitioners just practice acupuncture or herbal therapy, while others combine them. Acupuncture is often accomplished with *moxibustion,* burning the herb mugwort close to the skin. Note that other needle therapies exist that do not follow the rules of Chinese medicine.

Antitumor Actions

There are no definitive studies that show acupuncture or the use of Oriental herbs to be effective in the treatment of cancer. Acupuncture, however, is useful for treating nausea. It can also increase immune system activity, but whether this is related to the treatment of cancer is not clear.

Many Oriental herbs are very high in antioxidants, immune stimulants, and literally every kind of potential mechanism for anticancer activity seen in the Western botanicals.

Other Actions

For thousands of years, acupuncture and Oriental medicine have been used to treat literally every human condition. The last decade has seen a marked increase in scientific studies to confirm whether these ancient treatments really work. Although some studies support its use and others do not, acupuncture definitely seems to have a value as a treatment.

Toxicity

Acupuncture brings with it some risk for infection, especially when reusable rather than disposable needles are used. Immune-suppressed people may be at risk even when proper sterile technique is followed.

Acupuncture can result in pain at the treatment site, damage to blood vessels and nerves, or a burn from moxibustion. Such occurrences, however, are rare with trained, licensed, and experienced providers.

While few safety controls are in place for Western herbs in North America and Europe, even fewer safety measures exist for Oriental herbs manufactured in Asia. As a result, one cannot always be confident that what is on the label is in the bottle or that there are no added drugs or noxious elements in the bottle. Over the years, U.S. Customs Service has reported Oriental herbs with a number of serious contaminants. In some cases, little is known about the actions of certain ingredients in Oriental herbal products.

> Acupuncture is worthwhile for treating nausea that lasts more than a few days.

Suggested Use

Acupuncture is worthwhile for treating nausea that lasts more than a few days. Oriental herbs introduce risks that make them not recommended until such time that there are reliable, independent quality standards.

ALKYLGLYCEROLS

CATEGORY: COMBINATION OR MISCELLANEOUS SUBSTANCE

Antitumor Actions

Alkylglycerols are chemicals that occur naturally in humans and animals. The alkylglycerols sold in some health food stores are made from shark liver oil. Alkylglycerols are believed to have immune-stimulating action.

Other Actions

None known.

Toxicity

No formal toxicity studies are available, but alkylglycerols are believed to be toxic at high dosages.

Recommended Use

There is very little to support the use of alkylglycerols as an anticancer agent.

ALOE (Aloe vera)

CATEGORY: BOTANICAL

Antitumor Actions

Aloe has potent bone-marrow stimulation and antioxidant actions. It is approved for treatment by injection for some animal cancers. Studies suggest that it has some anticancer activity in humans.

Other Actions

Aloe is a laxative when taken orally. It has been used successfully as a topical (on the skin) cream for the treatment and healing of burns.

Toxicity

In its oral form, high doses can result in severe diarrhea with cramping. It can also precipitate spontaneous abortion during pregnancy.

Suggested Use

Aloe may have some benefit in the treatment of cancer but should be used carefully, especially if there are digestive problems. Oral adult dose is 4 g of dried herb or 1 teaspoon of tincture, three times per day.

AMERICAN BIOLOGICS

CATEGORY: PROPRIETARY TREATMENT

American Biologics' program incorporates a diet that avoids sugar, stimulants, and high protein consumption. Live cell therapy, laetrile, and enemas are also used. The stated objective is to support immune function and destroy tumor cells. Definitive, independent scientific human studies are needed before this treatment can be better evaluated.

ANGELICA (*Angelica species,* including *acutiloba, archangelica, atropurpurea sinensis,* and *sylvestris*)

CATEGORY: BOTANICAL

Antitumor Actions
Angelicas have plant-derived hormones called phytoestrogens, which, when taken internally, can mimic human estrogen. Angelicas can stimulate an increase of white blood cells and, in addition, contain antioxidant compounds. Angelica has some cancer-protective value, which may be from any one or a combination of these actions. A growing number of studies shows its potential use as a protective agent.

Other Actions
Angelicas also relax smooth muscles and act as painkillers. Because of these actions, they have been used traditionally for menstrual and other female reproductive complaints. Angelicas can have a mild laxative effect.

Toxicity
Very few studies have been done. Traditionally, the herb is considered to have low toxicity. High doses may increase skin sensitivity to the sun.

Suggested Use
As a preventive, angelica can be taken as a strong tea three times per day or as dried herb capsules 1 to 2 g per day.

ANTINEOPLASTIN THERAPY

CATEGORY: PROPRIETARY TREATMENT

Also known as the Burzynski Treatment, this treatment claims to "normalize" cancer cells by repairing damaged DNA. This method is currently being studied with permission from the U.S. Food and Drug Administration. Definitive, independent scientific human studies are needed before this treatment can be better evaluated.

ARGININE

CATEGORY: NUTRITIONAL

Antitumor Action
This amino acid can act as an immune system stimulator, increasing white blood cell production. No definitive human data suggests that it has any significant anticancer activity.

Other Actions
Arginine is not an essential amino acid, which means that the body can manufacture it. It is an important part of the biochemistry necessary for human growth.

Toxicity
Arginine is not considered toxic at normal human dosages. Arginine can, however, aggravate herpes virus outbreaks, which may be a problem for immune-suppressed people.

Suggested Use
Arginine is abundant in many foods, including almonds, pistachios, meat, eggs, and dairy products. Little evidence supports using additional supplementation for anticancer activity.

ASCORBIC ACID (*see* Vitamin C)

ASPIRIN

CATEGORY: COMBINATION OR MISCELLANEOUS SUBSTANCE
Yes, common aspirin has been suggested as reducing the incidence of colon, rectal, and lung cancer in several studies.

Antitumor Actions
Aspirin is believed to block the production of compounds in the body that allow tumors to grow.

Toxicity
Aspirin use can cause stomach bleeding; birth defects during pregnancy; blood sugar problems; and heart, thyroid, prostate, and other complications. It can also interact with and worsen side effects from many conventional treatments. Asprin should be used only if your team of health care providers decides that potential benefits outweigh risks.

ASTRAGALUS (*Astragalus* species, including *membranaceus*)

CATEGORY: BOTANICAL

Antitumor Action
Astragalus is an herb originally used in Chinese medicine. It has been shown to stimulate bone marrow activity. It may also have antioxidant activity. Studies suggest that it has anticancer activity in humans.

Other Actions
Astragalus has been used traditionally as an antibiotic and general tonic. It is referred to in scientific botanical literature as an *adaptogen*, which means that it tends to normalize human functions.

Toxicity
Astragalus has not demonstrated any toxic activity at normal traditional dosages.

Suggested Use
Astragalus is a safe herb to use when immune stimulation is a treatment objective. The normal adult dosage is 1 g of the herb four times per day in tablets or a tea.

BARBERRY (*Berberis vulgaris*)

CATEGORY: BOTANICAL

Antitumor Actions
Barberry contains potent bone marrow stimulation constituents that increase white blood cells. Animal studies suggest anticancer activity.

Other Actions
Barberry has been traditionally used as an antibiotic, as a liver tonic, and as a laxative.

Toxicity
Barberry has not demonstrated toxicity at normal doses.

Suggested Use
This is a relatively safe herb where bone marrow stimulation is indicated. Normal adult dosage is 15 drops of the tincture three times per day.

BEET ROOT (*Beta vulgaris*)

CATEGORY: BOTANICAL

Antitumor Action
Beet root in the form of a juice has been used traditionally as a cancer treatment. It contains antioxidants. Anecdotal evidence (but no conclusive formal studies) supports this use.

Other Actions

Beet juice has been used traditionally to stimulate bile production in the liver, ostensibly to speed the liver's detoxification of chemicals in the body. This use is supported by numerous, apparently reliable, anecdotal evidence.

Toxicity

Some individuals may experience digestive discomfort and diarrhea at high dosages.

Suggested Use

Beet juice in moderate quantities (8 ounces per day) may have some benefit in cancer prevention and during the recovery from certain conventional treatments.

BETA-CAROTENE

CATEGORY: NUTRITIONAL

Antitumor Actions

In humans, beta-carotene is a precursor of vitamin A. It is a powerful antioxidant and is capable of affecting all of the biochemical pathways in the body that can be affected by vitamin A. Studies have shown that beta-carotene protects against lung, stomach, and cervical cancer.

Beta-carotene is available in the natural *cis-* and synthetic *trans-* forms. These different versions of beta-carotene act differently in the body. A recent controversial study showed trans-beta-carotene to have a negative effect on certain individuals with lung cancer, causing the cancer to worsen. The mechanism of action of beta-carotene appears to be its antioxidant activity. The activities of cis- and trans- are known to be different, and this may account for the differences seen in outcome between the two.

Beta-carotene converts to vitamin A in the body in a rate-limited process, which means that it converts slowly enough not to have the same toxic side effects as high-dose vitamin A. Studies suggest that beta-carotene has cancer-protective activity in addition to that of vitamin A. Be certain to use only the natural cis- variety of beta-carotene.

Other Actions

Beta-carotene's actions in the body are a result of its conversion to vitamin A. See vitamin A in this chapter.

Toxicity

Studies of high doses of beta-carotene in normal individuals have not demonstrated toxic side effects. At high doses, the pigment of beta-carotene will temporarily add an orange tint to the skin. For this reason, beta-carotene has been marketed as a tanning agent.

Suggested Use
Natural (cis-) beta-carotene is a useful nutrient in the diet for all the reasons that vitamin A is important, including its antioxidant effects. Adult dosage levels up to 25,000 IU are ample when antioxidants are appropriate. Synthetic (trans-) beta-carotene is less effective in humans and may increase cancer risk in high dosages.

BROMELAIN (*Ananas comosus*)

CATEGORY: BOTANICAL

Antitumor Actions
Bromelain is an extract from the stem of the pineapple and contains enzymes that digest protein. Studies suggest that bromelain may have an anticancer activity against lung, skin, and ovarian tumors, as well as some leukemias. These are predominantly animal and test tube studies, however, and are without significant human confirmation.

Other Actions
Bromelain is used as a digestive aid, as an antibiotic, for the treatment of bronchitis, and to prevent blood clots. It may have other actions, including antioxidant and/or bone marrow stimulating activities.

Toxicity
Bromelain is not toxic at normal human dosages. Some individuals may be allergic to bromelain.

Suggested Use
Bromelain is a relatively safe herb. Adult dosage is 600 mg of the dried herb per day. It should be taken between meals for its potential anticancer effect.

BURDOCK (*Arctium lappa*)

CATEGORY: BOTANICAL

Antitumor Actions
Burdock appears to stimulate white blood cell production when taken orally. In addition, it has some antioxidant activity. No conclusive studies indicate its potential use as a cancer treatment, but anecdotal evidence of unknown reliability exists.

Other Actions

Burdock has been used as a diuretic to stimulate urination, as an antibiotic, as a fungicide, as a digestive stimulant, and to lower blood sugar. Once again, available studies and anecdotal evidence are suggestive but not conclusive.

Toxicity

There is no indication that this botanical is toxic at traditional dosage levels.

Suggested Use

Anecdotal evidence suggests that this herb is a useful cancer treatment. Some of its actions are potentially useful, and it will probably do no harm. Adult dosage is 60 drops of the tincture two times per day.

BURZYNSKI TREATMENT (*see* Antineoplastin Therapy)

B VITAMINS (*see also* Vitamin B$_6$)

CATEGORY: NUTRITIONAL

The B vitamins include thiamine (B$_1$), riboflavin (B$_2$), niacin (B$_3$), pantothenic acid (B$_4$), pyridoxine (B$_6$), cobalamins (B$_{12}$), biotin, choline, and folic acid. Together, they are known as B-complex and are necessary for proper function of the immune system, metabolism, and growth. Individually, vitamin B$_6$ has been shown to have anticancer activity.

CALCIUM

CATEGORY: NUTRITIONAL

Antitumor Actions

Studies suggest that calcium intake protects against colon cancer.

Other Actions

Calcium is essential for proper function of the nervous system, as well as for bone development and maintenance.

Toxicity

Toxicity from excess calcium in the blood can cause severe problems in children. It has been suggested that high calcium levels in the blood are the result of excessive calcium in the diet or, possibly, the result of too much vitamin D, which is necessary for absorption of calcium. There is no evidence that high oral doses of calcium in adults can result in high blood levels, but increased oral calcium can cause constipation in some individuals.

Suggested Use
Calcium is a necessary nutrient. Oral doses up to 2,000 mg per day for adult women and 1,200 mg per day for adult men are adequate. Calcium should be taken with magnesium and vitamin D for optimum effect.

CANCELL

CATEGORY: PROPRIETARY TREATMENT
Cancell is a combination of chemicals including inositol, nitric acid, sodium sulphate, potassium hydroxide, sulphuric acid, and others. The stated objective of this treatment is to eliminate tumor cells. Definitive, independent scientific human studies are needed before this treatment can be better evaluated.

CARNIVORA (*see also* Venus's-Flytrap)

CATEGORY: PROPRIETARY TREATMENT
Carnivora is the processed juice of the Venus's-flytrap plant. The stated objective of this treatment is to eliminate tumor cells.

CELANDINE (*see* Tetterwort)

CHAPARRAL (*Larrea tridentata*)

CATEGORY: BOTANICAL

Antitumor Actions
Chaparral contains a potent antioxidant constituent that probably accounts for its observed anticancer action. Chaparral has been the subject of a few studies that have resulted in both tumor regression and tumor stimulation.

Other Actions
Chaparral has also been used as an antihistamine and as an anti-inflammatory.

Toxicity
Chaparral is toxic to the liver. It can also cause nausea, vomiting, loss of appetite, and stomach pain at high dosages.

Suggested Use
Chaparral is not recommended for use, based on its potential for stimulating tumor growth and its liver toxicity.

CHLORELLA (*Chlorella pyrenoidosa*)

CATEGORY: BOTANICAL

Antitumor Action
Chlorella is an algae and may have a protective benefit against the recurrence of brain tumors. Studies, however, are far from conclusive. Chlorella's activity is probably a combination of antioxidant and bone marrow stimulation.

Other Actions
Chlorella has been used traditionally as an anti-inflammatory.

Toxicity
Little specific data is available regarding toxicity. Studies using normal human doses did not report toxicity.

Suggested Use
Chlorella may have some effectiveness but very little is known about it.

CHROMIUM

Some treatment programs suggest that tumor growth may be increased in the presence of high blood sugar.

CATEGORY: NUTRITIONAL

Antitumor Actions
Some cancer treatment programs suggest that tumor growth may be increased in the presence of high blood sugar. Chromium is one of a number of nutrients necessary for the body to control blood sugar properly.

Other Actions
Chromium's role in blood sugar metabolism is its principal use in human nutrition.

Toxicity

Chromium is not toxic in normal nutritional doses. Chromium is available in nonmedical form as an inorganic salt, however, which can be very toxic and should not be used. Use only chromium sources that are intended for human consumption since industrial grades of chromium can be extremely toxic.

Suggested Use

Chromium is a necessary part of the diet. Adult dosages from 120 mcg to 1,000 mcg are useful.

CLARK (Hulda)

CATEGORY: PROPRIETARY TREATMENT

The Hulda Clark "Cure for All Cancers" assumes that cancer is associated with parasites and offers diet and treatments to destroy the parasites.

CLEANSING DIET (*see* Acid/Alkaline Cleansing Diet)

COENZYME Q10

CATEGORY: NUTRITIONAL

Antitumor Actions

Coenzyme Q10 (also known as CoQ10) is a powerful antioxidant and is suggested to be effective against breast cancer. It is an immune system stimulant and has been shown to function in lieu of vitamin E.

Other Actions

Ongoing studies suggest that CoQ10 may have additional useful antioxidant actions in the body.

Toxicity

There have not been any toxic side effects identified at dietary doses.

Suggested Use

CoQ10 is manufactured by the body and is also available from numerous dietary sources. An effective dose appears to be 10 mg per day. It is recommended that CoQ10 be used with other antioxidants, not alone.

COLEY'S TOXINS

CATEGORY: PROPRIETARY TREATMENT

This treatment is the combination of toxins from several kinds of bacteria that are injected into the body. They have an immune-stimulating effect as the body responds to their presence. The objective of this treatment is to kill tumor cells. Definitive, independent scientific human studies are needed before this treatment can be better evaluated.

COLLOIDAL SILVER

CATEGORY: PROPRIETARY TREATMENT

Just as it sounds, colloidal silver is a liquid suspension of the metal silver. It is marketed by a number of companies for a variety of uses, including as an antibiotic and anticancer agent. There is no reliable human evidence that this is an effective cancer treatment.

COLONIC THERAPY

CATEGORY: PROCEDURE

Also known as enemas, colonics are a gentle infusion of water with herbs, salt, and, more popularly, coffee.

Antitumor Actions

Colonics are claimed to stimulate the liver and thus improve the body's detoxification. Coffee is used because of its stimulating action. Colonics are usually employed as part of a larger plan, such as the Gerson or Kelley therapies. No scientific evidence exists that they have any antitumor activity, directly or indirectly.

Colonic therapy should only be done by a licensed provider who has specific training and modern equipment.

Other Actions

Colonics can temporarily relieve constipation.

Toxicity

When done incorrectly, colonics can drain the body of important nutrients, including minerals and vitamins. They can also result in serious dehydration. There are reports of colonics causing significant infections and, when performed improperly, even some cases of perforation of the bowel. Chronic colonics can also create a dependency much the same as chronic use of laxatives.

Suggested Use
Colonic therapy should only be done by a licensed provider who has specific training and modern equipment. When used safely and carefully, colonics can provide important temporary relief of constipation and, as a result, improve the body's natural and important detoxification system. Chronic use is discouraged. Colonics should never be a substitute for getting the body's natural bowel function working properly.

COPPER

CATEGORY: NUTRITIONAL

Antitumor Actions
Very small amounts of copper are believed to be necessary for immune system function.

Other Actions
Copper is considered an essential nutrient for bone, blood, nervous system, and cardiovascular health.

Toxicity
Copper is not considered toxic at doses up to 20 mg per day for persons with normal copper metabolism. Copper can be a pro-oxidant, however, causing generation of free radicals in excess amounts.

Suggested Use
It is usually not necessary to supplement the diet with copper. A normal Western diet provides 2.5 to 5 mg per day and the prevalence of copper water pipes adds to that.

COQ10 (*see* Coenzyme Q10)

COTTONSEED OIL (*Gossypium species*)

CATEGORY: BOTANICAL

Antitumor Actions
Cottonseed oil has been used traditionally as an anticancer agent, but limited human studies indicate that it does not have anticancer activity. A little anecdotal evidence exists.

Other Actions
Cottonseed oil has been used traditionally to induce menstrual flow.

Toxicity
Cottonseed oil can induce a spontaneous abortion with pregnancy.

Suggested Use
Cottonseed oil is not suggested as an anticancer agent since there is no evidence that it works. It should never be used if pregnancy is even remotely possible. Adult dose is 20 drops of the tincture three times per day.

DHEA (Dehydroepiandrosterone)

CATEGORY: HORMONE

Antitumor Actions
DHEA has been suggested as a treatment for cancer in studies that are not definitive.

Other Actions
DHEA is a precursor to both estrogen and testosterone. It has been proposed as a treatment for heart disease, diabetes, high cholesterol, obesity, Alzheimer's disease, memory loss, fatigue, osteoporosis, and HIV. The studies are weakly suggestive.

Toxicity
Studies suggest that DHEA supplementation may cause certain cancers. In addition, DHEA can accelerate bone marrow production and worsen some cancers.

Suggested Use
DHEA may have some benefit against cancer, but it also has significant risks that, in some views, outweigh the potential benefits. DHEA is not recommended for use, based on the risks. If it is used, a complete review of your individual risks should be reviewed first.

DIET (*see* Acid/Alkaline Cleansing Diet, Grape Cure, Macrobiotic Diet)

DONG QUAI (*see* Angelica)

DYHYDROEPIANDROSTERONE (*see* DHEA)

ECHINACEA (*Echinacea species,* including *angustifolium, purpurea,* and *pallida*)

CATEGORY: BOTANICAL

Antitumor Actions
Echinacea has the ability to increase a wide variety of white blood cells. This mechanism of action is well studied, but the studies of its ability to actually create a significant antitumor effect are weak. Its immune-stimulating action has formed the basis for its traditional use as an anticancer agent. Inconclusive studies suggest it may be active against lymphocytic leukemias and certain sarcomas.

Other Actions
Echinacea is a well-studied antibiotic for both bacterial and viral infections. The mechanism of action is once again the herb's ability to stimulate an immune response of increased white blood cell production.

Toxicity
Both studies and anecdotal evidence suggest that echinacea's immune-stimulating action can become immune-suppressive with continuous use. It appears that use should be for no longer than two weeks at a time. During use, echinacea can cause dry mouth and throat, headache, and indigestion.

Suggested Use
Equal parts of each variety of echinacea should be used. Immune stimulation has not conclusively been shown to inhibit tumor growth in humans, but, when used carefully, the lack of significant side effects makes its potential benefits greater than its potential risks. Dose should be 100 mg of each variety four times per day.

EFA (*see* Essential Fatty Acids)

ENZYME BALANCING

CATEGORY: ENZYME

Antitumor Actions
Enzyme balancing is practiced by a number of providers, using very different methods. The theory is that cancer can grow because the immune

system is not functioning properly, either as a result of enzyme imbalance and/or because the enzymes that attack and control tumor tissue are not available in the body in proper amounts.

Determining enzyme imbalance is accomplished differently, depending on the provider. Some use a questionnaire, some use physical examination, and others use blood, hair, skin, and other tests to determine the enzymes needed. Some providers use the same formula of enzymes for all individuals without testing.

The enzymes administered are usually digestive enzymes, including protease, which digests protein; amylase, which digests carbohydrates; lipase, which digests fats; cellulase, which digests fiber; hydrochloric acid, which provides acidity in the stomach for the initial digestive process; and combination enzymes, including the European brand Wobenzymes. The enzymes are given in various schedules to affect digestion or to bypass digestion and be ostensibly absorbed into the bloodstream. Some are administered intravenously.

In the digestive tract, enzymes can aid in the digestion and absorption of nutrients, some of which are necessary for proper function of the immune and other systems. The enzymes can affect the pH of the body, creating an environment that is less friendly for the tumor cells. Most practitioners try to make the body more alkaline, some make it more acid, and others use measurements to determine what is needed.

Nonconventional providers propose that, in the bloodstream and tissue, enzymes remove the "coating" of tumor cells, thus allowing the immune system to destroy them. Some providers "balance" the body's key enzymes by manipulating nutrients as well as adding enzymes. This process is supposed to improve all the body's functions, including the endocrine (hormone), immune, digestive, and nervous systems.

No definitive studies show that any of these procedures are effective for the treatment of cancer, but there is ample anecdotal evidence. Many of these programs use high levels of useful nutrients along with enzyme manipulation. As a result, the nutrients may contribute to some of the positive reports.

Other Actions
Some of these programs have the added effect of improving nutrition, digestion, and other functions.

Toxicity
Toxicity potential is closely related to the particular program. The carefully planned programs use dosage levels of enzymes and nutrients that do not

The ABCs of Alternative Therapies

produce toxic, overdose results. Some other programs, however, use mega-doses of nutrients that can result in side effects and other problems.

Suggested Use

No definitive research exists to recommend any of the many enzyme treatment programs that exist. On the other hand, if the particular program you are interested in is considered safe and you can afford the cost of the treatment and follow-up nutrients, there may be no harm in trying as long as you understand that there is no scientific evidence to prove that it will work.

Too many varieties of enzyme programs are being practiced to be listed here, but you should find a provider you have confidence in and also have someone independently determine that the substances and dosages are safe for you.

ESSENTIAL FATTY ACIDS (EFA)

CATEGORY: NUTRITIONAL

Antitumor Actions

Essential fatty acids are oils that are necessary for proper immune system function. They are not manufactured by the body. The two classes of EFAs are the omega-three and omega-six. A third class of fatty acid, which is not considered essential but may be important, is omega-nine.

Studies suggest that essential fatty acids are protective against breast cancer and some other cancers.

Other Actions

EFAs have been shown to be necessary for cardiovascular health, including control of serum cholesterol.

Toxicity

Excess essential fatty acids can result in difficulty in blood clotting because of their effect on platelets. Excessive omega-six oils can promote inflammatory processes in the body.

Suggested Use

Omega-three fatty acids are considered by many to be the most positive and active in humans. They support the immune system, are anti-inflammatory, and have other functions. The omega-six oils are also important, but an excess promotes the inflammatory response known as the arachidonic acid pathway.

The most basic form of omega-three EFAs found in food is called alpha-linolenic acid (ALA). It occurs in many foods, including flax oil. It requires a number of steps to be processed by the body, however, before it becomes the more useful forms of eicosapentaenoic acid (EPA) and docasahexaenoic acid (DHA). Persons who have little of these processing enzymes may not be able to convert ALA to the more useful EPA and DHA and, as a result, may not have the positive benefits of omega-three nutrition. Fortunately, other foods, including many fish and fish oils, are high in EPA and DHA and do not require you to do the processing.

The most basic form of omega-six EFAs found in food is linoleic acid (LA). It also requires processing to reach the more important form of gamma linolenic acid (GLA) and dihommogamma linolenic acid (DGLA). For persons whose bodies may not produce enough of the processing enzymes, GLA and DGLA are available in some foods as well.

It is safest to use essential fatty acid foods and supplementation that include both the basic and more useful forms of the essential fatty acids. Your body may not be able to process the more basic forms of essential fatty acids when you are ill or in treatment.

The current wisdom is to use more omega-three than omega-six fatty acids, in order to emphasize the anti-inflammatory actions. A good start is to take 300 mg of omega-three oils with 50 mg of omega-six oils. Omega-nine oil, oleic acid, may also be useful for immune system and other functions. Olive oil contains a high amount of oleic acid. Using 1 teaspoon of olive oil per day or simply cooking with it should be ample.

ESSIAC TEA

CATEGORY: COMBINATION OR MISCELLANEOUS SUBSTANCE

Essiac tea is the name of a Canadian nurse, Rene Caisse, spelled backward. Caisse prepared a number of traditional herbs that were used for the treatment of cancer, which have some anecdotal evidence to back up their effectiveness. Before her death she licensed a formula to a company in Canada, but many other manufacturers also started producing it. Considerable controversy exists over whether any of the manufacturers produce the tea as it was originally made by Caisse.

The formula is believed to be 6.5 cups of *Arctium lappa* (burdock), 16 ounces of *Rumex actosella* (sheep sorrel), 1 ounce of *Rheum palmatum* (turkey rhubarb), and 4 ounces of *Ulmus fulva* (slippery elm bark). There are a number of other purported formulas, but most of the debate lies with how the herbs were processed.

Antitumor Action
There are no conclusive human studies to confirm the use of Essiac tea as a cancer treatment, although the constituent herbs have antioxidant and other mechanisms that may be useful.

Other Actions
Essiac is not marketed for any other purpose.

Toxicity
No direct toxicity studies have been conducted, but the combination should not be toxic at normal doses of the constituent herbs.

Suggested Use
Little evidence suggests that the commercial preparations of this tea will actually have a positive anticancer effect, but there are few risks in trying it, other than the cost, as long as antioxidant and immune-stimulating action is appropriate.

EURIXOR (*see* Mistletoe)

EVERS THERAPY

CATEGORY: PROPRIETARY TREATMENT
This program uses live cell therapy, chelation, nutrition, oxidative treatments, and antioxidants. In addition, laetrile, shark cartilage, and magnet therapies are also used. The objective of this program is to support and stimulate the immune system while killing tumor cells. Definitive, independent scientific human studies are needed before this treatment can be better evaluated.

EXERCISE

CATEGORY: PROCEDURE

Antitumor Actions
Aerobic exercise—using your muscles, lungs, and cardiovascular system—improves blood and lymph flow, improves oxygen absorption and distribution in the body, increases white blood cell production, helps control weight (if you are overweight), and improves muscle mass and

tone. Studies suggest that exercise and its results have a positive cancer-preventive action.

Other Actions
Exercise improves your sense of well-being and your daily ability to function. When done judiciously, exercise benefits literally every body system.

Toxicity
Exercise programs that are too strenuous can have the opposite of their intended effect. Over-training can break down muscle and cause excess fatigue. Obviously, some forms of high-impact exercise, such as football and soccer, raise the chances of physical trauma.

Suggested Use
Some form of exercise is indicated for everyone, whether they are ill or not. Aerobic forms of exercise, where you breathe hard and perspire for at least twenty minutes every other day, are best. If conditions do not permit this level of activity, start slowly with swimming, walking, or simple physical therapy exercises. The aerobic component, however, should not be left out because of its obvious benefits. Since there may be specific times when you should not exercise, such as after certain types of treatment, check with your medical specialist before starting any exercise program.

Choose a form of exercise that you enjoy so you can keep it up. It should be a joy, not a burden.

Exercises that put stress on your bones, such as jogging and weight training (even light weights), will also strengthen your bones, whereas exercises that do not stress your bones, such as swimming, will not improve bone strength. Aerobic programs, including aerobic dance, are tailored from low to high impact and from low to high stress. Such programs can be very useful, good fun, and even a pleasant social encounter.

Consult your providers and a competent physical therapist or exercise trainer for a program that works for you. Since many jurisdictions do not train and license exercise trainers, get a referral from your health care team to be certain you are getting someone good.

FLAVONOIDS

CATEGORY: NUTRITIONAL

Antitumor Actions
These brightly colored chemicals, found in many fruits and vegetables, are powerful antioxidants that also have the ability to make other nutri-

ents, such as vitamin C, more effective. Nutritionists suggest that they inhibit stomach cancer and also suspect that they protect against a number of other cancers.

Other Actions
Flavonoids are usually found in compounds containing a wide variety of nutrients, with an equally wide variety of actions.

Flavonoids are unquestionably useful, based on studies demonstrating how a healthy intake of fresh fruits and vegetables can help prevent many cancers.

Toxicity
Flavonoids have not been shown to be directly toxic, but some have been suspected teratogens, harming a fetus when the mother takes large quantities.

Suggested Use
Flavonoids are unquestionably useful, based on studies demonstrating how a healthy intake of fresh fruits and vegetables can help prevent many cancers. The best source for these chemicals is from the actual fruits and vegetables where they are found, preferably fresh and organic.

The best-known flavonoids include hesperidin, rutin, quercetin, citrin, and anthocyanins, including proanthocyanins.

GARLIC (*Allium sativa*)

CATEGORY: BOTANICAL

Antitumor Actions
The incidence of cancer is lower in areas where garlic consumption is high. Garlic's benefits are believed to be the result of antioxidant activity, of its ability to stimulate white blood cell production, or of its ability to inhibit chemicals that are suspected in cancer growth—or possibly all three.

Most of the anticancer associations studied are with digestive cancers such as of the stomach, colon, and liver. Garlic oil has also been used as a topical agent (applied directly on the skin) as a treatment for skin cancer.

Using garlic as an antitumor agent dates back to Hippocrates. Most of the evidence is anecdotal. Newer studies, however, suggest a positive association with reduced cancer incidence but do not demonstrate that garlic is either a cure or predictable treatment.

Other Actions

Garlic can reduce blood pressure, serum cholesterol, and the blood's ability to form clots. It is an antibiotic, effective against certain bacteria, viruses, parasites, and funguses. Garlic reduces blood sugar and is taken as a digestive aid. When used on the skin, it is an irritant, causing redness.

Toxicity

Excess doses of garlic can possibly irritate or interfere with liver and kidney function, cause increased white blood cell production, and cause excess bleeding.

Suggested Use

Garlic makes more sense as an addition to the diet than as a direct medicine. Raw garlic has been shown to contain more active ingredients than cooked. High garlic intake can cause breath and perspiration odor, which can be a blessing or a curse, depending on your views. Garlic with the odor removed has been heavily marketed, but its use is still controversial.

If using garlic interests you, five cloves of raw garlic or the equivalent should provide maximum benefit. If garlic is not your favorite food or aroma, pass this one by. Many other good choices exist.

GERMANIUM

CATEGORY: NUTRITIONAL

Antitumor Actions

Germanium is a trace mineral that seems to have both oxygen-enhancing and antioxidant qualities. It is suggested for use with chemotherapy to treat certain forms of lung cancer, but studies are far from conclusive.

Other Actions

No additional definitive studies exist regarding the use of germanium in humans.

Toxicity

No definitive studies exist regarding the toxicity of germanium in high doses.

Suggested Use

There is not enough suggested benefit from germanium to suggest its use at this time.

The ABCs of Alternative Therapies

GERSON THERAPY

CATEGORY: PROPRIETARY TREATMENT

This program was initially started by Max Gerson, M.D., and is now carried on by his family. The therapy includes a specific diet with a focus on juicing and using fruits high in digestive enzymes. The program also includes nutritional supplements and coffee enemas. Definitive, independent scientific human studies are needed before this treatment can be better evaluated.

GINSENG (*see* Siberian Ginseng)

GOLDENSEAL (*Hydrastis canadensis*)

CATEGORY: BOTANICAL

Antitumor Actions
Goldenseal contains potent bone marrow stimulation constituents that increase the number of white blood cells. Animal studies suggest anti-cancer activity.

Other Actions
Goldenseal has been traditionally used as an antibiotic and in the treatment of diabetes.

Toxicity
Goldenseal can cause very low blood pressure and convulsions at high doses, although it is considered safe at normal traditional doses.

Suggested Use
This is a relatively safe herb at normal doses where bone marrow stimulation is indicated. Normal adult dosage is 1 teaspoonful of the tincture three times per day.

GONZALEZ PROGRAM

CATEGORY: PROPRIETARY TREATMENT

The Gonzalez program uses detoxification, supplemental nutrition, enemas, and enzyme therapy. There is also a diet component. The objective is to support the immune system and kill tumor cells. It is very similar to the Kelley program. Definitive, independent scientific human studies are needed before this treatment can be better evaluated. Initial studies have begun.

GRAPE CURE

CATEGORY: STRATEGY

This diet involves fasting, enemas, raw foods, and lots of grapes. It is claimed to have anticancer activity, but there is no formal evidence to support this claim. Grapes are high in antioxidants and therefore could have some positive benefits. If this diet interests you, consult with a licensed provider to be certain that you will be getting adequate nutrition.

GREEN TEA (*Camellia sinensis*)

CATEGORY: BOTANICAL

Antitumor Action

Green tea comes from the same plant as black tea, but the difference in preparation significantly changes the activity of the tea. The black tea leaves are allowed to ferment, and black tea can actually increase the risks of certain cancers.

> Green tea has significant antioxidant activity.

Green tea has significant antioxidant activity. It may have estrogen-blocking and bone marrow-stimulation actions as well. Green tea shows prevention activity against many different kinds of cancers, probably as a result of its antioxidant actions.

Other Actions

Green tea traditionally has been used as a general tonic.

Toxicity

Some green tea preparations can have enough caffeine to interrupt sleep.

Suggested Use

Green tea is a good addition to the diet at times when high antioxidant intake is appropriate and as long as it does not interfere with sleep. One to three cups per day is common.

HOMEOPATHY

CATEGORY: PROCEDURE

Homeopathy is a treatment system developed by the German physician Samuel Hahnemann in the nineteenth century. In brief, homeopathy uses extremely diluted substances to generate a response, often similar to the symptoms of the malady being treated. The theory is that the body's response to disease was the correct one and the homeopathic remedy is being used to fortify that response. Considerable variation exists between schools of thought, which may account for the lack of consistent study results.

Homeopathy may not be effective during conventional treatment.

Antitumor Actions

Homeopathy has been used for the treatment of cancer since the nineteenth century. There is anecdotal evidence, both positive and negative, but no definitive studies. If homeopathy does have some antitumor activity, it probably occurs when used by itself as opposed to being used with conventional therapies. It has been suggested and observed that conventional therapies interfere with the body's ability to respond appropriately to homeopathic treatment.

Other Actions

Homeopathy is used traditionally for the treatment of a wide variety of maladies. There is much anecdotal evidence, both positive and negative.

Toxicity

The use of high dilutions can produce an extreme reaction in particular individuals. Most of the data and techniques are the result of observation rather than controlled studies.

Suggested Use

Despite the fact that there is no hard science to support it, homeopathy has been used by conventional physicians in Europe for many years, with many satisfied patients. It is relatively risk-free when applied by a trained provider. If the concept of homeopathy appeals to you, it is probably worth a try following conventional treatment but may not be effective during conventional treatment.

HOXSEY FORMULA

CATEGORY: COMBINATION OR MISCELLANEOUS SUBSTANCE

The Hoxsey treatment consists of several herbal remedies along with diet, nutritional supplementation, and some psychosocial treatment. The herbal treatments, known as the Hoxsey formula, are the best-known part of the method.

There are two formulas. The first contains potassium iodide, licorice, red clover, buckthorn bark, burdock, stillingia, berberis, pokeweed root, cascara amarga, and prickly ash bark. The second contains potassium iodide and a protein-digesting enzyme, elixir lactate of pepsin. The formulas are usually adjusted for the specific individual.

Antitumor Action
Supporters claim that the program interferes with the spread of cancer and normalizes the metabolism of cancer cells. No definitive studies have been performed, but informal review of data suggests that the program has some preventive activity. This may be a result of the antioxidant activity of some of the formula ingredients, as well as the other nutritional supplements.

Other Actions
None claimed or known.

Toxicity
No formal toxicity studies are available. Since the formula is variable, the individual herbs should be considered in combination.

Suggested Use
Properly used, the Hoxsey formula and other principles of the method can be safe and may offer some potential benefit.

HUANG QI (*see* Astragalus)

HYDROTHERAPY

CATEGORY: PROCEDURE

Antitumor Actions
Classic hydrotherapy, using alternating hot and cold treatments with or without electrical stimulation, has been shown in uncontrolled studies to increase immune system (white blood cell production) activity. This response has been proposed as an anticancer mechanism. No definitive studies exist, but anecdotal evidence from North America and Europe, spanning over a century, is mostly positive.

Other Actions
Hydrotherapy can be very relaxing. The increased perspiration and fluid loss is proposed as a means of detoxification.

Hydrotherapy can be very relaxing. The increased perspiration and fluid loss is proposed as a means of detoxification.

Toxicity

Hydrotherapy can cause electrolyte (mineral) loss, seizures, dehydration, increase or decrease in blood pressure, and aggravation of diabetes.

Suggested Use

Carefully done with trained and licensed supervision, hydrotherapy can be safe. There is no positive scientific evidence that it works against cancer. The positive anecdotal evidence combined with the fact that, for individuals who like physical treatments, it can be comforting, make it worth a try for those who find the procedure appealing.

HYPERTHERMIA

CATEGORY: PROCEDURE

Antitumor Actions

Increasing the body's temperature has been used as an anticancer treatment. The theory is that the tumor cells, which cannot survive at temperatures much higher than normal body temperature, will be destroyed when body temperature is increased. Studies suggest that hyperthermia is useful when combined with conventional radiation therapy.

Other Actions

Hyperthermia has been used as a means to control infection and is proposed to increase the activity of the immune system.

Toxicity

Hyperthermia can cause electrolyte imbalance, a loss of essential minerals and fluid through perspiration. It can be harmful or fatal to vulnerable individuals, including those with heart disease, temperature regulation problems, blood sugar metabolism problems (including diabetes), liver disease, nervous system disease, and a number of other conditions. Hyperthermia should not be used during pregnancy.

Suggested Use

Hyperthermia can be induced by immersing the entire body into hot water or hot air, such as a sauna. It can be induced by oral or intravenous administration of substances such as diaphoretics that increase body temperature. Hyperthermia can also be induced locally by diathermy, radiation, ultrasound, and hot packs.

Hyperthermia may actually be useful, but no studies clearly suggest this. Hyperthermia has clear toxicity risks. If used carefully, the risks can be minimized to the point where even the speculation of benefit may outweigh the risks. Hyperthermia should only be done under the supervision of a provider licensed and experienced with this procedure.

IMMUNO-AUGMENTIVE THERAPY (IAT)

CATAGORY: PROPRIETARY TREATMENT

This program analyzes the person's blood for the purpose of determining the status of four proteins. If "lack of equivalence" is found, then these proteins are injected into the individual. The objective of this program is to support immune function.

INDIAN HEMP (*see* MARIJUANA)

INOSITOL (INOSITOL HEXOPHOSPHATE, IP-6)

CATEGORY: NUTRITIONAL

Antitumor Actions

Inositol hexophosphate has been suggested to have antitumor action by virtue of its immune-stimulation action, increasing certain kinds of white blood cells in a manner similar to some herbs. The studies are far from definitive in humans, but additional studies are in progress for the hexophosphate form.

Other Actions

Inositol is a sugar like nutrient, sometimes mistakenly described as a member of the B-vitamin family. It is a lipotropic, aiding in the control and metabolism of fat. It helps the body produce lecithin and works with the B vitamin choline to help prevent hardening of the arteries. In humans inositol is needed by the liver

Toxicity

There is no known toxicity for inositol in its dietary form. Little is known about human toxicity for patented variations.

Suggested Use

Inositol is abundantly available in the diet from meats, vegetables, and fruits; no known minimum requirement exists for humans. Definitive, independent scientific human studies are needed before this treatment can be better evaluated.

IODINE

Antitumor Actions
Because iodine is necessary for proper functioning of the thyroid gland and thus control of the body's metabolism, nutritionists propose that it is useful as a cancer preventive.

Other Actions
Iodine has a suggested antibiotic activity.

Toxicity
Large doses of iodine over long periods can interfere with thyroid function. Doses greater than 300 micrograms per day can be toxic.

Suggested Use
Salt in most countries is fortified with iodine to a level satisfying human needs. Supplementation is rarely necessary for normal function. Data are not definitive enough to suggest using supplements for iodine's antibiotic effect.

IPE ROXO (*see* Pau d'Arco)

ISSELS' WHOLE BODY THERAPY

CATEGORY: PROPRIETARY TREATMENT
Also known as *ganzheitstherapie,* this therapy uses a combination of dental work (removing diseased teeth and mercury fillings); avoidance of coffee, tea, tobacco, and other substances of concern; psychotherapy; and oxygenation. Vaccines and hyperthermia are also sometimes used. The objectives of this program are immune support and stimulation as well as tumor cell destruction. Definitive, independent scientific human studies are needed before this treatment can be better evaluated.

ISCADOR (*see* Mistletoe)

KAMPO

CATEGORY: COMBINATION OR MISCELLANEOUS SUBSTANCE
Kampo describes the Japanese adaptation of traditional Chinese herbs. There are three specific herbal combinations used to treat cancer: *Juzen-Taino-To, Shi-Un-Kou,* and *Sho-Saiko-To.*

Antitumor Actions

Juzen-Taino-To is claimed to act as an immune system stimulator as well as an antioxidant. *Shi-Un-Kou* is claimed to inhibit tumor formation, and *Sho-Saiko-To* is claimed to increase natural interferon production. There is no definitive evidence that these combinations have significant anticancer activity in humans, although the constituent herbs do have immune-stimulating , antioxidant, and other useful qualities.

Other Actions

None known or claimed.

Toxicity

There are no formal toxicity studies. Large doses of *Sho-Saiko-To* can cause dizziness, erratic pulse, and confusion.

Suggested Use

Kampo should only be used with the services of a licensed and trained provider. Done correctly, it is reputed to be safe.

KELLEY NUTRITIONAL METABOLIC THERAPY

CATEGORY: PROPRIETARY TREATMENT

This program uses detoxification and a diet with emphasis on vegetables, fruits, and grains. High protein intake is avoided. Manipulation therapy is employed for stimulation. The Kelley program also uses enzyme supplementation and enemas. The program is designed to support the immune system and kill tumor cells. It is very similar to the Gonzalez program. Definitive, independent scientific human studies are needed before this treatment can be better evaluated.

LAETRILE (*Amygdalus persica*)

CATEGORY: BOTANICAL

Antitumor Actions

Laetrile has been suggested as a cancer cure when an extract is administered intravenously. Anecdotal evidence and suggestive studies support both its use and its lack of effectiveness, but nothing is conclusive.

Other Actions

It has been used traditionally as an oral treatment to relieve nausea and vomiting.

It is difficult to recommend laetrile's use, especially considering its potential toxicity and the fact that other natural therapies are better studied and show more promise.

Toxicity

No studies are available. Reported toxicity includes nausea, vomiting, headache, and dizziness. There are also reports of cyanide poisoning.

Suggested Use

Laetrile is not suggested, even by its advocates, to have significant antitumor effect when taken orally, and intravenous administration is not available legally in the United States. Without solid positive evidence, it is difficult to recommend laetrile's use, especially considering its potential toxicity and the fact that other natural therapies are better studied and show more promise.

LA PACHO (*see* Pau d'Arco)

LIVE CELL THERAPY

CATEGORY: PROPRIETARY TREATMENT

Cells from the fetuses of animals are injected directly into the body as an anticancer treatment. Usually, the animal cells are from the same source as the individual's cancer. For example, liver cells would be injected into a person with liver cancer. The procedure is done in the hospital over a period of one to three weeks. Advocates of live cell therapy claim that the procedure results in anticancer activity, but no definitive human studies support this. Side effects such as severe infections and allergic responses have been reported.

LIVINGSTON THERAPY

CATEGORY: PROPRIETARY TREATMENT

The Livingston therapy consists primarily of a diet plus additional nutritional supplementation designed to support the immune system. Definitive, independent scientific human studies are needed before this treatment can be better evaluated.

MACROBIOTIC DIET

CATEGORY: STRATEGY

The macrobiotic diet is a mostly vegetarian diet that emphasizes whole grains, organic foods, soy products, and attention to acid/alkaline considerations and psychosocial issues. Nutritional supplements are discouraged.

The term *macrobiotics* has been adopted and abused by many, but the original protocol, as practiced and taught by the Kushi and Aihara (Vega Institute) teachings, has resulted in considerable anecdotal evidence and some mildly suggestive studies of its anticancer activity.

The diet requires some cooking skills that can be easily learned. This program is best learned with a skilled and experienced teacher. Weight loss can occur, but this is minimized with knowledgeable instruction. If this diet interests you, consult a licensed provider to be certain that you are getting adequate nutrition.

MANIPULATION

CATEGORY: PROCEDURE

Manipulation is the act of moving the joints of the body. In some cases they are moved beyond the normal range of motion, moved very rapidly, or moved and stretched with the aid of a machine. Some methods are very gentle and low force, in which the joint motion is not perceivable. Manipulation is practiced mostly by the osteopathic, naturopathic, and chiropractic professions, each with its own philosophy. Other licensed providers are also trained to perform manipulation, depending on the jurisdiction.

A number of theories explain the usefulness of manipulation in humans. The two most predominant ones are (1) that the joint is mobilized where it was once "stuck" by muscle spasm or some other condition, thus allowing it to return to its normal position and function, and (2) the joint is adjusted from an incorrect position to a correct position by the force of the manipulation. In either case, especially where the bones of the spine are concerned, the manipulation is seen to remove pressure on surrounding nerves and other structures, thus allowing normal function to return.

Antitumor Actions

The theory for the use of manipulation in the treatment of cancer assumes that the resumption of normal function aids in the body's innate healing ability. No definitive studies have been conducted on the use of manipulation with cancer, but there is significant anecdotal evidence from people who report feeling much better.

Other Actions

Manipulation has been shown to definitively reduce pain and improve function in individuals with a wide variety of physical complaints.

Toxicity

The greatest risk with manipulation is the potential for damaging a bone, blood vessel, or other body structure. The prolonged use of manipulation, especially when it is forceful, has been associated with an increasing need for the therapy, ostensibly a result of stretching the connective tissue that holds bones in place.

People being treated for cancer may be at additional risk for harm if they have a bone lesion or reduced bone strength as a result of their disease.

Suggested Use

A scientific correlation between manipulation and cancer may not exist, but there is a good case for positive benefit in quality of life, especially for individuals having muscular and skeletal complaints. Before using this therapy, it is important to get approval from your oncologist, which, depending on the circumstances, may require a bone scan or other diagnostics. If your oncologist has a good reason to discourage the treatment, you should pass this method by. In any event, it is not advisable to risk forceful treatment but instead use the gentle ones, which often get equal results.

MARIJUANA (*Cannabis sativa*)

CATEGORY: BOTANICAL

Antitumor Action
None known.

Other Actions

When smoked and inhaled, cannabis has been shown in a number of studies to relieve the nausea and vomiting side effects of some chemotherapy regimes. It has also been used as a narcotic and a sedative. The specific mechanisms of action of all its constituents have not been well studied.

Toxicity

As with powerful narcotics, marijuana presents the danger of being addictive as well as seriously affecting consciousness, motor skills, and judgment. When used medically for symptomatic relief, rather than for recreation, it is proposed to have a much less addictive effect. However, considerable controversy about the use of marijuana continues.

Suggested Use

Cannabis appears to be reasonably safe and useful for the control of nausea, but its other effects are not well known. Smoking with careful and knowledgeable medical guidance appears to be safe and effective.

MARSHMALLOW ROOT (*Althea officinalis*)

CATEGORY: BOTANICAL

Antitumor Actions

None known.

Other Actions

Marshmallow root is most useful in cancer treatment for its soothing action on the digestive and urinary tracts. Most of the data available on the use of althea is anecdotal, although chemical analyses of its constituents have been done scientifically. In the first half of the twentieth century, althea was known as a pharmaceutical necessity for the treatment of irritation.

Marshmallow root is most useful in cancer treatment for its soothing action on the digestive and urinary tracts.

Toxicity

None known.

Suggested Use

Althea is useful after treatments that have irritated the urinary or digestive tract. Brew it as a tea or take three 100-mg capsules of the dried herb every three hours.

MASSAGE

CATEGORY: PROCEDURE

Antitumor Actions

Massage therapy increases white blood cell production, which suggests an anticancer action, but no definitive studies indicate that massage has a direct effect on cancer. Massage also reduces stress and improves the relaxation response for individuals who enjoy it. It also can increase local blood flow.

Toxicity

Massage therapists have long been taught that massage is contraindicated in cancer when there is a possibility that massage could increase spread of the disease by moving lymph and blood. A clear understanding of human physiology and tumor cell activity indicates that the chances of such spread are, in most cases, minimal. There are some exceptions in which massage therapy should not be used. Massage should not be applied directly over a tumor or in the immediate vicinity of skin lesions. Special attention is necessary if the person has structural damage, such as bone lesions. Other specific situations exist in which massage can be irritating or create new problems, but they are rare. Your oncologist can tell you whether massage poses a potential risk for you.

Suggested Use

Massage therapy is a helpful, supportive method that has been used too seldom. If massage appeals to you, it is strongly suggested.

There are many types of massage, some very forceful and others very gentle. The gentlest forms, such as Swedish massage, suit most people. The more forceful methods may be fine for individuals who are large, have a lot of muscle mass, or simply enjoy the more forceful technique, but they can be painful and uncomfortable for others. Your conventional and nonconventional providers can help you decide which form of massage makes the most sense.

MELATONIN

CATEGORY: HORMONE

Antitumor Actions

Studies suggest that melatonin has a protective effect against some cancers. It is proposed that melatonin, when used as a sleep aid, can improve sleep patterns, which in turn has demonstrated a positive effect on cancer prevention. Melatonin also has a proposed antioxidant effect.

Other Actions

Melatonin is a hormone secreted by the pineal gland in the brain, which controls the timing and actions of many other hormones and functions in the body. Since it can sometimes cause drowsiness, it has been used as a sleep aid.

Toxicity

Melatonin can cause sleep disturbances and anxiety in some people. There are no long-term human studies examining either the direct effects of melatonin use or if its effects on other body hormones and functions can result in problems later.

Suggested Use

The benefits of melatonin use may not outweigh its risks. This powerful hormone does not have a lot of scientific studies to support its use as an anticancer treatment. If it is used, the person should be monitored carefully and the treatment discontinued if sleep disturbance or anxiety symptoms occur.

MENADIONE (*see* Vitamin K)

METABOLIC TREATMENT
(*see* Kelley Nutritional Metabolic Therapy)

MILK THISTLE (*Silybum marianum*)

CATEGORY: BOTANICAL

Antitumor Action

Milk thistle has not been shown to have definitive antitumor activity in humans.

Other Actions

Milk thistle contains powerful antioxidants that have been shown in definitive human studies to protect and aid in the repair of liver damage resulting from chemical, drug, and alcohol abuse. Milk thistle is also believed to increase the production of bile by the liver.

> Milk thistle is indicated for the protection and repair of liver damage from most causes, including chemotherapy.

Toxicity

High doses of milk thistle may result in loose stool, as a result of increased bile production. In addition, milk thistle may cause low blood pressure and low heart rate at high doses.

Suggested Use

Milk thistle is indicated for the protection and repair of liver damage from most causes, including chemotherapy. The active ingredient in *Silybum marianum* is silymarin. Adult dosage is 200 mg of silymarin three times per day.

MISTLETOE (*Viscum album*)

Antitumor Actions
Mistletoe preparations for cancer treatment are generally administered by injection. Potential anticancer activity has been shown in investigational studies, which is probably from its immune-stimulating action. It may also have antioxidant activity.

Other Actions
Mistletoe in oral form has been used traditionally for the treatment of high blood pressure.

Toxicity
The berries and herbal preparations can have significant toxicity at high dosages. Toxicity varies greatly with preparations.

Suggested Use
Considering its potential toxicity and the lack of data about it, considerably more research is needed before mistletoe can be recommended.

MOLYBDENUM

CATEGORY: NUTRITIONAL

Antitumor Actions
Molybdenum deficiency has been observed in cancer of the esophagus but has not been demonstrated as a cause of the disease.

Other Actions
Molybdenum is necessary for the proper metabolism of carbohydrates in the body.

Toxicity
Intakes of greater than 10 mg per day can result in painful joint symptoms, similar to gout.

Suggested Use
Intakes of 500 micrograms (½ mg) per day of molybdenum are useful for normal human function. Additional supplementation for anticancer activity is not recommended.

MUSHROOMS (including shiitake [*Lentinan edodes*], reishi [*Ganoderma lucidum*], coriolus [*Coriolus versicolor*], tremella [*Tremella fuciformis*], poria [*Wolfporia cocos*], maitake [*Grifola frondosa*], wood ear [*Auricularia auricula*], and other types)

CATEGORY: BOTANICAL

Antitumor Actions
Most mushrooms are believed to have cancer-preventive activity by a combination of antioxidant and bone marrow-stimulation actions.

Other Actions
Mushrooms have been used as general tonics and antibiotics (reishi, shiitake).

Toxicity
The nontoxic mushrooms are completely safe when taken at normal human doses. Don't try to pick mushrooms unless you are an expert, since some varieties are extremely toxic.

Suggested Use
Many of these mushrooms can be added to the diet. They are a useful adjunct when antioxidant and bone marrow-stimulating therapies are indicated.

NONI (*Morinda citrifolia*)

CATEGORY: BOTANICAL

Antitumor Actions
Noni juice is a traditional South Pacific remedy that has recently been marketed as a cure for cancer, based on studies that show it increases white blood cell activity. However, there are no human studies showing any definitive anticancer action.

Other Actions
Noni is promoted as a cure for everything from high blood pressure to menstrual cramps, but the only evidence of its usefulness is as an antibiotic. This accounts for much of its reputation as a traditional medicinal herb.

Toxicity

Very little information is available regarding toxicity. The manufacturers claim that it is nontoxic.

Suggested Use

Noni has very little evidence to encourage its use as an anticancer herb.

NUTRITIONAL METABOLIC TREATMENT
(*see* Kelley Nutritional Metabolic Therapy)

OREGON GRAPE (*Berberis aquifolia*)

CATEGORY: BOTANICAL

Antitumor Actions

Oregon grape contains potent bone marrow stimulation constituents that increase white blood cells. Animal studies suggest anticancer activity.

Other Actions

Oregon grape has been traditionally used as an antibiotic, as a digestive aid, and for the treatment of nausea.

Toxicity

Oregon grape has not demonstrated toxicity at normal doses.

Suggested Use

This is a relatively safe herb where bone marrow stimulation is indicated. Normal adult dosage is 20 drops of the tincture three times per day.

ORIENTAL MEDICINE (*see* Acupuncture and Oriental Medicine)

OXYGEN TREATMENTS

CATEGORY: PROCEDURE

Antitumor Actions

Some tumor cells do not grow as well in a high oxygen environment. The theory for oxygen treatments such as oral oxygen inhalation, hyperbaric (high pressure) treatment, ozone, and hydrogen peroxide is that they increase the oxygen environment of the tumor cells and thus destroy them.

Oxygen inhalation is administered with a conventional oxygen mask or nose cannula (tubes). Hyperbaric treatment places the person in a chamber where the pressure is increased above normal atmospheric pressure, thus increasing the density of the air and its oxygen content. Hydrogen peroxide is generally administered either in a specially dilute oral preparation or intravenously. Ozone is usually administered rectally, vaginally, intravenously, topically (with all but the head wrapped in a body suit pumped full of ozone gas), and subcutaneously (under the skin).

There is some anecdotal evidence to support the use of oxygen therapy but no definitive studies have been conducted.

Other Actions
Oxygen treatments have an antibiotic effect in some instances.

Toxicity
Oxygen treatments tend to increase free radicals in the body, which increases cancer risk, thus making this treatment method controversial. Excess oxygen, especially from oral oxygen, can cause oxygen sickness, with breathing distress as well as nervous system, heart, and kidney effects. Hyperbaric treatment, if the pressure is reduced too quickly, can cause the bends (a painful and dangerous condition in which gas bubbles form in the blood) as well as sinus problems for susceptible persons. Depending on the route of administration and concentration, both ozone and hydrogen peroxide treatments can cause burning and discomfort at the point of administration, as well as metabolic imbalance.

Suggested Use
Little scientific evidence supports the use of oxygen treatments in the treatment of cancer, but, notwithstanding the long list of toxicity risks, it can be administered safely. The mechanism of action of free radicals parallels certain chemotherapy regimes, even though the free radical concentration is much less with the oxygen treatments, based on cellular response.

The careful use of mild doses of oxygen treatments may be worth a try as long as you understand this is a shot in the dark. If this therapy appeals to you, be certain the provider is knowledgeable and experienced in the therapy, use of the equipment, and the potential side effects. The use of a lot of antioxidants prior to and during the treatment will reduce whatever tumor-killing

The careful use of mild doses of oxygen treatments may be worth a try as long as you understand this is a shot in the dark.

ability the treatment has. However, replacement of antioxidants following the treatment is probably advisable.

PANCREATIC ENZYME

Category: Enzyme

Antitumor Actions

Pancreatic enzyme is given orally between meals or intravenously. The theory is that it will enter the bloodstream and attack the surface of the tumor. While no definitive or even suggestive studies prove that this procedure works, there is a lot of anecdotal evidence.

Other Actions

Pancreatic enzymes will break down food that remains in the small intestine, which will probably not be noticeable.

Toxicity

Taken between meals, high doses may cause stomach discomfort.

Suggested Use

There is no evidence that this procedure works, but, on the other hand, there is little risk other than the cost of the tablets. Pancreatin dosages of 100 mg to 1,000 mg have been used.

PAU D'ARCO (*Tabebuia* species, including *avellanedae, ipe, cassinoides,* and *ochracea*)

Category: Botanical

Antitumor Actions

Tabebuia, the bark of a South American tree, has a long folk history of use as an anticancer herb. Both anecdotal evidence and studies suggest that it has anticancer activity in humans. However, since the botanical has both pro-oxidant activity, where it creates free radicals, as well as antioxidant constituents, there is no agreement on mechanism of action.

Other Actions

Tabebuia has been shown in studies to have definitive antibiotic action against certain bacteria, parasites, and viruses in humans.

Toxicity

No toxicity has been demonstrated in humans using the entire bark. When its most active ingredient, lapachol, is isolated and given without the other fifteen or more constituents of the bark, extended use can result in anemia. It is theorized that the other active ingredients of the bark have a protective effect.

Suggested Use

The potential benefits, as described in suggestive studies and much ostensibly reliable anecdotal evidence, make the use of the whole herb worth consideration. Dose should be based on the amount of lapachol contained. Suggested adult dosage is the whole bark containing $1/2$ gram of lapachol three times per day. This can be taken in whole herb capsules, in glycerite extract, or in a strong tea. Do not use the extract lapachol by itself.

PC-SPES

CATEGORY: PROPRIETARY TREATMENT

Antitumor Action

This combination of Chinese herbs interferes with testosterone's ability to stimulate prostate cancer cells. It functions much like estrogen and is high in phytoestrogens.

Other Actions

PC-SPES is presumed to have many of the other hormone actions of estrogen.

Toxicity

As with other estrogens, it can cause breast enlargement and impotence in men.

Suggested Use

Early studies suggest that PC-SPES is effective in reducing prostate cancer cell growth. As with other hormone therapies, it may only work for a limited period of time. Definitive, independent scientific human studies are needed before this treatment can be better evaluated. There are ongoing studies that should provide more guidance.

PEACH TREE (see Laetrile)

PINEAPPLE (see Bromelain)

PHYLLOQUINONE (*see* **Vitamin K**)

PHYTOESTROGENS

CATEGORY: HORMONE

Antitumor Actions

These plant chemicals, which act like estrogen, are proposed to have a protective effect against breast cancer. These weak estrogens purportedly occupy the estrogen receptor sites on breast cancer tumor cells, thus preventing human estrogen from reaching the receptor and stimulating the tumor growth.

This proposed mechanism for phytoestrogens was modeled after the actions of the drug tamoxifen. Plant and food sources of phytoestrogens, such as soy, have been shown to have a protective effect against breast cancer.

There is, however, some controversy over the theory and the reasons for the results. Soy and other foods that have been tested as anticancer elements also have significant antioxidant activity and it has been proposed that it may be the antioxidant activity rather than the phytoestrogens that are protective. In fact, it has been suggested that the phytoestrogen activity can stimulate some cancers but that the antioxidants present may counter the negative effects of the phytoestrogen.

> Foods containing phyto-estrogens, including soy, are probably helpful in protecting against cancer and are worth including in the diet.

Other Actions

Phytoestrogens have been shown to have significant estrogen effect to the extent that they can act as birth control in animals and probably humans at high dosages.

Toxicity

Phytoestrogens have not been shown to be toxic at normal food dosage levels with soy. Isolated phytoestrogen products, especially those that have modified or eliminated the antioxidant component that originally existed in the source foods, may introduce an unwanted risk, especially for women with breast cancer who have positive estrogen receptors.

Suggested Use

Foods containing phytoestrogens, including soy, are probably helpful in protecting against cancer and are worth including in the diet.

PHYTONADIONE (*see* Vitamin K)

POLARITY THERAPY

CATEGORY: PROCEDURE

Polarity therapy is founded on the belief that your body is a magnet with an electrical field surrounding it. When that field is impaired or blocked, it can interfere with health. The polarity therapist seeks to reestablish the magnetic field using diet, nutrition, exercise, special yoga positions, psychosocial counseling, fasting, and colonics.

No studies demonstrate that this therapy has any measurable anticancer activity, but most of its individual parts should have general health benefits. Practitioners advise against the use of polarity therapy during pregnancy.

POLY MVA

CATEGORY: PROPRIETARY TREATMENT

MVA is an acronym for minerals, vitamins, and amino acids, including the metal palladium. The manufacturers claim that this oral supplement kills tumor cells.

PURPLE CONEFLOWER (*see* Echinacea)

PYRIDOXINE (*see* Vitamin B$_6$)

QIGONG

CATEGORY: PROCEDURE

Qigong (pronounced "chee gung") is a system of slow, gentle motions developed and practiced in Oriental medicine. These exercises are intended to have many of the effects of traditional exercise, such as increasing blood and lymph motion, but in a calming and relaxing environment. Qigong means to literally support the body's vital energy, called *qi*.

Antitumor Actions
No definitive studies demonstrate the anticancer effects of qigong, but there is ample anecdotal evidence. The potential mechanisms of anti-cancer action would be similar to conventional exercise, with emphasis on stress reduction.

Other Actions
Qigong has been used for centuries in Asia. It probably has a positive effect on any malady that can be helped by reducing stress.

Toxicity
There is no known risk with qigong when done with a trained instructor.

Suggested Use
Done properly and carefully with a trained instructor, qigong is gentle, although certain individuals may not be able to do the motions. Check with your health care team to find out if it might be useful in your particular situation.

RED CLOVER (*Trifolium pratense*)

CATEGORY: BOTANICAL

Antitumor Action
Red clover has a long folk history as an anticancer herb. It contains phytoestrogens and antioxidants, which have suggested antitumor action. No definitive studies exist for the use of red clover as a cancer treatment in humans.

Other Actions
Red clover contains coumarin, which slows the blood-clotting process in humans. It is also a diuretic and has been used traditionally as a sedative.

Toxicity
Because of its coumarin content, trifolium can make bleeding disorders worse.

Suggested Use
Trifolium is a worthwhile botanical to consider but only when its coumarin constituent is accounted for. Suggested adult dosage is 15 drops of a fluid extract three times per day.

REVICI THERAPY

CATEGORY: PROPRIETARY TREATMENT

The Revici program uses lipids (dietary fats) and minerals, including antioxidants, to reach a "balance" of the body's biochemistry. The objective is to support the immune system. Definitive, independent scientific human studies are needed before this treatment can be better evaluated.

ROSEMARY (*Rosmarinus officinalis*)

CATEGORY: BOTANICAL

Antitumor Actions

An animal study using grocery store rosemary was shown to interfere with the development of breast cancer. A mechanism of action has not been determined.

Other Actions

Rosemary is a traditional herb used as a stimulant and liver cleanser.

Toxicity

High doses of rosemary can interfere with sleep.

Suggested Use

Rosemary is an excellent spice with meals. As a tincture, the adult dose is 30 drops three times per day.

SAW PALMETTO (*Serenoa repens*)

CATEGORY: BOTANICAL

Antitumor Actions

Saw palmetto's use with prostate cancer is apparently the result of its ability to reduce prostatic hypertrophy, swelling of the prostate. In prostate cancer, this action is proposed to reduce the pressure on the capsule of the prostate, thus reducing the chance for the carcinoma to escape the capsule and spread. Saw palmetto also has some suggested immune-stimulating activity.

Other Actions

By the same mechanism of controlling prostate swelling, saw palmetto has been used to treat other, noncancerous conditions such as prostatitis. Saw palmetto has a mild diuretic action.

Toxicity

In studies, saw palmetto has not been demonstrated to have toxic side effects.

Suggested Use

Saw palmetto is a safe and effective herb. Normal dosage is 160 mg two times per day.

SELENIUM

CATEGORY: NUTRITIONAL

Antitumor Actions

Selenium is a potent antioxidant. Clinical studies suggest that it is protective against lung, colon, rectum, prostate, and skin cancer.

Other Actions

Selenium is a necessary component in the body's system for protecting itself against toxins. It protects against heart disease, cataracts (where the lens of the eye gets clouded), anemia in newborns, infections, infertility in both men and women, liver disease, pancreatic disease, and sudden infant death syndrome (SIDS).

Selenium is a necessary component in the body's system for protecting itself against toxins.

Toxicity

Adult doses above 400 micrograms can result in hair loss, skin color change, digestive problems, garlic breath, and tooth decay.

Suggested Use

Selenium is a necessary nutrient. Supplementation levels up to 200 micrograms per day are reasonable during times when antioxidants are appropriate.

714X THERAPY

CATEGORY: PROPRIETARY TREATMENT

This treatment involves the injection of 714X, a mixture of camphor, alcohol, salts, and water, into the lymph nodes of the groin. The 714X is claimed to attract cancer cells and both mobilize and unclog the immune system. Definitive, independent scientific human studies are needed before this treatment can be better evaluated.

SHARK CARTILAGE

CATEGORY: COMBINATION OR MISCELLANEOUS SUBSTANCE

Antitumor Actions

Shark cartilage is advertised as an antiangiogenesis agent—that is, it cuts off the blood supply to the tumor, causing it to die. However, there is no conclusive evidence that shark cartilage has any anticancer activity in humans.

Other Actions

Fish connective tissue, including shark cartilage, has been used for the treatment of arthritis.

Toxicity

There are no conclusive toxicity studies with humans.

Suggested Use

Shark cartilage can be very expensive. Very little evidence supports its use as an anticancer treatment. Definitive, independent scientific human studies are needed before this treatment can be better evaluated. Several studies have been initiated.

SIBERIAN GINSENG (*Eleutherococcus senticosus*)

CATEGORY: BOTANICAL

Antitumor Actions

Siberian ginseng is legendary among herbs. It has well over thirty physiologically active constituents, including vitamins, minerals, sugars, and plant chemicals. Paradoxically, it is both a stimulant and a calming agent. Studies suggest that it can inhibit the growth of certain tumors, but definitive human studies are lacking. The active constituents of Siberian ginseng include some with antioxidant activity, which may result in an antitumor effect.

Other Actions

Siberian ginseng is referred to in scientific botanical literature as an *adaptogen,* which means that it tends to normalize human functions. Studies suggest human use of Siberian ginseng for normalizing adrenal gland function, thyroid function, kidney function, blood sugar, cholesterol, and stress by a variety of physiological mechanisms. It has been used extensively as a stimulant as well.

Toxicity
High doses can result in excessive stimulation, causing anxiety, irritability, depression, and insomnia. These side effects have not been shown at standard doses.

Suggested Use
The large number of active constituents and variability in the plant kingdom raise concerns about the predictability of commercial Siberian ginseng as a cancer treatment. The botanical industry often standardizes some of the ingredients, but until they are all standardized and categorized, the risks for side effects need to be a prime consideration.

Normal adult dosage is 2 to 4 g of the dried root per day. If side effects are noted, use should be reduced or discontinued.

TABEBUIA (*see* Pau d'Arco)

TAHEEBO (*see* Pau d'arco)

TELLURIUM

CATEGORY: NUTRITIONAL

Antitumor Actions
No studies show this mineral to have definitive anticancer action in humans, although tellurium has demonstrated some immune-stimulating activity.

Other Actions
None known.

Toxicity
Tellurium can be very toxic. There are no comprehensive human studies of the toxicity of tellurium. Certain organic forms are less toxic but toxicity is still a problem with higher dosages.

Suggested Use
Given the minimal information regarding tellurium's safety and usefulness, it is not recommended.

TETTERWORT (*Cheledonium majus*)

CATEGORY: BOTANICAL

Antitumor Actions
Also known as celandine, tetterwort has been used to stimulate the liver's production and elimination of bile. In addition, the active constituents of the herb are thought to have antioxidant effects. These actions are not well studied but may form the basis for its traditional use as an anticancer agent.

Other Actions
Tetterwort has been used traditionally as a diuretic, as a laxative, and as a sedative. These actions are also not well studied but have been the subject of much questionable anecdotal evidence.

Toxicity
Large doses can produce nausea, vomiting, severe diarrhea, dehydration, liver pain, shortness of breath, chest pain, and shock.

Suggested Use
Considering the potential toxic side effects and limited potential benefit, this botanical is not recommended as an antitumor treatment.

THERAPEUTIC TOUCH

CATEGORY: PROCEDURE
Therapeutic touch functions on the belief that a trained practitioner can "transfer energy" into the body of the individual where it is needed. A typical twenty-minute session involves the practitioner reaching a meditative state, with the intent of healing the individual, and then holding his or her hands just above the individual's skin. The practitioner senses the person's energy, detects areas of blocked energy flow, and resolves them.

Therapeutic touch is not claimed to have anticancer activity but is believed by some to improve the body's healing processes. Anecdotal evidence indicates that after a session, people who believe in the process often feel better.

TOLPA TORF PREPARATION

CATEGORY: BOTANICAL

Antitumor Actions
Tolpa torf preparation (or TTP) is a European drug extracted from peat that increases white blood cell counts in humans. Studies suggest that it has some antitumor activity based on this mechanism.

Other Actions
None known.

Toxicity
This drug is reported to have toxic side effects, but they are not defined in reliable studies.

Suggested Use
There is no conclusive evidence that this drug will work in humans. For adults, the drug is administered orally at 5 mg per day for three weeks. It is only available in some countries. It may be worth consideration if reliable, independent human studies are conducted to define effectiveness and safety.

TURMERIC (*Curcuma longa*)

CATEGORY: BOTANICAL

Antitumor Actions
Turmeric has a powerful antioxidant effect in humans. Studies suggest that it has anticancer activity, especially for persons exposed to tobacco smoke.

Other Actions
Turmeric has been used traditionally as an antibiotic and a painkiller.

Toxicity
Turmeric has not been reported as toxic in traditional use.

Suggested Use
As an anticancer agent, this is a safe and potentially useful herb. Adult dosages are 200 to 400 mg three times per day.

VENUS'S-FLYTRAP (*Dionaea muscipula*)

CATEGORY: BOTANICAL

Antitumor Actions
Anecdotal evidence exists regarding the use of *Dionaea*, but studies have not supported its use as an anticancer agent. It is generally administered by injection.

Other Actions
Venus's-flytrap is not a commonly used medicinal herb.

Toxicity
There is no definitive information regarding toxicity. Clinics using this treatment do not report significant toxicity.

Suggested Use
Based on the lack of evidence, Venus's-flytrap does not appear to offer any specific anticancer benefit for humans.

VITAMIN A

CATEGORY: NUTRITIONAL

Antitumor Actions
Vitamin A is a powerful antioxidant. It has been found to have a protective role against certain skin and lung cancers.

Other Actions
Vitamin A is essential for normal vision, body growth, bone growth, normal development, health of skin and mucosa, normal hormone functions, and normal cell division.

Toxicity
Excess dosages of vitamin A can result in a condition known as hypervitaminosis A, with physical symptoms including drowsiness, loss of appetite, headache, blurred vision, irritable behavior, diarrhea, nausea, hair loss, flaking and itching skin, and swelling over bones of the arms and legs, as well as over the liver and spleen. Hypervitaminosis A can interfere with liver function.

Normal adults do not experience hypervitaminosis A until dosages of 50,000 IU per day are reached, but persons with compromised liver function or metabolism may experience these toxic side effects at lower doses.

Recommended Use
Vitamin A is an essential nutrient. Adult dosages up to 10,000 IU per day are ample when other conditions are appropriate.

VITAMIN B$_{17}$ (*see* Laetrile)

VITAMIN B$_6$ (Pyridoxine)

CATEGORY: NUTRITIONAL

Antitumor Actions
Vitamin B$_6$ has the greatest antioxidant activity of the B vitamins. Studies suggest that it is helpful in preventing the recurrence of bladder cancer.

Other Actions
Vitamin B$_6$ is essential for the metabolism of proteins, fats, and carbohydrates. It is especially important in the function of the nervous system and the blood's ability to carry oxygen.

V itamin B$_6$ has the greatest antioxidant activity of the B vitamins.

Toxicity
High doses of vitamin B$_6$ may produce fatigue and become habit-forming over long periods of time but have not demonstrated any other toxic activity.

Recommended Use
Vitamin B6 is an important part of the diet and probably offers some benefit with cancer prevention. Adult dosages of 100 mg per day are ample.

VITAMIN C (Ascorbic Acid)

CATEGORY: NUTRITIONAL

Antitumor Actions
This most famous and often studied vitamin offers a definitive protective effect against many kinds of cancer. Anecdotal evidence and some studies

also suggest that at higher doses, Vitamin C may have a role as a cancer treatment.

At normal physiological doses of 500 to 3,000 mg per day, vitamin C is a powerful antioxidant, quenching free radicals, which probably explains at least part of its cancer-protective activity. At higher doses it can become a pro-oxidant, creating free radicals rather than quenching them, especially in the presence of iron. Just as some chemotherapy treatments kill tumor cells with free radicals, it has been proposed that this same mechanism explains how vitamin C can attack cancer. This proposal is, to say the least, controversial.

Other Actions

Vitamin C is essential for strong and healthy walls of blood vessels and is required for the metabolism of certain nutrients, including fats, some amino acids, and folic acid. It is also necessary for maintaining strong bones and teeth.

Toxicity

At adult doses greater than 8,000 mg per day, vitamin C can cause nausea, diarrhea, and stomach cramps. At these doses it may also interfere with the formation of red blood cells and bone, as well as with the absorption of other nutrients.

It has been proposed that the diarrhea resulting from increased doses of vitamin C is a "bowel tolerance" measure—in other words, the body absorbs as much as it "needs" and then creates diarrhea when more is taken. This theory is also controversial.

Suggested Use

Vitamin C is an essential nutrient required by all humans. Adult dosages ranging from 500 mg to 3,000 mg per day appear to be more than ample, based on current studies. Using vitamin C in much higher doses is an individual decision that should be made based on all available information and with the assistance of a qualified nonconventional provider.

VITAMIN D (Cholecalciferol)

CATEGORY: NUTRITIONAL

Antitumor Actions

Vitamin D has been shown to inhibit possibly precancerous genetic damage, as well as the growth of some tumor cells. It reduces the risk of colon cancer. Vitamin D is necessary for proper function of the immune system.

Other Actions

Vitamin D is a necessary part of the body's utilization of calcium and phosphorus for building and maintaining bones and teeth.

Toxicity

Excess dosage of vitamin D can result in a condition known as hypervitaminosis D. Physical symptoms include loss of appetite, nausea, vomiting, excessive urination, and alternating diarrhea and constipation. Toxic symptoms can occur with sensitive individuals at dosages as small as 10,000 IU (50 micrograms) per day when used over long periods.

Suggested Use

Vitamin D is an essential nutrient required by all humans. Supplement levels of 400 IU to 1,000 IU per day are more than adequate.

VITAMIN E

CATEGORY: NUTRITIONAL

Antitumor Actions

Vitamin E is a powerful antioxidant that is believed to help prevent a wide variety of cancers by virtue of its ability to scavenge free radicals and thus reduce their potential for causing precancerous cellular damage.

Vitamin E has been suggested for use with radiation therapy to increase the actions and tolerance of the radiation. However, it also may reduce the ability of the radiation to prevent a future recurrence. Definitive, long-term studies are necessary before this use of vitamin E can be considered to be without risk of interfering with the long-term benefits of the radiation.

Other Actions

Vitamin E is believed necessary for the proper function of red blood cells. Its powerful antioxidant effects also suggest that it may be useful in preventing atherosclerosis, the buildup of plaque in arteries.

Toxicity

Vitamin E can increase bleeding time by slowing the effects of platelets but has not been shown to be toxic in high doses.

Suggested Use
Vitamin E dosages ranging from 400 IU to 1,600 IU have been suggested as useful.

VITAMIN K, AS K-1 (Phylloquinone or Phytonadione) or K-3 (Menadione)

CATEGORY: NUTRITIONAL

Antitumor Actions
Vitamin K-3 has been suggested to have some anticancer action by supporting immune system function. Unfortunately, K-3 is a more toxic version of vitamin K.

Vitamin K-1 may also have some cancer-preventive activity, but the studies are not definitive.

Other Actions
Vitamin K is essential for proper blood clotting and bone development.

Toxicity
Vitamin K can cause excess clotting for persons with liver disease.

Suggested Use
Vitamin K is an essential nutrient. A daily oral dose of 1 mg is adequate for a normal adult.

WHEATGRASS

CATEGORY: BOTANICAL

Antitumor Actions
Wheatgrass juice is made from wheatberry seeds. It is claimed that wheatgrass detoxifies the body, provides nutrition, helps oxygenate cells, and reduces cell mutations that could be precancerous. It is believed to have anticancer activity, although there are no strong human studies to support this. It is also believed that the juice is high in chlorophyll, enzymes, vitamins, minerals, and antioxidants.

Other Actions
None known.

Toxicity
There are no toxicity studies, but anecdotal reports state that it is not toxic.

Suggested Use
Wheatgrass juice is available from most health food juice bars, as well as in formal treatment programs. It is probably safe in moderate (one or two glasses per day) amounts orally. It is also used in colonic therapy with unknown results.

WHOLE BODY TREATMENT (*see* Issels' Whole Body Therapy)

ZINC

CATEGORY: NUTRITIONAL

Antitumor Actions
Zinc is an essential nutrient for proper immune system function. It has numerous functions in the body, including some antibiotic effects. Contrary to some claims, there are no definitive studies showing anti-cancer activity but it is still an important nutrient.

Other Actions
Zinc is a necessary component for healthy bones, teeth, skin, and hair. It is a critical part of many human enzyme systems and organ functions, including the control of blood sugar.

Toxicity
Adult dosages above 150 mg can result in toxicity, including interference with copper and iron utilization. Toxicity symptoms include anemia, stiffness, bone loss, and reduced appetite.

Suggested Use
Adult dosages of 50 mg per day are more than ample.

Special Cases: When "Average Person" Doesn't Apply

M ost diagnostic and treatment plans are designed for the "average" person: a 150-pound adult who is not pregnant and has a single, well-defined illness. The real world, however, is not so average. Real people often have needs that are remarkably unlike the statistically average person. If you or your loved one simply does not fit into the average category, this chapter will show you how to get the best results with your unique circumstances.

The special cases we'll discuss include the following.

- Children
- The elderly
- Pregnant women
- Multiple tumor types
- The recurrence of cancer

CHILDREN

Children are not merely scaled-down adults. They have a different metabolism and a different tolerance for treatments. In addition, diagnosis is often more difficult because children do not have the skills for communicating symptoms and events. As with adults, it's essential that you consult with both your conventional and nonconventional practitioners before proceeding with any treatments.

Children often make a valiant effort to act grown-up during treatment, but they do not have the age and perspective to process and understand why they are in this situation, something that is especially critical when the disease or treatment has a lot of side effects.

When treating children, parents and caregivers must also be considered. If your child has been diagnosed with cancer, it is likely that you're experiencing significant stress.

> Children are often able to tolerate much higher levels of chemotherapy than adults.

A Child's Tolerance for Treatment

Children are often able to tolerate much higher levels of chemotherapy than adults. The therapeutic plans for children, which describe the particular treatment and timing, are often remarkably more complex than those for adults.

It is important to be certain that a particular treatment is appropriate for children. Many drugs and other treatments list children's dosages. When that information is not available, it can be estimated by the ratio of your child's weight as follows:

$$\text{Child dosage} = \frac{\text{Adult dosage} \times \text{child's weight in pounds}}{150 \text{ lb.}}$$

For example, if your child weighs seventy-five pounds and the adult dosage is 300 mg:

$$\text{Child dosage} = 300 \text{ mg} \times 75 \text{ lb.}/150 \text{ lb.} = 150 \text{ mg}$$

Never self-treat with nutrients or herbs, and make certain that both your conventional and nonconventional providers agree on the safety of any combination.

Some children do not do well with pills. Often the best strategy is to empty capsules and grind up tablets as finely as possible. This can then be mixed with juice or food. You should check with the provider who prescribed the medication before grinding the pills, however, since some, such as certain digestive enzymes, should not be ground up.

Some nutrients should not be used with certain children. It all depends on the diagnosis, the patient's condition, and the treatments. Nutritional supplementation for children is a fairly complex medical subject—one that should be addressed by your child's conventional and nonconventional care providers.

Don't attempt temperature therapies with children without expert help. A child's internal thermostat and tolerance for heat and cold are not like those of an adult. In addition, a child's lower body mass can respond more quickly to temperature changes than an adult. Hyperthermia treatments may result in excessive body temperature and convulsions. Hypothermia (cold) treatments can result in pneumonia.

Fasting should also be avoided in children because it can potentially interfere with growth and development.

Communication Issues with Children

Children don't always know how to communicate what they are feeling. It can be difficult for a child to differentiate an important symptom from "just feeling bad." Most children have not yet developed the vocabulary or understanding of their bodies to be able to describe their experiences or symptoms as well as an adult. As a result, making a diagnosis based on a child's report can be difficult, even for an experienced pediatrician.

Children, especially those who have endured a lot of treatment, may fail to report important symptoms. It is often necessary to have a child in a more controlled, in-patient environment for closer monitoring.

A simple solution to working with children's communication issues is to allow plenty of time. As a parent, you can improve the situation by asking questions about how your child is feeling, helping your child articulate to the doctor what he or she is experiencing, and taking notes of significant events between provider visits.

Children are sometimes hesitant to report symptoms because they fear the treatments. Your child should be assured that the treatment, in the long run, is better than the symptoms.

Time and patience are the best insurance that all of the important symptomatic information needed from the child has been received.

Psychological Issues in Children

Cancer treatment can be an unforgettable trauma for any child. Some children respond aggressively while others withdraw. Whatever the

Children, especially those who have endured a lot of treatment, may fail to report important symptoms.

response, it is safe to assume that the child is going through much more than he or she has the experience and coping skills to endure.

Whenever possible, I would recommend that if your child is undergoing cancer treatment, that you arrange some form of counseling. A counselor can help bring perspective to the situation much more easily than you because the counselor is not as close. Children's hospitals now include a counseling and psychiatric staff trained to deal with these issues.

Your child may respond to the trauma and insecurity of a cancer diagnosis and treatment with atypical behavioral patterns, such as loud outbursts, periods of crying, coarse language, or even withdrawal. A sudden change in behavior should be acknowledged and dealt with early. It is often a way of asking for help. Once again, it is important to take advantage of the trained hospital or clinic staff since they deal with these kinds of issues every day.

Parents' Issues

Having a sick child can be the most terrifying experience in a parent's life. When the diagnosis is cancer, the situation is even more difficult. The treatments are so complex that you may feel as though you've lost control of what's happening with your child. When there are crises, you may stay up with you child for days or even weeks at a time, getting little or no sleep and living in a state of constant anxiety.

As parents, your child's sickness can wear you both down and even threaten your relationship.

However, it is important for you to pay attention to your own physical and emotional health. As parents, your child's sickness can wear you both down and even threaten your relationship. If your child is in the hospital, you should take time away from the hospital room on a regular basis. Go out for a meal someplace other than the hospital cafeteria, see a movie, or just take a nice long walk. The hospital is more than able to take care of your child for that time, and your physical and mental health will benefit immeasurably.

And now for the most important part: Do not take any guilt with you when you take your time away. It may take some practice, but you will be better able to function as parents when you get some relief. This is why baby-sitters have been part of the earliest recorded civilizations.

If you've been at the hospital constantly, your child may be upset the first time you leave but once it is understood that this is a predictable event (for example every night from six until eight) and that you always return, it will become easier. Do not give up just because your child became upset the first time you left, and you felt guilty and wretched.

If you and your spouse have problems during this time, do not assume that something is fundamentally wrong with your relationship. Marital difficulties are common for parents with a child undergoing cancer treatment. Make use of the parental counseling services at the hospital or in their referral network. Do this earlier rather than later, before a problem gets more difficult to mend.

THE ELDERLY

As we grow older, we experience changes in the way we respond to treatments such as drugs, surgery, and radiation. Our response to nonconventional treatments also changes.

The psychological and emotional issues for elderly persons with cancer are also different. Illness and treatment affect elderly people in ways not usually seen in younger populations.

Tolerance for Treatment in the Elderly

Seniors do not tolerate treatment the same as middle-aged or younger adults. Differences in metabolism, hormone levels, and organ function can introduce significant variability.

As we grow older, the drug level that is needed to get a specific therapeutic result can increase, while the amount that causes unacceptable side effects can decrease.

Drugs and botanical medicines are often described in terms of their *therapeutic window*, which is the size of the dose that provides an acceptable result. If the dosage is "inside the window," the treatment will work and toxicity will be absent or tolerable. Dosages "below the window" will not produce the desired result. Dosages "above the window" will be too toxic.

The size of the therapeutic window for many substances changes with age. As we grow older, the drug level that is needed to get a specific therapeutic result can increase, while the amount that causes unacceptable side effects can decrease, in effect narrowing the therapeutic window. As the window gets narrower, finding the appropriate dosage gets more challenging. For this reason, the dosage and side effects must be monitored more carefully with elderly persons to be certain that the drug or botanical is doing what it was intended to do and also that it isn't producing unacceptable side effects.

Seniors do not always respond the same way to treatments. Reduced muscle mass; decreased total body water; and reduced heart, lung, kidney, digestive, and other body system activity can change elderly patients' responses to many treatments. Their sensitivity to heat, cold, and pain are not as acute; as a result, they will not report discomfort as quickly when the treatment is too strong.

An elderly person's reflexes may also be diminished. Complications, such as pneumonia, may not produce the same response in an older patient that would be expected in a younger one, thus requiring greater vigilance.

Allow extra time for healing with elderly patients. Their bodily repair mechanisms are not as rapid and their risk for complications is greater.

Psychosocial and Environmental Issues in the Elderly

Older people can be influenced more seriously by a cancer diagnosis and treatment. Being removed from their usual environment when undergoing treatment can reduce or eliminate positive social contacts. At a time when isolation and separation from friends and loved ones is already a reality, changes such as a move to a care facility or hospital may seem like the realization of an elderly person's worst nightmare.

Every effort should be made to provide familiar surroundings and familiar faces. Home-health care and home-hospice care can do wonders, delaying or eliminating the need for a nursing care facility in some cases. The security of familiar surroundings can remarkably improve the patient's mental status and probably has a positive effect on healing as well.

Have a trained and licensed provider do a functional assessment, such as the *Katz index of independence Activities of Daily Living* (ADL), to judge the person's status and to determine what is needed in his or her environment. Functional ADL tests consider the person's ability to accomplish normal functions such as bathing, dressing, and going to the toilet. The ADL assessment can be repeated as necessary to review the adequacy of the environment. How well elderly persons can function on their own can be improved by making their environment more user-friendly.

Take the time and effort to make the living space user-friendly. Home-health care experts and books on the subject of caring for the elderly will tell you how to remove such dangers as loose carpets, how to add good lighting, and how to provide all the extras that can change an individual's status from dependent to independent.

If it becomes necessary for the patient to be moved to a new location, you can take several steps to make the move as easy as possible. Bring familiar items, such as family pictures, to the room. Familiar clothing, familiar toilet items, and even familiar music and aromas can help. Familiar faces and voices are also helpful. Even if it means that you must act as a shuttle service or provide for cab fare, arranging for visits from old friends and acquaintances can do wonders for elderly persons with cancer.

The combination of illness and treatment, along with a new location, can create confusion. This confusion is usually worse at night, when it can be difficult to find anything recognizable. This phenomenon, known as *sundowning,* can be very disturbing for an elderly person. Until they have gained some familiarity with their new surroundings, the best solution is to make certain that lighting is good and that familiar faces are present at night.

Both during and after cancer diagnosis and treatment, attention to these issues can make the difference between a positive and negative outcome.

PREGNANT WOMEN

A cancer diagnosis during pregnancy adds to the equation the considerations of another life. Many conventional and nonconventional therapies can harm both mother and fetus. Competent, licensed providers can ensure that such interactions do not occur within their own specialties, but little is known about combinations of conventional and nonconventional treatments when applied to pregnancy.

The fetus has its own blood circulation system, protected to a limited extent from the mother's blood system by the placental barrier. The placental barrier is not much of a barrier, however. It allows many substances through, including not only vitamins, minerals, and other needed nutrients but also some drugs and toxins. Some, but not all, drugs, herbs, and nutrients have been evaluated for their ability to cross the placental barrier and, if they do, for their potential effect on the fetus.

The best strategy for treatment during pregnancy is to use the minimum necessary treatments and not to use anything that you are not absolutely sure about. *Never self-treat with nutrients or herbs and make certain that both your conventional and nonconventional providers agree on the safety of any combination.* Many nonconventional treatments are known to be safe during pregnancy, while others can harm the fetus or result in spontaneous abortion.

Maintain good nutrition during pregnancy with the assistance of an experienced specialist. Pay particular attention to vitamins, including folic acid, minerals, and essential fatty acids. When drugs or other treatments are known to deplete nutritional stores, these nutrients should be replaced when it is safe to do so.

Many women have used conventional and nonconventional treatments for cancer during pregnancy and have had healthy, happy, normal babies—and so can you.

MULTIPLE TUMOR TYPES

When you have two different kinds of cancer at the same time, both your conventional and nonconventional treatment plans are affected. Although having multiple tumor types complicates the possibilities for interactions, combining conventional and nonconventional treatments can still be done.

The conventional treatment protocols should be reviewed for both diagnoses. Naturally, the best situation is when one treatment can be found that works for both types of cancer. If that is not possible, compatible programs should be developed to the extent that is possible.

Although having multiple tumor types complicates the possibilities for interactions, combining conventional and nonconventional treatments can still be done.

The nonconventional programs should be developed taking into account the two diagnoses and the two conventional treatments. Once again, compatibility must be assessed.

Finally, *multiple interaction pathways* must be considered. That is, all conventional treatments and nonconventional treatments must work together. The good news is that, with careful planning, this can be accomplished. It is more work but is well worth the effort.

With multiple diagnoses, the greatest challenge is usually communication between providers. Conventional issues and treatments can change with little notice, and the nonconventional treatment plan must respond accordingly. Motivating your busy conventional provider to communicate in a timely way with your nonconventional provider will be a challenge. Short delays may occur in the process, but timely communication will ensure that you get the best treatment.

THE RECURRENCE OF CANCER

A recurrence means that the original treatment did not eliminate all of the tumor cells and/or whatever caused the cancer the first time has caused it again. If the recurrence is from leftover cells that the immune system was not able to finish off after treatment, the cells may well have mutated. *Mutation* means that they may have changed their character, so that they will not reproduce or respond to treatments the way they did the first time around.

A recurrence brings with it feelings of disbelief, disappointment, fear, and anger. Try to move past these feelings as quickly as you can to get through this event victoriously. Many people who've experienced recurrences have been successfully treated and have spent the rest of their lives cancer-free.

> A recurrence brings with it feelings of disbelief, disappointment, fear, and anger.

Recurrences can be more difficult to resolve than a first occurrence, but the good news is that new, more effective conventional treatment protocols exist. Other promising new clinical trials are being conducted. Shop around for a second opinion to be certain that you are getting the best treatment available. (See chapter 2 for a guide in selecting a second opinion.)

Conventional treatment for recurrence can mean higher dosages, which makes it an especially good time to consider nonconventional strategies as well. Nonconventional therapies can help you better tolerate the conventional treatment and therefore give it the opportunity to eliminate more tumor cells. At the same time, exercise explicit care to ensure that the nonconventional treatment does not interfere with your conventional treatment. This will enable you to get the maximum benefit available from the conventional treatment. Another benefit of using nonconventional treatment during recurrence is the addition of a preventive element to help stop yet another recurrence.

Cancer survivors with special circumstances are often concerned that they may not receive proper treatment. In fact, these individuals often get extra attention and even better service from providers. If you have special circumstances, don't be dismayed, but instead look at this as an opportunity to get special treatment. The technology and willingness exists in health care to make the best of circumstances that are not the norm.

10

Prevention Strategies

Most of us are delivered into this world without cancer. Most babies are healthy, happy, and disease-free. With the passage of time and the stresses of our culture, however, some individuals will eventually develop cancer. We don't know all of the reasons why cancer occurs. What we do know is that cancer does not normally arise from a single event but is instead the result of a combination of factors, many of which can be avoided. Furthermore, most of the cancer survival statistics are for individuals who did not use preventive strategies, giving those of us who focus on prevention even better odds.

We face cancer risks every day. Carcinogenic (potentially cancer-causing) chemicals are in our diet and our environment, and we are frequently exposed to a variety of forms of radiation. These factors cause nearly continuous cellular damage in our bodies and these damaged cells can become cancerous if our bodies are not able to repair or remove them. Each day of our lives, such microscopic battles are normally fought and won by our immune systems.

However, if the damage occurs too quickly or if our immune systems are not strong enough, the result can be cancer. The good news is that most of the factors that increase our risk for cancer are avoidable.

Prevention is a critically important part of any cancer survival plan. Whatever the reasons that your cancer may have developed, you'll want to do everything within your power to reduce or eliminate the chances of a repeat performance.

In order to keep potentially cancer-causing damage from overwhelming your body's natural defenses, your prevention strategies should have two major objectives:

- To reduce external risk factors
- To support and improve your immune system

REDUCING EXTERNAL RISK FACTORS

Ample evidence exists showing that outside factors influence the development of cancer. As early as the eighteenth century, the surgeon Percival Pott observed that the incidence of scrotal cancer was much higher in chimney sweeps than in the general population. Other clear, unambiguous historical observations include the discovery of increased bladder cancer with aniline dye workers and increased lung cancer with cigarette smokers and with shipbuilders (when asbestos was commonly used).

Other studies support the fact that cancer is often an environmental, and therefore preventable, disease. First-generation Japanese women who emigrated to the United States have a remarkably lower incidence of breast cancer than the average American woman. Third-generation Japanese-American women, however, who've been exposed to the Western diet and environment, have essentially the same incidence of breast cancer as other American women. Debate is ongoing over whether these differences are a result of the Japanese diet, which is higher in fish, essential fatty acids, and soy and lower in meat, or if it is the fact that Japan has been significantly more responsible about limiting pollution. Japan, for example, has air quality standards for the inside of office buildings.

Prevention is a critically important part of any cancer survival plan.

Cancer risks occur in many places. It is important to remember that although virtually everyone is exposed to these factors, not everyone gets cancer. Since it is not possible to eliminate all of the risk factors, your objective will be to reduce them significantly. It is the *amount* of exposure that you should be concerned with.

Many of us were ignorant of potential carcinogens and as a result did not take steps to avoid them. It's important that you now have the opportunity to reduce your exposure to these potentially dangerous substances. Now that you are becoming aware of cancer risks, however, don't go to the other extreme and assume that exposure to any of these risk factors will automatically cause cancer, because that is not the case. In fact, the stress of worrying may be almost as bad as the risks themselves, since stress itself is a risk factor for cancer.

Once you've taken steps to effectively reduce the following risks, you can relax, smile, and be happy. You'll have done what you could and it will be time to let your well-supported immune system deal with the leftovers.

Common Sources of Cancer Risks

- Diet (including carcinogens in the foods we eat)
- Carcinogens in the environment
- Ionizing radiation
- Non-ionizing radiation
- Lifestyle

Diet

Our eating habits affect us in many ways. They can change the speed and effectiveness of our digestive systems; they determine the nutrients we receive; they can affect our hormones and biochemistry; they can change our energy level, sleep patterns, and weight; and they can introduce food additives and nonfood chemicals into our bodies.

In this section, we will review the areas where risk factors can be improved in general.

Eat Your Vegetables

Vegetables should be included in at least one meal per day and preferably all your meals. Use organic vegetables whenever possible, because these will be free of the pesticides, fertilizers, and other possibly carcinogenic chemicals used in agriculture. Raw vegetables are better than cooked, but raw vegetables can be difficult to digest. Steamed vegetables are a good choice if you need to eat them cooked. Boiling veggies, however, is not recommended since many of the nutrients are left in the water.

Making vegetable juices and vegetable smoothies is also popular. There is some debate about which is better, since with juicing, the fiber and some of the nutrients of the vegetable are thrown away with the pulp. Whether you juice or puree, the concentration of nutrients can potentially interfere with some conventional medical treatments. They may also be a little hard on your digestion. Eating cooked, whole vegetables the old-fashioned way still works well.

Eat a variety of vegetables.

Eat a variety of vegetables, with emphasis on the ones that you like the best. Yellow and green veggies contain many of the antioxidants and flavonoids that have significant cancer-fighting activity. The fiber portion of vegetables adds important roughage, which also helps prevent many kinds of cancer. A variety of vegetables keeps meals more interesting and provides you with a broader spectrum of protective nutrients.

Cut Back on Sugar

Sugar has been suggested as a factor supporting tumor cell growth, so be sure to reduce the amount of sugar in your diet. Sugar reduction has been part of a number of cancer-prevention studies. These include studies of traditional macrobiotics, which has a good record of anecdotal successes.

Be aware that the sugar in your diet comes not only from sweets but also from many prepared foods. Be careful about what you eat. Make it a habit to read labels and to learn what you are really consuming.

If you crave sugar, other factors may be at play with your body chemistry. Your cravings should be considered by a competent medical provider.

Eat Fish Regularly

Fish is an excellent source of protein and essential fatty acids. Oily fish, such as salmon and cod, are the best choices, although most fish varieties are healthful. Shellfish has more fats and calories and is not as good for you. Avoid eating fried fish and overly processed fish. Cooking it almost any other way is preferable to fried: baking, broiling, poaching, grilling, or steaming.

If you cook your fish in foil, use stainless steel foil (available in some specialty cooking and health food stores), rather than aluminum foil, because of the risks associated with excess aluminum in the diet. Fresh fish are the best, and line-caught fish are better than farm-raised or frozen. Even canned fish can be a good food source, but this leaves you with less control about which fish and which parts of the fish you are actually eating. It's also important to read the label carefully, looking for chemical additives and added fat content.

Eat Only Moderate Amounts of Meat

Meat and poultry are good sources of protein but may also create an increased risk for certain kinds of cancers. These animals may have been raised in pens literally the size of their bodies, under questionably sanitary conditions. They may have been treated with antibiotics, hormones, and god knows what else to artificially increase their weight.

Meat and poultry can cause constipation, which may increase the risk of some cancers. Meat can also be difficult to digest.

Many cancer-prevention strategies advise total avoidance of meat and/or poultry. While this may work, it may not be completely necessary. The other alternative is to use small amounts (less than four ounces per servings) of certified free-range, grain-fed, chemical-free meat and poultry, which are increasingly available from a number of food stores.

Be Careful with Dairy Products

Dairy products, which include cow's milk and cheeses, can be a problem for adults. Dairy proteins and fats are often difficult to digest. Dairy products can cause constipation and may pose a risk for colon cancer. In addition, persons of all ages can be seriously allergic to dairy products.

I recommend that you substitute soy, rice, almond, or goat's milk for cow's milk. Alternative cheeses are also available, made with goat's or sheep's milk as well as soy and other vegetables. These substitutes are actually quite good and can help reduce your cancer risk.

Watch Your Water

Drinking water isn't what it used to be. Water supplies are commonly treated with controversial chemicals such as chlorine and fluoride. The cleanliness of major water systems has been increasingly in question. Having your own well can be fine in some areas but a problem in others, as we continue to contaminate groundwater reserves. It is possible to have your well water tested for contaminants.

If you think that the pricey designer water you buy in the market is any better, you may be surprised to learn that some of these products are nothing more than bottled city water with perhaps a bit of filtration and a fancy label.

The most straightforward solution to finding pure drinking water is to purchase a water filter that will remove the chlorine, fluoride, and other potentially harmful chemicals. Make sure to clean or replace your filter regularly; otherwise, you may end up drinking water contaminated with bacterial buildup. There are reliable sources for good bottled drinking water as well. Your local water supply may be one of those rare systems that does not need to be chemically altered, but if that is not the case, an alternative water source is a good idea.

Playing It Safe with the Foods You Eat

In order to survive, you must consume balanced amounts of protein, carbohydrates, and fats. Eat moderate amounts and avoid eating too much of any one category. Eat three meals per day when possible. The largest meal of the day should not be dinner, since you may be (inadequately) digesting it all night. Always have your last meal at least three hours before going to bed. Eat a wide variety of foods and try not to repeat any single food every day. Don't eat any food that gives you a headache, indigestion, or bothers you in any other way.

Avoid extremely hot (temperature that is) foods and beverages since they can increase the risks for certain kinds of cancers. It may also be wise to avoid obvious chemical foods such as soft drinks, chewing gum, and other products with strange fluorescent colors. And, in case you were wondering, chewing tobacco is not a food.

> Avoid extremely hot (temperature that is) foods and beverages since they can increase the risks for certain kinds of cancers.

When purchasing frozen, canned, or prepared foods, take a few seconds to read the labels, so that you can avoid unknown food additives, dangerous chemicals, added fats and sugars, and surprise ingredients. Many good books on this subject are available to help you decipher the multitude of chemicals commonly found in foods, some of which are known carcinogens.

The safest method for controlling this area of risk is to avoid foods with artificial colors, preservatives, and other unnatural ingredients. Many prepared foods, such as delicatessen meats, may be treated with chemicals without a warning label. If you can't see the original package, it's best to move on. Avoid "mystery foods," such as hot dogs, sausage, and hamburgers. You simply can't know for sure what's in them.

The good news is that food cooperatives and health food stores are becoming available in many areas. Often, they provide outstanding selections of good foods. In addition, conventional supermarkets are getting on the bandwagon with both chemical-free meats and produce as well as a variety of safe and healthfully prepared foods. The availability of safe and healthful foods is constantly increasing.

A craving for certain foods may be a sign that you are allergic to them. Many books describe strategies for eliminating allergenic foods from the diet, but people invariably do better working with a health professional who is experienced and trained in this area.

There are countless diet strategies for preventing cancer. Before trying any one of them, I encourage you to discuss it with your nonconventional provider to ensure that it is safe, healthful, and the best course of action for you.

Carcinogens in the Environment

Chemicals are in the air you breathe, the water (including rain) you come in contact with, the clothes you wear, and virtually all of the products you use in daily life, from shampoo to newspaper print. In addition, there are both natural and man-made radiation, neither of which you can see or feel.

To minimize the possibility of cancer, you'll want to reduce these risks as much as possible. Once again, it's important not to be paranoid but instead to take practical, reasonable steps to limit your exposure to these factors, which can increase the load on your immune system.

The air we breathe outdoors in cities and developed areas usually includes vehicle exhaust, ozone, and a variety of other chemicals, some of which are proved or suspected carcinogens. We usually think we are safer in rural areas, but that air often contains dust, pesticides, fertilizer residues, and other questionable chemicals.

The outdoor air in cities is usually worst during rush hour, times when the area is downwind of heavy air polluters, or times when the air is stagnant, such as during a temperature inversion. The outdoor air in rural settings is most polluted when wind is blowing up dust, when you are downwind of sprayed crops, or when the air is stagnant. During those times, you should limit your time outdoors or at least avoid strenuous outdoor activity, since that increases the amount of air your lungs use.

Because we are exposed to so much pollution when we are in our automobiles, you'll want to keep the polluted air out of your car as much as possible. The normal safety warnings, such as being certain that you don't have any exhaust or fuel leaks, apply here. Keep your windows closed in heavy traffic. In addition, many automobiles have a recirculate function with the heating and air-conditioning controls. This will reduce the outside air and pollutants brought into the car.

Check with your mechanic or dealer if you are unable to figure out this feature with your car.

The air in your home can be as bad as that outdoors. It is best to keep your windows closed if pollution outside is high, and I recommend the use of a good air filter system for the rooms where you spend most of your time, such as the bedroom and family room. If you have central forced-air heating, it is possible to get a central filter system as well. Be certain that whichever system you use has the ability to remove pollutants and not just dust.

Air in the workplace can be an even greater challenge. Office buildings, large and small, recycle air to save on heating and air-conditioning costs. Even with filtration, this often causes higher levels of carbon dioxide and other gases, some of which are toxic gases emitted by office equipment. If you are in a smaller area, such as a single office, a room air filter can remove many of these recycled pollutants. Reducing the air flow into the space may also help, as long as you can maintain a comfortable temperature and still have some air circulation. If you work in a large open area, the only relief may be to have a small room air filter blowing in your direction. This may be seen as extreme by some of your colleagues, but it can limit your exposure to toxins.

> I recommend the use of a good air filter system for the rooms where you spend most of your time, such as the bedroom and family room.

Some office buildings have windows that open, which is, paradoxically, usually a good idea since the air inside many office buildings may well be worse than the air outside. Indoor air can be affected by the *off-gassing* of furniture and particle board, which occurs when toxic chemicals, such as formaldehyde, which is used in the manufacturing of these products, are released into the air. Off-gassing is greatest in the first few years of the product's life.

"Secondhand" tobacco smoke can be as dangerous as smoking. Don't allow smoking in your home. As much as possible, avoid places where you are likely to encounter tobacco smoke, such as bars or lounges. If you find that you must be in one, get as close as possible to where the air is entering the room, since the smoke is probably least offensive there. Ask if you can open a door or window and, if possible, take frequent breaks outside in cleaner air.

Travel is another important consideration. There isn't much data regarding buses and trains, but they seem to get enough air exchange to be safe. Airplanes, however, are a different story. Jet aircraft, especially the newer ones, recycle a significant amount of air, often without filtering it at all. In addition, to save fuel, airlines often limit the amount of new air they bring into the cabin. Unfortunately, the U.S. Federal Aviation Administration and other government bodies have for decades refused to correct this problem, even though they have the information and authority to do so.

If you must travel by aircraft, try to find a flight that is not full. Some of the older aircraft do not recirculate air and, from that perspective, may be a better choice. Traveling first-class may also provide cleaner air, since there are fewer persons in that area of the plane. Since ventilation varies greatly from one kind of aircraft to another, sitting in one part of the plane is not predictably better than another.

Ionizing Radiation

Ionizing radiation gets its name from the fact that it is so strong it can knock an electron clear off an atom, creating a charged particle known as an ion. The most common ionizing radiation sources are medical and dental X-rays and cosmic radiation.

Because of more sensitive films and better aiming techniques, X-ray technology has improved in terms of requiring less radiation exposure, but it is still a potential cause for cancer. If other diagnostic sources are available, insist on them. Since X-rays can often provide important information not available from other sources, it may not be practical to avoid them altogether. If you need the X-ray and there is no other good option, just do it. It is extremely unlikely that cancer can result from just a few X-rays.

Cosmic radiation is always with us. It is greater in some locales than in others but is impossible to avoid as long as we live on this planet. Cosmic radiation is higher, however, when flying in commercial jet aircraft. The newer, higher-flying aircraft are exposed to even more radiation than lower-flying aircraft. The best strategy is to choose the older, lower-flying airplanes whenever possible. This will reduce exposure.

Antioxidants in the diet from food and supplementary antioxidants can significantly reduce but not eliminate the damage from ionizing radiation. If you are exposed to extra radiation from X-rays, flying, or some other source, it is worth taking extra antioxidants. If you are currently undergoing conventional cancer treatment, however, consult with your practitioners because antioxidants can interfere with the treatment's effectiveness.

Non-Ionizing Radiation

The magnetic field that surrounds power lines, electrical wires in your home, and any electrical conductor that is carrying current is called *non-ionizing radiation*. This field cannot knock an electron off an atom, but it does have effects that have been associated with a number of diseases, including some cancers.

Electromagnetic fields, also known as EMF, have been the subject of a controversy that began more than fifty years ago when Russian children living close to power lines were found to have a higher incidence of leukemia. Some recent studies have shown a definite connection with EMF and cancer, while others have not.

I recommend that you avoid EMF exposures whenever possible. As with many other risk factors, a single or even a few exposures are not likely to cause cancer, whereas regular exposures are more of a potential risk.

> Electromagnetic fields, also known as EMF, have been the subject of a controversy that began more than fifty years ago.

The easiest way to check for EMF exposure in your home is to request that your local power company come out to measure the levels. This service is usually free. If they won't do it, many private contractors can. When the test is conducted, be certain that everything electrical in the house is on. This includes the washer, dryer, dishwasher, heat, air conditioner, refrigerator (open the refrigerator door until the compressor turns on), and lights.

Be certain that they measure the areas where you spend the most time, such as the bedroom or family room. There are experts who will help you interpret the results, since no specific, universally accepted guidelines exist. The readings will be in milligauss (mG). In general, readings less than 1 mG are considered fine; readings less than 5 mG are higher than you want but probably not a great concern; and readings over 10 mG are considered unacceptable.

There is plenty of debate about these levels. If the readings are high, a qualified electrician or licensed EMF expert can help you track down the offending source. If it comes from house wiring, you can often reroute the high-current wire to a less troublesome location. If the source is outside your house, such as power lines, then you may want to relocate.

Lifestyle

Some behaviors, especially when done to excess, can increase the risk for cancer. These risks can be lessened by simply reducing or avoiding these behaviors.

Avoid alcohol. It is associated with a number of cancers, in addition to having other undesirable physiological effects, which can include dehydration, constipation, and sleep disturbance.

Get regular exercise and stay active. A sedentary lifestyle is associated with a number of cancers, including those of the breast and colon.

Avoid being overweight. Obesity is associated with breast, endometrial, and colon cancers. When you lose weight, do it in a program that maintains muscle mass and builds endurance. Avoid on-and-off dieting that produces a "yo-yo effect" with your weight.

Eat a high-fiber, lowfat diet with lots of vegetables. Such a diet has been suggested to prevent nearly every type of cancer. High fat and low fiber are associated with a long list of cancers.

Avoid excess (more than two cups per day) coffee. High coffee intake has been associated with pancreatic cancer and is suspected with others.

Get at least eight (and preferably nine) hours of restful sleep each night. If your sleep patterns become a problem, deal with them. Consult a professional if need be.

Avoid the unnecessary use of drugs, including hormones, since they can sometimes increase cancer risk and may have other undesirable effects.

Certain occupations increase the risk of cancer. If you are in one of these professions, this does not mean you need to quit, but you should take extra precautions to limit your exposure risks. The more common professionals experiencing an increased incidence of cancer include workers exposed to petroleum, tar, and soot; workers in the boot and shoe industry; furniture and cabinetry workers; chemists; pilots and flight attendants; rubber industry workers; foundry workers; painters; printers; and textile workers. The U.S. government keeps comprehensive lists of cancer incidence by profession.

UNIQUE RISK FACTOR REDUCTION STRATEGIES

For some types of cancers, you can do specific things to reduce your chance of a recurrence. In addition to the general preventive strategies that we've already discussed in this chapter, it's worth taking the extra effort to follow these risk-avoidance strategies for your particular diagnosis.

Adrenal Tumors

Avoid steroid hormones. Research has not yet defined other risk factors.

Breast Cancer

Avoid long-term use of high-dose estrogen therapies. Avoid high alcohol intake. If you are more than 20% above your ideal weight or are in poor physical condition, start an exercise program and maintain close to ideal weight. Avoid fatty and fried foods. Avoid radiation exposure. Studies suggest that a tight bra might increase the risk for breast cancer, indicating that a looser bra or none might be better.

Carcinoid

If you have frequent indigestion, pernicious anemia, or reduced stomach acid, have them resolved with the assistance of a health professional. Avoid using the drug omeprazole (Prilosec) for stomach problems.

Colon and Rectal Cancer

Eat a lowfat, high-fiber diet. Avoid constipating foods, including cheese and cow's milk. If you experience frequent constipation, resolve it with dietary changes. Avoid excessive calcium supplements, including some antacids. Avoid aspirin and nonsteroidal, anti-inflammatory drugs. Avoid alcohol.

Esophageal Cancer

Avoid foods containing nitrates and nitrite preservatives. Avoid eating very hot (temperature that is) foods and liquids. Avoid alcohol use. If you have difficulty swallowing or have regular heartburn, see your conventional provider.

Genitourinary Cancers

Avoid hormone treatments. Avoid local radiation.

Gynecological Cancers

If you are more than 20% above your ideal weight or are in poor physical condition, start an exercise program and maintain close to ideal weight. Avoid fatty and fried foods. Avoid having multiple sexual partners. Avoid industrial pollution. Avoid estrogen use (combination oral contraceptives are okay). If you have high blood pressure, correct it. If you have diabetes or other serum glucose metabolism problems, be certain they are controlled. Check with your provider before starting long-term tamoxifen use.

Gliomas

Avoid radiation. Research has not yet defined other risk factors.

Head and Neck Cancers

Avoid tobacco smoke. Don't use chewing tobacco. Avoid mechanical irritation such as smoking a pipe. Avoid alcohol. Avoid very hot foods and drinks. Avoid high-alcohol (greater than 25%) mouthwash. Maintain good oral and dental care. Avoid exposure to airborne toxins such as heavy metals (nickel, cadmium, etc.), small fibers such as are used in textile manufacture, and wood dust.

Hodgkin's Disease

If you have chronic fatigue syndrome or Epstein-Barr virus, be certain that you treat it with the assistance of a health care professional. Avoid both ionizing and non-ionizing radiation exposure.

Leukemias

Avoid both ionizing and non-ionizing radiation exposure.

Liver, Gallbladder, and Biliary Cancers

Avoid liver stressors such as alcohol and drugs. If you have a treatable liver disease, seek professional care. Avoid exposure to radiation. Avoid the use of steroid hormones. Avoid exposure to arsenic. If you have a parasitic infection of any kind, be certain to treat it to the extent it can be resolved.

Lung Cancer

Avoid all tobacco smoke. Avoid all airborne pollution. Avoid exposure to heavy metals such as arsenic. Avoid radiation. Avoid small airborne fibers such as asbestos. Avoid radon gas in your home. Avoid industrial chemicals such as chloromethyl ether.

Myeloma

Avoid radiation exposure, especially ionizing radiation. Avoid chronic immune stimulation from allergies and immune-stimulating herbs. Avoid exposure to pesticides. Avoid exposure to paints. Avoid exposure to chemical solvents.

Non-Hodgkin's Lymphoma

If you have chronic fatigue syndrome or Epstein-Barr virus, be certain that you treat it with the assistance of a health care professional. Avoid both ionizing and non-ionizing radiation exposure.

Pancreatic Cancer

Avoid cigarette smoke. Avoid alcohol. Avoid coffee. Avoid exposure to solvents such as benzidine and beta-napthylaminex, which are frequently found in cleaning products. If you have pancreatitis, have it treated.

Sarcomas

Avoid exposure to chemical toxins. Avoid radiation. Avoid exposure to industrial chemicals such as polyvinyl chlorides (PVC). Avoid exposure to toxins such as arsenic. Avoid excess iron in the diet.

Skin Tumors

Avoid direct exposure to the sun, especially if you have light skin or burn easily. Avoid tobacco smoke. Avoid exposure to heavy metals such as arsenic. Avoid industrial chemicals such as polycyclic aromatic hydrocarbons.

Stomach Cancer

Avoid cigarette smoke. Avoid alcohol, coffee, and tea. If you have frequent indigestion or inadequate stomach acid, have that resolved with the assistance of a health care practitioner. Avoid any foods that cause indigestion. Avoid aspirin and nonsteroidal, anti-inflammatory drugs.

Thyroid Tumors

Maintain adequate iodine nutrition. Avoid head and neck radiation.

IMMUNE SYSTEM SUPPORT

Supporting the immune system means providing the nutrition and lifestyle necessary for your immune system to function at its maximum potential. Immune support is not the same as immune stimulation, which provokes the immune system to produce more white blood cells. Immune support can be accomplished with good nutrition and by making some lifestyle changes.

Ensuring Good Nutrition

The immune system is a complex series of cells and processes that work in harmony with many other body systems. The immune system depends on an wide variety of nutrients, including vitamins, minerals, and essential fatty acids. The most effective preventive nutrition strategy is to get good overall nutrition and to identify any particular nutritional deficiencies and resolve them. This is best done with the assistance of a health care professional.

Persons with certain lifestyle behaviors have a greater tendency toward nutritional deficiency. In some cases, the typical deficiencies are specific and in others more general. The following list may help you identify potential nutrient deficiencies. If you are receiving a conventional cancer treatment, check chapter 7 to be certain that supplementation does not interfere with its effectiveness. The following situations can lead to nutritional deficiencies:

Immune support can be accomplished with good nutrition and by making some lifestyle changes.

- Persons drinking more than three alcoholic drinks per week tend to be deficient in vitamins A, B_1, B_6, and D and folate.
- Persons exposed to tobacco smoke tend to be deficient in beta-carotene; vitamins B_6, C, and E; and folate.
- A general nutritional deficiency is more likely with people who are hospitalized; persons who have infectious or chronic diseases; persons with allergies and food intolerance; persons who have had recent surgery; pregnant women; and people who eat a high-fat diet or who are on a diet.
- Persons with osteoporosis can be deficient in calcium and vitamin D as well as other nutrients.
- Elderly people can be deficient in vitamins B_{12}, C, and D and folate.
- People using oral contraceptives can be deficient in vitamin B_6, folate, and beta-carotene.
- Teenagers can be deficient in vitamin A and folate.
- Athletes and heavy exercisers and persons under serious stress can be deficient in many nutrients, including B vitamins.
- Diabetics can be deficient in vitamins B_6, C, and D, as well as magnesium and chromium.
- Strict vegetarians can be deficient in vitamins B_{12} and D.

Lifestyle

The two lifestyle behaviors that improve immune system function without a doubt are exercise and stress reduction.

Moderate exercise, twenty minutes every other day at aerobic levels, will do the trick. You should be breathing hard and sweating. A casual walk around the neighborhood is good but will not provide the support that your immune system needs.

Reducing stress is also important. Maintain that warm, fuzzy feeling inside. Identify the signals that show you're under stress, such as clenching your teeth or tension in your neck or back. When you know that stress is coming on, take steps to avoid it. If you find that the stress signals are coming often, then it's time to review chapter 12.

Cancer prevention is the best deal in town. It almost always makes you feel better, has minimal side effects, and can provide remarkable benefits. Whatever else you do, I encourage you to make prevention a solid part of your life. The benefits can last a very long time.

11

Quality of Life: Making Every Day As Good As It Can Be

Agood quality of life is what we all strive for. Whether it's a new car, a vacation, or grandchildren, we spend much of our lives trying to achieve or maintain a quality of existence that makes us happy and contented people. Then along comes the cancer diagnosis, and with it the realization that our life spans are finite (which they always were) and the sense that we must try to make our remaining years and minutes as enjoyable as possible.

Cancer generally makes itself known by occupying space where it was not intended to be. The result is that the tumor interferes with normal body functions, which in turn impacts the quality of life. In addition, cancer is often treated without prioritizing quality-of-life issues. It simply doesn't have to be this way. A lot can be done with both conventional and nonconventional treatments to improve a person's quality of life without interfering with the best possible outcome. In fact, many of these considerations can potentially improve the results of conventional cancer treatments.

There are many strategies for maintaining a good quality of life before, during, and after cancer treatment. Surprisingly, most cancer survivors don't take advantage of them. In this chapter, we will review how your quality of life can be influenced by cancer and how you can reverse some of those effects.

Following a cancer diagnosis, your quality of life can be most affected by:

- Dealing with pain and discomfort
- Changes in your ability to perform functions of daily life
- Changes in your appearance
- Progress of other health issues
- Conventional treatments
- Nonconventional treatments
- Your personal attitude
- Your personal living situation
- Your personal financial situation
- Failure to thrive

DEALING WITH PAIN AND DISCOMFORT

Pain and discomfort are the most troublesome quality-of-life issues when dealing with solid tumors. For a treatment to be as effective as possible, it is important that the pain of cancer be recognized and defined as well as possible. For some people, the exact source of pain may be difficult even to identify. Others might resist talking about their pain out of fear of distressing loved ones or because they do not want to be seen as complainers.

If you are experiencing pain or discomfort, it is important to report it immediately to your health care provider. A good idea is to keep careful notes describing your particular discomforts. When did you first notice the pain? Did it occur only after meals, following a particular exercise or motion, or at a particular time of day? Is it sharp, dull, radiating?

Short questionnaires, known as *pain tools,* are available from your medical specialist or from a pain specialist. Pain tools will help you collect information for your providers so they can more effectively treat your pain. Take your time and fill out one completely. When completed, bring it to the doctor who provided it so that you can get the help you need to deal with your discomforts. There is no reason to endure pain unnecessarily.

A number of different strategies for controlling pain are available. You may wish to use more than one of these at a time and that's all right. Before you do, however, you should consult with your appropriate provider.

The strategies for controlling pain include

- Removing the source of the pain
- Deadening the pain
- Nutrition
- Hypnosis
- Biofeedback

Removing the Source of the Pain

Conventional medicine can sometimes remove the source of the pain with surgery, radiation, or chemotherapy (or a combination of treatments). Your medical specialist can inform you of the potential benefits and risks for your particular situation.

If the pain comes from a primary tumor (as opposed to a secondary, metastatic tumor), you've probably already considered removal. If the pain has become serious enough, however, you may want to consider removal again. If conventional treatment is unable to remove all of the tumor, you might wish to consider having only part of the tumor removed to ease pain and discomfort. This procedure is known as debulking.

If the pain is from a metastatic site, the new tumor may be a better candidate for removal than was the primary tumor. The earlier you report the pain, the better the chance that it can be resolved with removal of the tumor.

Surgery

Surgery to remove a tumor for pain control is controversial because of its potential side effects and risks. Experienced surgeons may discourage such an operation, fearing that surgery will worsen your quality of life. If you are thinking about this procedure, it is important to consider all of the factors, including the difficulty of the surgery, its potential for success and for adverse effects, and how long it will be before the procedure may be needed again. Listen carefully to your surgeon and don't be afraid to get a second opinion, as described in chapter 2.

Surgery to remove a tumor for pain control is controversial because of its potential side effects and risks.

Radiation

Radiation for pain control can be effective, especially for bone pain. Although radiation still carries with it some risk, it is usually less than the risks involved with surgery. When considering the use of radiation to treat pain, it is important to carefully weigh the same issues you did when considering surgery: the potentials for success, the procedure's adverse effects, and how long the positive effects can be expected to last. It is always important to consider a second opinion before making your final decision (see chapter 2).

Chemotherapy

Chemotherapy is rarely used for the sole purpose of pain control but it still remains a conventional option. The benefits and risks must be considered very carefully, but the result may be worthwhile if the agent is not a very toxic one.

Deadening the Pain

The body can be fooled into feeling less pain by a number of strategies that are worth consideration:

- Acupuncture
- Pain-Killing Herbs
- Pain-Killing Drugs
- Pain-Numbing Procedures

Acupuncture

Acupuncture can have a remarkable effect on pain reduction. The theory of acupuncture is that the needle creates a stimulus that activates the sensory nerve that is delivering the pain signal to the brain. Since a nerve can only carry one signal at a time, a "gate" closes behind the needle signal, thus blocking the pain signal. Acupuncture does not work every time and the results are temporary. When it does work, however, it can provide pain relief with a minimum of side effects.

If you don't get relief from the first acupuncturist you see, try a second one. There are significant differences in the style and training of these practitioners, especially between the Asian- and Western-trained acupuncturists. (This is not to say that one is better than the other but merely that they are different.)

Pain-Killing Herbs

A number of herbs have mild analgesic (pain-killing) effects. Since pain control depends not only on the strength of the painkiller but also on its particular chemical action, herbal painkillers are worth a try even if conventional painkillers were not effective. Keep in mind that these herbs may also have other actions. If they're used during conventional treatment, avoid using them during the protected zone.

Because of similarities in action, these herbs should *never* be combined with each other or with other painkillers of any kind.

BRYONY (*BRYONIA ALBA*)

Other Actions
Bryony has been used traditionally both to control fevers and as a laxative.

Toxicity
Large doses can cause diarrhea, nausea, vomiting, and stomach discomfort.

Suggested Use
Notwithstanding the toxicology risks, this herb can be an effective painkiller and is safe when administered by an experienced, trained, licensed provider. The adult dose for tincture is 5 drops every four hours.

CAYENNE (*CAPSICUM FRUTESCENS*)

Other Actions
Red cayenne pepper, also commonly called capsicum, is a traditional stimulant that has been used to increase digestive peristalsis and raise body temperature. It has also been used as an antidepressant.

Toxicity
Large doses can cause nausea, vomiting, and diarrhea.

Suggested Use
Capsicum can be effective as a painkiller at safe dosages. The adult dose is 10 drops of the tincture every four hours.

MONKSHOOD (*ACONITUM NAPELLUS*)

Other Actions
Monkshood can raise or lower body temperature, numb sensory nerves, and act as a sedative. It is also believed to act as an antibiotic.

Toxicity

Monkshood can be very toxic, even in small doses. It should always be used under the direct supervision of an experienced, trained, and licensed provider. With an overdose, monkshood can severely suppress heart and lung function. The first signs of toxicity are high or low temperature, numbness and tingling of the skin, difficulty breathing, and dizziness. In the event of overdose, emergency medical procedures should be started immediately. Monkshood's effects can combine with other painkillers and therefore it should not be used at the same time.

Suggested Use

This herb is usually prepared in an alcohol or glycerite tincture. The suggested adult dose is 5 drops every hour, but this can vary with the preparation. Toxic symptoms do not usually occur until 10 drops per hour are taken. Consult your provider and the manufacturer for the proper dose for individual products.

Even though this herb has significant toxicity, it can be effective when used with expert advice.

MOTHER'S WORT
(*LEONURUS CARDIACA*)

Other Actions

Mother's wort has been used traditionally to increase body temperature, as a laxative, and to increase menstrual flow.

Toxicity

With traditional use, Mother's wort has not been reported to have toxic side effects.

Suggested Use

As a tea, mix 2 teaspoons with a cup of boiling water. Steep fifteen minutes before taking two to three times per day.

PEPPERMINT (*MENTHA PIPERITA*)

Other Actions

Peppermint has been used traditionally as a bitter agent to improve digestion, as an antinausea treatment, and to stimulate the liver.

Toxicity
Peppermint can cause upset stomach in very large doses.

Suggested Use
Adult dose is $1/2$ teaspoon of tincture every four hours.

TURMERIC (*CURCUMA LONGA*)

Other Actions
Turmeric (also known as curcumin) is used as an anti-inflammatory and antioxidant.

Toxicity
Turmeric has not been found to have toxic effects in traditional use.

Suggested Use
Suggested adult dosage is 200 to 400 mg three times per day.

VALERIAN (*VALERIANA OFFICINALIS*)

Other Actions
Valerian has been used traditionally as a stomach stimulant, sedative, anti-hypertensive (to lower blood pressure), and antibiotic.

Toxicity
Valerian can have a sedative effect and can cause mild stomach discomfort in large doses. Effects may be exaggerated with alcohol.

WINTERGREEN (*GAULTHERIA PROCUMBENS*)

Other Actions
Wintergreen has been used traditionally as an antibiotic. It is believed to have pain-killing actions similar to aspirin.

Toxicity
High doses can cause sedation, stomach pain, and ringing of the ears. Overdose should be attended by emergency medical treatment.

Suggested Use

Wintergreen is safe when used in proper dosages. There is anecdotal evidence that wintergreen can relieve pain that is not relieved by other painkillers. Suggested dose is 30 drops of tincture every four hours. Reduce the dose if ringing in the ears is experienced.

Suggested Use

Adult dose is 500 mg of the dried herb every four hours.

Pain-Killing Drugs

The wide range of pain-relieving drugs can be both potent and remarkably effective. A skilled pain specialist has the ability to pick, choose, and combine these drugs to deal with a variety of circumstances.

> If pain-killing drugs did not work the first time, a revised prescription may be more effective.

Opioid drug painkillers have common side effects, which can include constipation, nausea, vomiting, slowed breathing and heart function, dizziness, mental clouding, depression, weakness, restlessness, agitation, sedation, and some others. A qualified pain specialist can often minimize these side effects and still provide effective pain relief.

If pain-killing drugs did not work the first time, a revised prescription may be more effective. It is not uncommon for patients to discontinue use of painkillers simply because the first prescription was not optimized. If your pain continues, consult with your conventional practitioner. Conventional painkillers may still have the answer even if the first prescription did not provide it.

Pain-Numbing Procedures

When pain cannot be controlled or when the side effects of treatments are unacceptable, there are procedures that can directly numb or sever the nerve carrying the pain message. Remarkably, this can be done with few adverse effects.

In some cases, the offending nerve can be injected with alcohol or other chemicals, which can deaden it for weeks, even months. The procedure depends on the location of the nerve and the pain, but is usually done without complications. Surgically cutting the nerve has the disadvantage that it may not be possible to reconnect it later, but if the pain cannot be controlled any other way, this may be a viable option.

New pain-control strategies are being discovered regularly. A medical pain specialist can keep you abreast of the latest treatments.

Nutrition

Much credible anecdotal evidence suggests that cancer patients whose total nutrition was optimized experienced little or no pain when conventional experience would have predicted otherwise. There is no mechanism to explain this phenomenon physiologically. The best of these unscientific reports used nutritional supplements with basic vitamins and minerals, as well as improving diet and digestion.

Hypnosis

Hypnosis is an effective, scientific treatment, unlike its portrayal in the movies. Hypnosis works by helping the mind interpret sensory signals, such as pain, differently. The physiological and chemical mechanisms are not well defined scientifically, but the results can be remarkable.

Hypnotherapists are licensed in many areas. If your state does not provide this level of public protection, consider a referral from your conventional or nonconventional provider. Hypnotherapy can be a useful treatment, even when other pain-control methods are being used. It is literally free of side effects and can provide some real relief.

Biofeedback

Biofeedback is a technique that enables us to teach our brains to control physiological functions (such as pain recognition) that we are not normally able to control consciously. Anecdotal evidence suggests that biofeedback can be used with some success for pain control. Although no definitive studies have been conducted, it may still be worth a try since there are no side effects other than a generally modest expense.

CHANGES IN YOUR ABILITY TO PERFORM FUNCTIONS OF DAILY LIFE

The progress of cancer can interfere with your physical strength, agility, endurance, and mental function, all of which can affect your ability to accomplish the normal activities of daily living. When this happens, your first response may be denial.

We would all like to continue functioning as though we were eighteen (with, we would hope, a little more common sense). As a result, we do our best to ignore these changes. This response, unfortunately, can make things even worse and, in some cases, can cause us to miss opportunities for better solutions.

Changes in our ability to function can also be accompanied by a sense of loss and dread. The effect of these changes on our mental, emotional, and spiritual well-being is of very real importance. It may seem trivial when someone else can no longer tie his shoelaces, but when it happens to us, it feels like a huge loss.

Remaining as independent as possible—within reason—is very important. For example, if being able to prepare your own meals is important to you, then it is far better that you are able to do it with whatever help is available, perhaps a special can opener designed for the physically challenged, rather than give up this basic level of independence.

Ability to function in daily life can be assessed by licensed providers using standardized tests. Most of your providers can arrange for such an assessment, which can be a valuable tool to help determine where extra help is needed.

Reduced Physical Function

If muscles, the nervous system, or blood flow are interfered with, the result can be a reduction of physical abilities. Useful strategies include:

- Physical devices to assist with function
- Nonconventional therapies to compensate for function
- Conventional treatments to compensate for function

Physical Devices to Assist with Function

Make the task as easy as possible. We've already mentioned devices to help open cans. Mechanical tools can assist with virtually all the activities of daily living. There are aids for everything from getting in and out of the bathtub safely to driving a car with the use of only one leg. Such appliances can be found through medical supply companies and businesses that specialize in geriatric supplies. Look in the Yellow Pages to see what's available in your area.

Using extra help to make life easier is not an admission of failure.

The secret to success is to introduce these devices early enough to allow their use to become second nature. As function is lost, so is the ability to learn the easier alternatives. Some resistance to these interventions is natural, especially for a proud and independent person. However, this needs to be put into perspective. Two principles will help.

First, using extra help to make life easier is not an admission of failure. We use power steering in our cars even though we are strong enough to turn the wheel without it. Driving is simply better with it, especially in a large car. Second, not everyone can do everything. There are peanut butter jars that 250-pound competitive weight lifters can't open. Everyone needs help with something. Perspective is important with such issues, especially when emotion and fear undermine logical thought processes.

Nonconventional Therapies to Compensate for Physical Function

Physical function can often be enhanced with physical treatment techniques, including physical therapy, manipulation, exercise, and, in some cases, botanical and nutritional medicine. For it to be effective and safe, the treatment must be carefully chosen to fit the individual. If quality of life is potentially affected, the situation may be so complex that you'll want to consult a licensed provider for appropriate referrals. See chapter 3 for strategies for finding the right referral.

Conventional Treatments to Compensate for Physical Function

As with compensation for pain, numerous conventional treatments, including surgery, radiation, and drugs, may have a useful role in retaining function. The challenge is to be certain that the treatments have more benefits than risks. A competent medical provider can usually give you the straight scoop. Chapter 3 describes methods for finding such a provider referral.

Reduced Mental Function

Cancer can interfere with brain function in many ways. Brain lesions, for example, can directly affect brain function and hormone-secreting tumors can change the brain's chemistry. Some cancers can restrict the transfer and transport of oxygen and nutrients, which, in turn, can restrict mental function. Other tumor effects, such as pain and loss of physical function, can indirectly affect mental function by creating distraction or even depression.

When reduced *mentation* (the ability to comprehend and process information) occurs, the first step is to identify the mechanisms at work. This will require the careful attention of both your conventional and nonconventional providers.

The potential solutions may be simple but can also be remarkably effective. Some answers are as simple as providing supplemental oxygen, fluids to treat dehydration, or improved nutrition. In cases of depression, pharmaceutical or herbal antidepressants can be helpful, as can counseling.

Mental exercises can also be of some benefit, whether they are as complex as crossword puzzles or as simple as reviewing the names of your children or grandchildren. The more brain cells that are used, the better. There's one important exception to this: Never attempt mental exercises in which failure is possible, since this may further undermine confidence and put a halt to progress.

CHANGES IN YOUR APPEARANCE

A tumor can change your physical appearance if its growth is visible. Secondary changes that accompany the tumor, such as those affecting weight, skin tone, and voice can also alter your appearance as well as your self-image.

Opportunities to maintain and improve your appearance are worth serious consideration.

Conventional treatment to correct your appearance is in many cases worthwhile. Surgical removal of visible tumors, especially when you are disturbed by them, should be considered if it is an option. People may dismiss such interventions as vain and unnecessary, but such corrective procedures are usually successful, cause only a minimal amount of discomfort, and can be affordable, if they are not covered by health insurance.

It is also possible to use makeup, clothing, and various accessories to minimize the visual effects of some tumors. Don't underestimate the positive effect these strategies can have on your mental status and self-image.

Sometimes people's concerns over changes in their appearance get out of proportion. Try to keep things in perspective. You are possibly being your own worst critic. What may be a huge disfigurement to you may not even be noticed by others. At the same time, your feelings should not be ignored. Opportunities to maintain and improve your appearance are worth serious consideration.

PROGRESS OF OTHER HEALTH ISSUES

When dealing with a cancer diagnosis, it's easy to forget everything else that's going on in your life. This includes other medical problems, ones you might have been tolerating easily before your cancer diagnosis.

Both cancer and its treatment can turn a tolerable physical problem into one that is disruptive, even unbearable. What was occasional constipation or indigestion in the past can, with certain cancer diagnoses and treatments, become debilitating. Previously mild symptoms of cyclic depression or anxiety can become overwhelming.

The best strategy is to make a list of all (emphasis on *all*) of your health complaints. Prioritize them, starting with the ones that bother you the most. Take this list to your conventional and nonconventional providers and, one by one, take steps to resolve them as much as possible. Go through the list item by item and be persistent. Don't give up if the first answer or first provider isn't productive. Use the referral and second opinion plans from chapters 2 and 3 to be certain you get satisfaction. Remember that one provider may be able to achieve what another cannot. You may not solve all your problems completely, but this strategy almost always provides some real, objective improvements in quality of life.

Although you have the option of self-treatment with self-help books, I caution against it. You will gain significantly greater benefit and will be infinitely safer if you're working with a skilled and experienced practitioner.

CONVENTIONAL TREATMENTS

Conventional treatments can produce a myriad of side effects that can significantly affect your quality of life. (These are described in detail in chapter 6.) The challenge is not only to consider quality of life seriously when planning and using these treatments but also to take care not to interfere with the treatment's ability to provide the best response.

If you have not already started treatment, be certain that you have considered all of the options available. If two different treatments can produce equivalent results, select the one that leaves you with the best quality of life. If there are small differences in treatment effectiveness and large differences in quality of life during or after treatment, make an informed decision about which is most important.

Once treatment begins, certain strategies can minimize side effects and help maintain quality of life. These include:

- Using conventional and nonconventional treatments to alleviate side effects
- Adjusting lifestyle and schedule to help you through your treatments
- Keeping a positive attitude about your therapy

Using Conventional and Nonconventional
Treatments to Alleviate Side Effects

Treatments, both conventional and nonconventional, are available to deal with virtually every problem from mouth sores to post-surgical infections. Some are very effective, others may only help a little. Many, however, can provide benefits without adding risks. Be sure to ask your conventional provider and his or her staff about the various strategies for dealing with the effects of your conventional therapy.

Often something as simple as a saline mouthwash to relieve mouth sores can reduce a major discomfort to a mild annoyance. Conventional and nonconventional strategies abound for relieving nausea, insomnia, and a host of other treatment-related ailments. Many of these will significantly improve your quality of day-to-day living.

Adjusting Lifestyle and Schedule to
Help You Through Your Treatments

Making small changes in your lifestyle or your schedule to accommodate your treatment can have both physical and emotional benefits. Avoid stressful activities during the times you will experience side effects. Give yourself a treat on treatment days as a reward for showing up but be certain it's a treat that you can fully enjoy. If you usually don't feel well immediately after treatment, have the treat before. Good choices include seeing a movie, taking a trip to your favorite bookstore or hardware store, or going to the park or the beach. Do whatever makes you happy. Dinner at your favorite restaurant may not be a good choice if your treatment affects your digestive system, unless, of course, it's a light and healthful meal.

Keeping a Positive Attitude About Your Therapy

Keep a positive view of your conventional treatment. Avoid difficult experiences and troublesome individuals during treatment times since they will only serve to bring you down at a time when you need to stay up. If you recuperate at home, put a "no solicitors" (or even a "no visitors") sign on your door to avoid interruptions and irritation. Let an answering machine or voice mail screen your calls.

Conventional treatments for cancer get a lot of bad press and criticism. Of course, many effective conventional treatments are toxic, but if you make an informed choice you will receive benefits that outweigh the risks and side effects. Accent the positive and think of the side effects as the price you must pay for the benefits. Take the best and minimize the rest (that was an unintentional rhyme). Your mental attitude will do much to improve your tolerance and quality of life during conventional treatment.

NONCONVENTIONAL TREATMENTS

Most properly implemented nonconventional treatments will not adversely affect your quality of life. The few exceptions are those with more than one effect or those for which the desired effect may include some discomfort.

Oral supplements can affect your quality of life by creating indigestion, nausea, or diarrhea. Assuming that the treatment plan is sound, the most likely reason for this might be too many pills to digest or an allergy-like response to a binder, filler, or other ingredient of the pills. If there are simply too many pills, you can grind the tablets with a mortar and pestle (which can be purchased inexpensively from most large department stores), empty the capsules, and mix them with juice or water. Before you do this, however, check with your nonconventional provider or pharmacist to be certain that you don't create a harmful combination. Liquid-filled gelcaps can sometimes be bitten to release the contents in your mouth (then you can spit out the pill). It is usually unwise to grind or empty enzymes. Once again, check with a licensed, knowledgeable provider before modifying the form of your medication.

If you have what appears to be an allergic or sensitivity response, contact your nonconventional provider at once. Either the culprit will be identified or your supplements will be discontinued. Afterward, you may be re-introduced to them one at a time, until the offender is found. Don't be surprised if a nutritional plan that bothered you becomes easier to digest after you take a break from it.

Physical modalities such as manipulation and physical therapy can leave you sore and uncomfortable. If so, your licensed provider should be notified immediately. Unless there is an overwhelming argument to the contrary, natural treatments that adversely affect your quality of life should be discontinued.

People often assume that everything natural is free of side effects, but this is not true. Nutritional supplements can sometimes have such side effects as nausea, dizziness, or fatigue. Most side effects are predictable;

some are unique. Your nonconventional provider can help you to identify those treatments that don't agree with you.

Your quality of life can be seriously affected by nonconventional treatments, especially if they are not the right ones for you. Use these therapies for their positive benefits and take care to avoid the potential risks.

YOUR PERSONAL ATTITUDE

Attitude has everything to do with quality of life, regardless of the diagnosis. Each of us responds to our environment based on the way we interpret and interact with it. I strongly recommend your concerted accent on the positive, regardless of how unfair or unreasonable the facts may seem.

If your objective is to improve your quality of life, all of the strategies in this chapter will be less effective if your attitude is negative. I don't want this to sound like a do-gooder lecture. Ignoring reality and acting like Pollyanna makes no sense, but allowing the pendulum to swing to the other extreme, in which everything is negative, is not useful either.

M̲ake the best of what you can make the best of.

Make the best of what you can make the best of. Improve your situation and life quality wherever you can and allow the improvements to work. Take joy in those small parts of life that retain their value and that have nothing to do with you being ill. Emotional support and useful resources are available through organizations such as Cancer Lifeline (www.cancerlifeline.org; phone 206-297-2500).

Sometimes counseling is worthwhile but, for it to be effective, you must want it to work. Regardless of how difficult things may be, any day that you wake up is a good day. See chapter 12 for additional strategies for dealing with stress.

YOUR PERSONAL LIVING SITUATION

Cancer diagnosis and treatment can affect your personal living situation in many ways. Finances can change, your work and social life can change, your schedule can change, and your ability to function can change. These things can have as profound an effect on your quality of life as the disease and its treatment. But rarely do these changes get the same attention. It is important that you get on with life despite the adversity.

Try to maintain an enjoyable social life. Visit with friends, take part in social activities that you enjoy, and make time for activities that are fun for you, even if you have to adjust them somewhat.

If your diagnosis comes at a time when you're experiencing other changes, such as personal separation or loss, changing jobs, or moving, find a support system to help (see chapter 12). Change itself can be traumatic and should be limited if possible.

Enjoying as many of the normal functions of life as you can is an important part of the healing process. With few exceptions (be sure to ask your licensed provider), laughter, fun, friends, and regular sex are just fine.

YOUR PERSONAL FINANCIAL SITUATION

Frankly, financial difficulties can affect your health. If your disease and treatment have had a serious impact on your finances, ask for help. Your conventional provider can tell you about the resources available for financial aid, low-cost loans, and even assistance with the cost of treatment. In addition, public service organizations can also provide financial advice. The services of a financial planner may also be helpful in getting you on your financial feet when this experience is over. Such a person can help you develop a strategic plan and give you the confidence to make it work.

Worry over finances shouldn't be a problem when you are ill, but unfortunately it can be. The less you have to worry about money, the faster you will heal and the better your quality of life will be.

FAILURE TO THRIVE

Few circumstances are more frustrating for providers and families than when a cancer patient does not improve. Failure to thrive often results from multiple factors that combine to create circumstances that an individual simply cannot overcome. Physical and emotional challenges can create a vicious cycle in which each reinforces the other. Or physical limitations can result in a sense of defeat, which in turn makes it more difficult to find the energy to deal with the physical problems.

Typical signs and symptoms include a lack of interest in the events of daily life, weight loss, poor appetite, and loss of muscle mass. This situation is not always easily diagnosed, and even when it is, the solution depends more on the individual's willingness to participate than on drugs, nutrients, or exercise.

Emotional, Psychological, and Spiritual Considerations of Failure to Thrive

Failure to thrive usually has as much to do with what's going on in a person's head as it does with his or her body. Efforts to solve this problem that understand this important factor are invariably more effective than those that do not.

Depression is not uncommon in people with cancer, even in those with a favorable long-term prognosis. A cancer diagnosis, fear of treatment, fear of finishing treatment, and concerns of mortality all enter into this equation. A person may feel dejected, without hope, and lacking joy in life. Efforts on the part of family and friends to cheer up the person are often ineffective.

Conventional medicine traditionally offers antidepressants and counseling. Both are worth considering. Antidepressants may take up to six weeks to be effective and do not work with everyone. When they do, however, the results are impressive. Interestingly, most medical oncologists have developed expertise in the use of antidepressant medications simply because they are faced with this problem so frequently.

Counseling also can be a useful treatment for depression. As a general rule, I recommend counseling whenever antidepressants are being taken. It is very important, however, to find a counselor who is a good match. Psychiatrists, psychologists, and other licensed counselors all have their own personalities and beliefs. The most effective treatment will come from a provider who can align closely with the person's needs.

Depression can also be caused by nutritional deficiencies. Vitamins, minerals, amino acids, and other nutrients are effective in treating depression and can reduce or eliminate the need for drugs. To get the best result, however, I recommend the services of someone expert in this area. An appropriate nonconventional provider such as a naturopathic physician, an orthomolecular psychiatrist, a psychologist, or another provider with specific expertise in dealing with depression will be the most helpful.

Certain treatments can make some people better and others worse. It almost always takes more than simply buying a bottle of St. John's wort at

> Depression is not uncommon in people with cancer, even in those with a favorable long-term prognosis.

the corner store. Keep in mind, too, that some over-the-counter remedies for depression can interfere with certain antidepressant drugs. Once again, for the best result, you need expert advice.

Known as the "fight-or-flight system," the sympathetic nervous system can also affect failure to thrive. This system is what helps our bodies respond to stressful situations by preparing them for action. Stress, episodes of panic, and anxiety attacks can set off a series of events that negatively affect the health of a person with cancer. This kind of response can cause the person to overreact to the situation, which in turn creates even more stress and thus a vicious cycle.

The sympathetic nervous system only operates effectively for a short period of time, just long enough to provide the adrenaline necessary to deal with an emergency, such as running away from a dinosaur or, in modern times, getting out of the way of a truck. Such emergencies are usually resolved in a short time. When stress and anxiety continue for longer than the short duration that the system was designed for, the state of high alert turns into irritability and fatigue.

The sympathetic nervous response has much to do with the way a person processes and deals with information. It can be made worse by pain and discomfort, fear, and nutritional deficiency. In fact, the fight-or-flight response can even *contribute* to nutritional deficiency.

The solution is usually a combination of counseling and nutritional support. If depression is also a factor, which is often the case, dealing with the depression will also help.

A good general nutritional supplement program can be helpful, but the outcome will almost always be better when enlisting the support of someone licensed and expert in this area.

When a person simply gives up, the result can also be failure to thrive. This can occur without signs of depression or other physical considerations. Reversing a failure to thrive requires the participation of the person with cancer.

Each of us has an internal need to survive and to thrive, but when that need can no longer express itself, the path to wellness becomes much more difficult. The interventions of family, friends, and providers are often rebuffed. This problem can be very difficult for caregivers. When there is no obvious cause for the person giving up, it is often productive simply to assume that the individual suffers from one or more of the factors discussed in this chapter, especially depression, and is hiding it. Treating presumptively can be successful although the person affected may put up a wall that may preclude further assistance. It is best in such circumstances to get as much expert help as possible to assess the problem, even if the advice is to do nothing further at this time. Remember, if the expert assessment doesn't ring true for you, find a second opinion. However, it is also important to honor the person's ability to determine his or her own destiny.

Failure to Thrive and Its Physical Considerations

Failing to thrive brings with it a variety of physical problems. Both conventional and nonconventional medicine can provide useful solutions for these problems.

Improving Weight and Muscle Mass

Weight control has probably been addressed by most if not all of the members of your health care team. The usual advice is to maintain a few extra pounds and to eat a high-calorie diet. If you've ever had to worry about being overweight, this may sound like a dream diet.

The reason for this advice, however, is because cancer patients often suffer severe weight loss during treatment. Cancer and many of the conventional treatments used to treat it tend to reduce appetite, interfere with digestion, and consequently, produce significant weight loss. If the weight loss is extreme, it can be life-threatening.

M uscle mass has been shown repeatedly to be among the most important indicators of long-term survival, regardless of whether or not you are ill.

Preventing excessive weight loss is an important issue when dealing with cancer, but of equal or greater importance is what the weight is made from. While having fat stores is important, maintaining muscle mass is vital.

Muscle mass has been shown repeatedly to be among the most important indicators of long-term survival, regardless of whether or not you are ill. It is muscle mass, not fat cells, that opens doors, climbs stairs, gets you in and out of the bathtub, and generally allows you to perform the daily activities of life.

Muscle mass provides the strength and endurance to respond to physical challenges, such as carrying a bag of groceries, opening a heavy car door, or catching yourself if you slip getting out of bed. Inadequate muscle mass can contribute to fatigue and discomfort when you are performing simple tasks.

Maintaining muscle mass requires two elements: having protein in your diet and using your muscles. Without both, muscle mass and strength will be lost.

We need carbohydrates, proteins, and fats for our bodies to function properly. Unfortunately, modern diets and quick-weight-gain programs often neglect protein. Protein, which is a combination of amino acids, must be present in the diet or in supplements. Once eaten, protein must be absorbed efficiently from the digestive tract into the blood system. After it is absorbed, protein provides nutrition for the muscles to grow and repair themselves.

Without protein, muscle mass and strength will simply decline. Adequate protein levels can be calculated for you by your provider, but 50 grams per day is a good starting point.

If you are having digestive problems, a nonconventional provider can tailor a program for you, ensuring that proteins are properly broken down and absorbed into the bloodstream and that they don't just take the scenic digestive tour, only to be discharged with the next bowel movement. As for diets, many excellent books (with recipes to provide some interest and variety) are available.

Muscles must be used in order to be maintained. The paradox here is that it takes muscle mass to exercise, so if muscle mass is low, it may be difficult even to begin muscle-building exercise. The good news is that an exercise program will get remarkably easier and even enjoyable once you begin.

For cancer patients suffering from reduced muscle mass, exercise might seem like an impossible challenge. Such a person might fear that exercise will bring on pain and disappointment at a time when he or she may not be able to endure either. As a result, of the very people who need such a program, most never start one.

The key to success often lies with two factors. First, with designing a program that will be successful, one having measurable results and with little chance of failure. Consult a physical therapist, licensed exercise physiologist, or someone who is trained and licensed in this field. This is not a plan you should try on your own, nor should you rely on your pal Big Gordo at the local gym.

Second, the program should use most muscle groups, with particular attention paid to lower body and leg strength. The program should have a structured feedback system. You will be more interested in continuing if your progress is measurable and acknowledged, even perhaps with some fanfare.

The objective is to develop functional muscle mass and maintain adequate weight. A few extra pounds is okay, whereas a lot of extra pounds is not, since the available muscle mass has to carry those fat pounds all over town. We're not talking about developing a physique like Arnold Schwarzenegger but rather developing the ability to physically accomplish the important tasks of daily life.

Maintaining Flexibility

Flexibility is an important part of physical function. The ability to reach, bend, and turn one's body as much as necessary to get in the car or to reach a bottle from the back of the refrigerator can, in some situations, be more important than strength.

Loss of flexibility can result from cancer, cancer treatments, and inactivity. The person with cancer may have always lacked flexibility but may have been better able to accomplish things before becoming ill. Whatever the circumstances, flexibility should be evaluated in a person with cancer who fails to thrive.

Every exercise program should include a gentle flexibility component, professionally designed specifically for that person. Once again, I strongly recommend the services of a licensed expert to develop a plan that will work.

Learning to Deal with Pain

Pain often contributes to failure to thrive. If pain has not been resolved satisfactorily after the first few tries, patients may give up on ever being pain-free. They may not even wish to discuss it, since talking about it draws attention to the pain. It may be more comfortable for them to avoid thinking about what they think may not be fixable.

Whatever the source, pain should and usually can be controlled.

At night, with fewer distractions, pain seems worse. Such discomfort will often interfere with sleep and cause fatigue and listlessness during the day, reinforcing the failure-to-thrive situation.

Pain caused by movement may be hard to pin down because it is transient. This kind of discomfort discourages the individual from attempting even modest exercise and movement, which results in a vicious cycle of reduced muscle strength, function, and avoidance of daily activities.

Whatever the source, pain should and usually can be controlled. The first option, as we discussed earlier in this chapter, is to remove the source of the pain when that is possible. If the pain is from an infection, poor surgical healing, or some other correctable source, a surgical or antibiotic intervention would be the place to start. If the pain is not identifiable or amenable to repair, then pain-control strategies are in order. Such techniques were discussed in detail previously.

Controlling pain can result in a remarkable improvement in a person's overall well-being. It may take some perseverance and the help of a pain-control specialist, but the results will more than reward everyone's efforts.

Personal Appearance Considerations

Any unwanted change in appearance can be traumatic, even if it is not visible to other people. We humans are not always able to deal easily with such change.

Cancer can often cause physical changes that tend to undermine one's self-image. This, in turn, can reinforce failure to thrive in several ways. When individuals with cancer become self-conscious about their appearance, they often avoid being seen. This may so limit their social contacts that they become reclusive. Such a lack of social stimulation can bring about many of the emotional issues we discussed earlier in this chapter.

A person's concern with appearance may even impact his or her nutrition. Avoiding being seen may include refusing to shop for food. As noted earlier, nutrition can play a significant part in failure to thrive, and appearance issues are not always admitted or recognized.

If a person's change in appearance is visible and disfiguring, correction should be a priority, if possible. Cosmetic surgery has advanced substantially. Where surgical resolution is not an option, many other strategies, such as makeup, clothing, or a wig, can help more than you might think.

If the change in appearance is minor or not noticeable, this might be a good time for counseling. A trained provider can help put things into perspective in a way that family and friends cannot.

All of our lives we tell our friends and loved ones that it's what's inside that really matters. The cancer patient is no exception to this tenet. Gently remind the person that this is still true without dismissing his or her feelings. It's acceptable to tell someone that he or she still looks good, but it is not supportive to say "Don't worry, it doesn't matter."

If failure to thrive is being affected by appearance and self-image, steps to improve these can be surprisingly effective.

Strategies for Improving Diet and Appetite

Although nutritional supplements can supply vitamins, minerals, and other nutrients, when it comes to getting basic nutrition, there's no substitute for good food. When someone fails to thrive as a result of poor appetite, altered taste sensation, or because of the physical discomforts of eating this should be addressed quickly. The greater the loss of weight and muscle mass, the longer and more difficult the recovery. A number of strategies have proved useful, including:

- Diet changes
- Botanicals (herbs)
- Drugs
- Nutritional supplementation
- Hydrazine sulfate (appetite stimulants)

Diet Changes

If you are helping a person, start with his or her favorite foods. These will produce the best responses, increasing the desire to eat and thus the body's production of digestive enzymes. Prepare the foods the way that the person likes them. If the aroma or taste is off because of altered taste sensation, try to identify exactly what is bothersome. Don't be afraid to experiment with salt, spices, herbs, and even sweeteners.

When it comes to sweeteners, white sugar might seem bitter and disagreeable to someone undergoing cancer treatments (you didn't actually expect me to say something nice about white sugar, did you?). Other sweeteners such as molasses and honey, however, may be more palatable.

> When it comes to sweeteners, white sugar might seem bitter and disagreeable to someone undergoing cancer treatments.

Experiment with new foods. Persons with cancer often develop new tastes. A good cookbook can help. Another useful strategy is to browse the supermarket shelves for international foods, produce you've never tried, and anything else that strikes your fancy. There may not be any rhyme or reason for the foods that turn out to be appealing, but when you find them you will know the joy of success.

Emphasis on protein and nutrition is important, but it is more important that the individual begin eating *something*, even if it is not the perfect food. Once food intake and appetite return to normal, there will be plenty of opportunities for more healthful eating. In most cases, no particular diet is required. However, you may find some general advice helpful.

Avoid foods that are potentially troublesome and difficult to digest, such as fried foods, rich foods such as cream sauces, and foods that have a history of causing digestive problems. If constipation or diarrhea are problems, avoid foods that make them worse. Cheese and rice are common causes of constipation whereas tomato products, raw fruits and vegetables, and fried foods are frequent causes of diarrhea.

Large meals may be more problematic than smaller ones, resulting in indigestion and a further loss of interest in eating. Don't encourage a person to continue eating when he or she is full. This can cause indigestion. The largest meal of the day should be lunch, rather than dinner. This will provide adequate time for digestion.

Try to eat at the same time each day. The body's internal clock will then anticipate eating times and actually prepare the digestive tract. Varying meal times can disrupt that process and interfere with digestion. Avoid eating late in the evening. To allow for proper digestion, the last meal of the day should be at least three hours prior to bedtime.

The assistance of a licensed dietitian or other trained individual to help with food choices may be useful. Many good cookbooks are available from a variety of sources, including, for example, the American Cancer Society. Foods that are laden with preservatives or artificially colored may be particularly distasteful to the patient and should be avoided.

Botanicals

The use of botanicals, including stomach bitters, can help with both appetite and digestion. These have been used traditionally, and anecdotal evidence supports their use. See chapter 8 for more details and consult a licensed, nonconventional provider for more specific advice.

Drugs

A number of drugs have been used to stimulate appetite. The hormone megastrol acetate has been successful. If more conservative approaches have not worked, this drug may be a good choice to at least get the process started.

Nutritional Supplementation

The body's system for stimulating hunger depends on a number of chemical reactions, which in turn depend on proper nutrition. It is sometimes useful to provide supplemental nutrition, such as a multiple vitamin and mineral tablet, to support that process. Supplemental amino acid combinations are also anecdotally reported to improve appetite and may be worth a try as well. These are usually found in the form of protein powders. Be certain that supplements do not interfere with the protected zone.

Hydrazine Sulfate

This chemical solvent has been promoted for a number of treatment objectives, but one thing it seems to do well is to increase the appetite of cancer patients. It has potential side effects but, in moderate doses, seems to be safe. The biggest problem is that, at this time, it is not available in most countries in a form approved for human consumption. It has been prepared and sold by companies who bypass FDA requirements for safety by labeling it "not for human consumption" or not labeling it at all. I hope both the product and the research will improve by the time you are reading this.

If loss of appetite is an issue, I believe that hydrazine sulfate is worth a try, but only when it is available in a form approved for human consumption and only with the assistance of a competent provider experienced with dosage and administration.

Lifestyle Considerations

Lifestyle can have a significant effect on a person's ability to thrive. The most common culprits are sleep habits and stressors. Poor sleep habits, insomnia, the use of stimulants such as coffee and tea, and other behaviors that reduce the quality of sleep can potentially interfere with the individual's ability to function during the day. The fatigue and irritability that result from inadequate sleep can aggravate failure to thrive.

Sleep problems should be dealt with immediately. Remove stimulants from the diet; be certain that the bedroom is very dark, that the temperature is comfortable, and that outside noises and distractions are minimized. Earplugs and eye shades may be necessary. Exercising a few hours before dinner may also be helpful. If problems persist, enlist the services of a provider experienced with sleep disturbances. If you suspect depression or some other factor, deal with it as well.

Stressors can also affect ability to thrive. Any person, place, task, or experience that is a negative for the individual is a stressor. Although not all stressors can or should be removed from a person's daily life, the ones that are troublesome should be dealt with, especially if they are affecting mood or sleep. While some factors that lead to stress, such as a problem boss or a rebellious child, can seem insurmountable, in fact, they usually can be dealt with. Oftentimes, a good counselor can help you sort through such circumstances, giving you the perspective and the ideas for a solution.

Dealing with failure to thrive is not a lost cause. Perseverance and the support of experts will make a real difference. You may not find a simple solution on your first try, but I urge you to hang in there. Reversing failure to thrive improves the individual's quality of life and chances for survival. It is always worth the effort.

12

The Mind-Body Connection: Relieving Stress, Getting Support

Often we're so busy dealing with the physical when treating cancer that we forget to nurture our spirit. As I discussed in the previous chapter, stress and lack of social contact can adversely impact our prospects for recovery. There's no doubt that the mind and the body share a common destiny and that each has a significant effect on the other. Both science and clinical experience continue to observe this phenomenon, even though we're just beginning to understand its significance. In this chapter I will discuss how to nurture your spirit and improve your health by learning to use this mind–body connection.

In addition, I will consider the common sources of support—including family, friends, and support groups—and discuss how to take advantage of them while avoiding common pitfalls. None of us is an island. As human beings, we are basically communal and tend to function best when in the company of those who support us. This is especially so in times of crisis. Doubtless, having cancer qualifies as such a situation. At times like this, we should clearly see that the support of others can make our journey more bearable.

HARNESSING THE POWER OF YOUR MIND

Some people still contend that the body is not affected by the mind and spirit, but this argument is increasingly difficult to defend. For example, the principles of biofeedback have shown us how the conscious mind can control heart function, body temperature, and even immune system activity. In human physiology, the autonomic nervous system, that part of our nervous system that separates "fight or flight" from "rest and relax" modes, can affect many parts of our basic function, once again including immune system activity.

Studies, including those by O. Carl Simonton, M.D., have shown promising results with the use of biofeedback to help resist cancer. The important message for cancer survivors is to make the best of this valuable information.

Biofeedback is a technique in which humans learn to control a variety of body functions by using only their brain power. Participants can tell how well they are doing by following their progress on an electronic measuring device. People have successfully controlled pain, headaches, stress, and other functions with mental images, progressive relaxation of muscles, meditation techniques, and other mental control strategies. Even in its infancy, biofeedback has shown beyond question the tremendous authority of the mind over the body.

Learning to Live with Stress

The importance of stress and mental status on human function can be explained by known physiological principles. The autonomic nervous system, the "control central" for our nervous system responses, has two parts, the *sympathetic nervous system*, also known as "fight or flight," and the *parasympathetic nervous system*, also known as "rest and relax." These separate systems allow us to respond appropriately to the varied situations we encounter.

The rest-and-relax system stimulates digestion, elimination, relaxation, sexual arousal, and the other bodily functions that are important when we are in comfortable surroundings. The fight-or-flight system, on the other hand, helps us respond quickly and forcefully to emergencies. This system helped our ancestors to run a little faster and escape hungry dinosaurs, and it still helps us by getting us quickly out of the way of an on-coming truck. The fight-or-flight system puts our energy into increased muscle strength, mental alertness, metabolism, and blood flow. It produces the adrenaline response that increases our ability to physically respond to challenges and also improves healing in case we are injured. At the same time, the fight-or-flight system tends to shut down the digestive system. The sympathetic nervous system assumes that if you are running away from a large animal that wants to eat you or are avoiding an oncoming tractor trailer, you will not stop at that moment to have lunch.

When your mother told you to be quiet and pleasant at the dinner table, she was actually promoting sound scientific information.

The sympathetic nervous system was designed to operate only for short periods of time, just long enough to deal with the situation at hand. In modern times, however, stress can activate the fight-or-flight response for much longer periods. When this happens, internal responses, such as increased metabolism and increased heart rate, begin to tire and literally wear down those systems. Adrenal insufficiency can result, which interferes with the body's ability to respond effectively. This wearing-down effect can impair the immune system's function as well.

Long-term stress, along with the fight-or-flight response, can also cause the digestive system to do a poor job of breaking down and absorbing nutrients, which can interfere with the body's nutritional status even if you eat a good diet. Since all human functions, including the immune system, require dietary nutrition, stress can have a negative effect on our ability to resist cancer. This is ironic when you consider how many of us, when we are under stress, tend to eat. It also puts a new light on the term "fast food." When your mother told you to be quiet and pleasant at the dinner table, she was actually promoting sound scientific information.

The strategies for using the mind–body connection to your advantage are straightforward:

- Control the stress and stressful events in your life.
- Use your mind's ability to control your body's responses.

Stress control starts with identifying the parts of your life that are stressful. These can be a job, boss, business partner, lingering stress from a past event, or anything else that keeps you from having that warm, fuzzy feeling inside. You can include your cancer diagnosis on that list.

We all have stress in our lives. It is impossible to live a stress-free existence, but we can deal with and limit the effect stress has on us. You can accomplish this on your own, which can be difficult; with the help of friends, which can be impossible; or with the services of a professional who is trained to help you accurately identify stressors and put them into perspective. I am not suggesting that you sign up for five years of intensive analysis to find out why you hate the color yellow. I am recommending, however, that you learn the techniques to effectively and quickly identify and resolve stress. Some people can do this on their own, but it is usually faster and more effective to take advantage of the training and experience of a professional. Chapter 3 can help you locate the right person.

Both massage and meditation can also help with stress reduction. Licensed massage therapists, as well as counselors specializing in meditation, can be found by referral and using the techniques in chapter 3. After a single session with either, people are often amazed that they are able to feel so good. Reliable studies have confirmed the positive effects of both these strategies.

Joy in life is important. One way of reducing stress is by staying in touch with those things that give you pleasure. Make a point of doing what makes you happy.

Prayer As a Cancer Treatment

The act of praying, for those who believe in it, can have a positive effect on stress reduction.

Prayer has been investigated in connection with cancer treatment. The act of praying, for those who believe in it, can have a positive effect on stress reduction even though there is some scientific debate over how this intervention actually takes place. In addition, studies have shown that others praying for you can improve your outcome. Those studies have been the subject of scientific criticism and controversy, but in the final analysis, if it might help and won't hurt, it's worth considering.

Using Visualization to Treat Cancer

The mind's ability to control the body has been applied to cancer treatment in the form of visualization. This is the process of forming a mental image of what your body is doing. An example would be visualizing white blood cells traveling through your bloodstream to the tumor, finding tumor cells, and eliminating them. Positive images may actually cause what is visualized to happen in the body. Positive images also have the effect of limiting stress and allowing the immune system to work better, and we know that is helpful, too.

Visualization is taught by the Simonton Institute, as well as by many trained counselors and therapists. The potential benefits are good, and literally no risk is associated with this practice other than the risk of smiling a little more often.

Making use of the mind is a strategy with many potential benefits. Learning to control stress and its effects on you will undoubtedly make you feel better, positively affect your nervous system function, and improve your quality of life. I strongly recommend that these strategies be adopted and used as often as possible.

MAKING THE MOST OF SUPPORT SYSTEMS

Scientific studies strongly suggest that cancer patients who use support systems have better outcomes than those who do not. Surprisingly, many cancer survivors fail to take advantage of the human support they have available. The most common support systems are:

- Family and friends
- Cancer support groups
- Cancer support organizations
- Counseling

Family and Friends

The helpfulness of family will depend on your particular family and how their support is provided. Family members can provide closeness, comfort, and the kind of selfless, limitless support that is rarely found elsewhere. Family support can also be too much. It can be smothering when you need some freedom. Family members sometimes also intervene in places where you don't want them to and can push you in directions you don't want to go.

You need to decide as early as possible exactly what kind of support you need from your family and make certain that your family members understand. Family members generally want to do what is best for you, but their interpretation of your best interests may not agree with yours.

Encourage family members and friends to schedule visits and not just drop in. Even when you're in the hospital there will be times you simply need to sleep or wish to be alone. Don't be afraid to ask unexpected visitors to wait in the waiting room rather than your room if you are undergoing a procedure you don't wish to share.

Tell visitors beforehand how long you can tolerate a visit before you get tired. Be kind, yet firm. If the visit is lasting too long, start yawning or simply remind the visitors that you need your beauty rest.

Be direct about your needs. Whether you need a ride to the doctor or the dog fed at home, be as clear and as detailed as possible. Your family may know you well but may not understand the details of your life that they are now assisting with.

Don't be afraid to let your family and friends do things for you. They feel the need to help and will usually appreciate the opportunity to be part of your support system. If you are normally very self-sufficient, this can be the time to relax a little and concentrate on your healing.

Finally, remember that even family and friends have limits. Be respectful of their other commitments and responsibilities even when their offers are without limits. Work, taking care of children, and other important activities can only be ignored for so long before resentment begins to sneak in. Express your appreciation even when they didn't quite figure out what you wanted. Never take their kindness for granted.

Cancer Support Groups

Cancer support groups are available in almost every community. There are support groups for specific diagnoses, for persons who practice a particular religion, and ones just for men or just for women. Some are managed by trained providers such as nurses or social workers, some are more social, and others are just loosely organized for general conversation. Some support groups are uplifting while others are serious. And some have a strong educational component while others focus on social events.

The secret to finding a support group that really helps is to shop around.

Some patients feel that their cancer support group is the best thing that ever happened to them, providing a place where information and feelings can be shared and their needs can be filled. These things, they claim, simply can't happen anywhere else. Other patients have found support groups to be contrary to their needs, making them feel worse rather than better.

The secret to finding a support group that really helps is to shop around. You can attend a few meetings with each group until you find one that makes you click your heels. You may also feel that you don't want to participate in a group, but you won't really know until you try.

Many of the strongest supporters of cancer support groups are survivors who started out saying they wanted nothing to do with them.

Try out a few groups before deciding. You may do just fine without one but finding the right group can add a great deal to the quality of your life. It is definitely worth a try.

Cancer Support Organizations

Cancer support organizations can provide an abundance of information for cancer patients and are especially helpful when you're feeling confused or at a loss. Their staffs are professionally trained so that the information they provide is well organized and valid. Want a second opinion? Curious about an unusual treatment? Cancer support organizations can be an excellent place to begin your quest. Some raise funds for cancer research and create social events for cancer survivors. Some are psychosocial support organizations such as Cancer Lifeline. This organization provides telephone support twenty-four hours a day, answering questions and helping people deal with personal crises. Most of the organizations with telephone help lines raise funds from sources other than from callers, so you will not be asked for money. Get to know the organizations in your area and don't hesitate to use them when you need them.

Counseling

Counseling is another valuable support system that should not be overlooked. In addition to having therapeutic benefit, counseling can also be a great emotional support. There are many different kinds of counselors, each with his or her own training and priorities. If you decide to use counseling services, I urge you to take the time to find a counselor who fits your personal needs. Counseling support services are also available to help with financial and family issues. Your conventional and nonconventional providers can help you find the counseling services that you need.

Support systems are available at every level, providing every conceivable service. You never have to be alone. A whole world of caring people is out there, including all of your providers, their staffs, and the caring people who run the many support programs. All of them want to help you survive and thrive. All you have to do is to take the first step and the support will be there. I strongly encourage you to take full advantage of these services even if you tend to be a loner. You might be surprised by how good you can feel.

Caffeine-Containing Foods and Medications

Coffee

Black tea

Green tea

Chocolate, including milk chocolate, chocolate candy, baking chocolate, cocoa

Some herbal tea (read the label)

Some soda pop, especially colas (read the label)

Some processed fruit juice preparations (read the label)

Many diet pills and preparations (read the label)

Many stimulants (read the label)

Some pain relievers (read the label)

Some cold and allergy medications (read the label)

Some over-the-counter medicines (read the label)

APPENDIX

2

Diuretics

Common Foods

Coffee
Tea, including many herbal teas
Apple juice
Alcohol (including wine and beer)
Excess sugar for some individuals
Watermelon juice

Herbs

Equisetum arvense, a.k.a. shavegrass, horsetail
Hernaria, a.k.a. smooth rupturewort
Juniperus communis, a.k.a. juniper berries
Ononis, a.k.a. spiny restharrow
Petroselinum, a.k.a. parsley, parsley seed
Phaseolus, a.k.a. haricot bean, green bean seed
Serenoa repens, a.k.a. saw palmetto
Taraxacum officinale, a.k.a. dandelion
Urtica dioica, a.k.a. nettles
Scilla, a.k.a. squill

Common Antioxidants

Beta-carotene
Vitamin A
Vitamin B_6
Vitamin C
Vitamin E
Many minerals, including zinc and selenium
Bioflavonoids
Superoxide dismutase (SOD)
Glutathione
Taurine
Most herbs (*Note:* Many of the constituents of medicinal herbs have not been well studied, so when in doubt, it is safest to assume that some antioxidant activity exists, so avoid using in the protected zone.)

A P P E N D I X

4

Pressors

Pressors are foods that should be avoided when using drugs that have monoamine oxidase–inhibiting actions.

Aged cheese
Aged meat
Salami
Dried sausage
Soy products, including soy sauce, miso, soy paste, and so forth
Fermented foods
Fava and broad beans
Snowpeas
Sauerkraut
Beer
Yeast products
Banana peel
All cooked cheese products, including pizza, quiche, and casseroles
Wine
Caffeine-containing foods (see appendix 1 for a complete list)

Common Liver Stressors

Alcohol

Excess vitamin A

Excess synthetic (not natural) vitamin K, a.k.a. menadione

Herbs. Most herbs are processed by, and therefore increase the stress on, the liver. Only the most common herbs that can be toxic to the liver are listed here.

Allium Sativa, a.k.a. garlic, in large doses

Cheledonium, a.k.a. tetterwort, celandine

Citrullus, a.k.a. watermelon

Hydrastis, a.k.a. goldenseal

Larrea, a.k.a. chaparrel

Senecio, a.k.a. ragwort, life root

Drugs. Some drugs, including both prescription and over-the-counter, are toxic or increase the stress on the liver. These include some painkillers, cold and allergy remedies, and so forth. Always consult a pharmacist or provider if there is no warning on the label, since liver function effects may not be mentioned.

GLOSSARY

2'-deoxycoformycin. (*see* pentostatin)

5-Fluorouracil. Also known as 5-FU, an antimetabolite class of chemotherapy drug.

5-FUDR. (*see* floxuridine)

6-MP. (*see* mercaptopurine)

6-TG. (*see* thioguanine)

ablative oophorectomy. Surgery that renders the ovaries inactive.

ABVD. A combination of the chemotherapy drugs doxorubicin, bleomycin, vinblastine, and dacarbazine.

acupuncture. A branch of Oriental medicine that involves the use of needles, electrical voltage, or pressure to stimulate "meridians of energy flow" in the body.

adaptogen. A substance, usually an herb, that is thought to normalize human functions.

adenopathy. Swelling of lymph glands.

adrenal cortical carcinoma. Cancer of the adrenal gland.

Adriamycin. (*see* doxorubicin)

aflatoxin. A fungus found on certain edible plants, including peanuts, which can cause liver cancer.

Aldesleukin. Also known as interleukin, this is a biological agent chemotherapy drug.

alkaloids. Medicinal ingredients found in herbs and other plants.

alkylating agents. A class of chemotherapy drugs that attacks cancer by creating substances known as free radicals.

allergy. An immune response to an allergen. Allergens are numerous and can include foods, pollen, chemicals, dust, fibers, and many other substances. Different individuals can have allergies to different allergens.

allogeneic transplant. Using someone else's cells for a bone marrow transplant. (*See also* bone marrow transplant)

altretamine. Also known as Hexamethylmelamine, this is an alkylating agent class of chemotherapy drug.

amino acids. The chemical building blocks that make up a complete protein. There are nine essential amino acids that must be in the diet since they cannot be synthesized by the body, as well as thirteen nonessential amino acids, which can be synthesized by the body.

aminoglutethimide. Also known as Cytadren, this is a hormonal class of chemotherapy drug.

Amitriptyline. A tricyclic antidepressant drug that is sometimes used to treat cancer pain.

analgesic. A type of painkiller that includes both drugs and herbs.

anemia. A condition in which the blood has too few red blood cells and/or reduced hemoglobin. Anemia can result in reduced ability to carry oxygen from the lungs to the tissues needing it. Symptoms can include fatigue and pale skin.

anthracyclines. A subclass within the antitumor antibiotic class of chemotherapy drugs.

antibiotic. A drug that helps to eliminate agents such as bacteria, viruses, and funguses that can cause infection.

antibody. A protein in the body usually developed by the immune system to respond to and destroy a particular foreign substance, or antigen.

anticonvulsant. A drug that relieves or prevents convulsions.

antidepressant. A drug for the relief of depression. Subclasses of antidepressants include selective serotonin re-uptake inhibitors (SSRI), monoamine oxidase inhibitors (MAOI), and tricyclics.

antigen. Any substance, usually foreign to the body, that evokes a defense response from the immune system. Antigens can include chemicals, foods, bacteria, and toxins.

antimetabolite. A class of chemotherapy drugs that interferes with the metabolism and reproduction of tumor cells.

antineoplastic agents. These are drugs that inhibit or prevent the development of tumor cells. Chemotherapy drugs are antineoplastic agents.

antioxidant. A substance that quenches free radicals in the body. A free radical that has been quenched by antioxidants is no longer capable of damaging cells in the body. Antioxidants include certain vitamins, minerals, herbs, and other substances.

antipsychotic. A class of drugs used for the treatment of psychiatric disorders.

antitumor antibiotic. A class of chemotherapy drugs whose chemical structure resembles traditional antibiotics. Like alkylating agents, most antitumor antibiotics create free radicals that attack rapidly dividing tumor cells.

apoptosis. Programmed cell death.

arginine. A nonessential amino acid.

ascorbic acid. Vitamin C.

asparaginase. An enzyme that breaks down the nonessential amino acid asparagine. Asparaginase is also a drug known as L-asparaginase or ELSPAR, which is an antimetabolite class of chemotherapy drug.

astrocytoma. A tumor of the nervous system, which includes the brain.

autologous transplant. Using the patient's own cells for transplant.

Bacillus Calmette-Guerin (BCG). A biological agent class of chemotherapy drug. It is a live bacterial strain that is administered directly to the site of certain urinary tract cancers.

BCNU. (*see* carmustine)

beta-carotene. The precursor to vitamin A.

BFM. An intensive combination of chemotherapy drugs used for the treatment of leukemia.

BiCNU. (*see* carmustine)

biliary system. A system of tubes connecting the liver and pancreas to the small intestine. Bile from the liver as well as pancreatic enzymes flow through these tubes to the small intestine, providing digestive enzymes as well as eliminating toxins. The biliary system also includes the gall bladder, which stores bile until needed.

bioflavonoid. Also known as vitamin P, these are yellow pigments found in fruits, vegetables, and grains. Nearly 1,000 varieties have been identified. They have not been shown to be essential in human nutrition but do improve the function of vitamin C and have suggested anticancer activity.

biological agent. A class of chemotherapy drugs that are living organisms or act like parts of living organisms such as chemicals normally found in the body.

biopsy. Procedure for obtaining a tissue sample for analysis and diagnosis.

bleomycin. An antitumor antibiotic chemotherapy drug.

blood chemistries. Blood tests that examine a variety of enzymes, hormones, and other chemicals.

bone marrow. The cells inside bones that manufacture many but not all the cells of the immune system and blood.

bone marrow suppression. Reduction of the ability of the bone marrow to produce adequate white blood cells and/or red blood cells and/or platelets. In some cases, suppressed marrow may produce adequate numbers of cells but with cells that do not perform properly.

bone marrow transplant. The process of eliminating the existing bone marrow with very high dose conventional cancer treatments such as chemotherapy and/or radiation and replacing with bone marrow from the patient (autologous) or from another person (allogeneic). Bone marrow damage may be secondary to treatment or purposeful to eliminate defective marrow function.

brachytherapy.   The process of implanting radioactive "*seeds*" within or very close to a tumor. The *seeds* release a slow, steady dose of radiation. Brachytherapy has the advantage of being very specific and localized, thereby reducing damage to healthy tissue.

Burkitt's lymphoma.   A type of lymph system cancer.

busulfan.   An alkylating agent chemotherapy drug.

camptothecan.   (*see* irinotecan)

cannabinoid.   A drug or substance that acts like cannabis, such as marijuana.

carboplatin.   An alkylating agent chemotherapy drug.

carcinogen.   A substance that can cause cancer.

carcinoid.   A hormone-producing cancer.

carcinoid syndrome.   A condition caused by carcinoid tumors that includes hot flashes, diarrhea, breathing difficulty, and heart problems.

carcinoid tumor.   A cancerous tumor that secretes hormones. When the tumor is located on the liver or a vulnerable part of the digestive system or some other rare site, the secreted hormones can create carcinoid syndrome.

carcinomatosis.   The condition of widespread cancer throughout the body.

cardiac toxicity.   Damage to the heart.

carmustine.   Also known as BCNU, an alkylating agent chemotherapy drug.

CAT scan.   (*see* computerized axial tomography)

central nervous system.   The brain and spinal cord and the nerves that emanate from them.

Cerubidine.   (*see* daunorubicin)

chelation therapy.   The use of drugs in the blood that bind to and remove unwanted substances. Most commonly used with the drug EDTA (ethylenediamine-tetraacetic acid) to remove plaque from arteries of patients with cardiovascular disease.

chemoprevention.   The use of dietary and other substances to prevent cancer.

chemoradiotherapy.   The combination of chemotherapy and radiation at the same time, used usually for the purpose of intensifying the actions of both.

chemotherapy.   The use of any chemical to treat any disease. The term has been used more narrowly to describe drugs used for the treatment of cancer.

chiropractors.   Practitioners providing chiropractic adjustment, a form of manipulation of the spine.

chlorambucil.   An alkylating agent chemotherapy drug.

CHOP.   A chemotherapy drug combination.

cisplatin.   Also known as Platinol, an alkylating agent chemotherapy drug.

cladribine.   An antimetabolite class of chemotherapy agent.

clear margin.   When a tumor can be removed with a measurable margin of tissue that has no visible cancer. Clear margin usually means the entire tumor has been removed.

CNS.   (*see* central nervous system)

codeine.   A pain-killing drug. An analgesic.

cognition.   Awareness of surroundings, perception, and memory.

colonoscopy.   Visual inspection of the inside of the colon.

colony stimulating factors.   Drugs that mimic naturally occurring chemicals in the body that stimulate bone marrow manufacturing of certain cells.

colostomy.   Surgery to make the bowel exit the body into an appliance rather than the anus.

complementary medicine.   Combining conventional medicine with alternative medicine.

computerized axial tomography.   Radiographic technique that provides a three-dimensional view of the body and its internal parts.

constipation.   Bowel movements that are infrequent, hard, or require straining for elimination.

CSF.   (*see* colony stimulating factors)

Cushing's syndrome.   The result of excess secretion of the adrenal glands or high doses of corticosteroid drugs such as prednisone. Symptoms include puffiness, fatigue, weakness, loss of periods, and sometimes other symptoms, depending on dose and condition.

CVP.   A chemotherapy drug combination.

cyclophosphamide. Also known as Cytoxan, an alkylating agent chemotherapy drug.

cystitis. An infection or inflammation of the urinary bladder.

Cytadren. (*see* aminoglutethimide)

cytarabine. An antimetabolite class of chemotherapy drug.

Cytosine arabinoside. (*see* cytarabine)

cytotoxic. Capable of killing cells. In the case of cancer treatment, capable of killing cancer cells.

dacarbazine. Also known as DTIC, an alkylating agent chemotherapy drug.

dactinomycin. An antitumor antibiotic class of chemotherapy drug.

Daily Recommended Value. Also known as Daily Value, DRV, and DV, this is the level of oral nutrients such as vitamins and minerals recommended by the U.S. Food and Drug Administration. These replace the recommended Daily Allowance or RDA.

daunorubicin. Also known as Cerubidine, an antitumor antibiotic class of chemotherapy agent.

DCF. (*see* Pentostatin)

debulking. Process by which size of a tumor is reduced prior to surgery. Debulking usually involves chemotherapy or radiation.

dementia. Term used to describe the general loss of mental function including memory, judgment, abstract reasoning, and personality.

DES. (*see* diethylstilbestrol)

dexamethasone. Also known as Decadron, a steroid drug with many uses including controlling swelling and pressure from brain tumors.

DHAP. A chemotherapy drug combination.

diabetes. A disease marked by inability to control blood sugar (glucose), inadequate insulin production or utilization, and excessive urination.

diarrhea. Stool that is watery or very frequent.

dietary fiber. (*see* fiber)

diethylstilbestrol. Synthetic estrogen, also known as DES.

Dilantin. Anticonvulsion drug.

docetaxel. Also known as Taxotere, a plant-derived class of chemotherapy drug.

doxorubicin. Also known as Adriamycin, an antitumor antibiotic class of chemotherapy agent.

DRV. (*see* Daily Recommended Value)

DTIC. (*see* dacarbazine)

DV. (*see* Daily Recommended Value)

EAP. A chemotherapy drug combination.

EBV. (*see* Epstein-Barr virus)

ECOG. The Eastern Cooperative Oncology Group.

edema. Also known as dropsy and anasarca, the local accumulation of body fluids resulting in puffiness. Edema can be a side effect of some drugs and also a sign of other processes in the body that warrant attention.

effusion. Escape of fluid into part of the body.

electromagnetic field. Also known as EMF. The field around an electrical wire such as a power line or house wiring that develops when the wire is carrying electrical current. EMF exposures have been associated with certain cancers.

ELF. Extremely low frequency, describing the magnetic field created by house wiring and power lines.

EMF. (*see* electromagnetic field)

encephalopathy. Any disease of the brain.

endocrine. Having to do with the hormone system.

endometrium. The inside lining of the uterus.

engraftment. The process of transplanted bone marrow cells settling back into the bone and generating new blood cells.

enteral. Within the small intestine.

enzyme. A chemical that can change other cells or molecules without being changed itself.

epirubicin. An antitumor antibiotic class of chemotherapy.

epithelium. Layer of cells on the surface such as skin or the surface of organs and blood vessels.

EPO. Evening primrose oil, a source for essential fatty acids.

EPO. (*see* epoietin)

epoietin. A hormone that stimulates the growth of red blood cells.

Epstein-Barr virus. Also known as EBV, a virus associated with infectious mononucleosis, chronic fatigue, Burkitt's lymphoma, and nasopharyngeal carcinoma.

esophagus. The tube that carries food from the throat to the stomach.

essential fatty acids. Oils needed by the body for many physiological functions and which must be attained from the diet since they cannot be manufactured by the body.

estrogens. Female hormones.

ether. A gas used as an anesthetic.

etoposide. Also known as VePesid, a plant-derived class of chemotherapy drug.

external beam. A type of radiation therapy.

Ewing's sarcoma. A kind of cancer, usually involving bones of children and adolescents.

FAM. A combination of the drugs 5-fluorouracil, doxorubicin, and mitomycin C.

FAMTX. A combination of the drugs 5-fluorouracil, doxorubicin, mitomycin C, methotrexate, and leucovorin.

fats. A class of required nutrients in the diet.

fatty acids. A class of dietary fats.

Fentanyl. A drug for controlling pain.

fiber. In the diet, necessary elements that have no nutrient value but absorb fluid and add bulk and softness to the stool.

fibrosis. The formation of fibrous tissue, such as scar tissue, in places where it doesn't normally occur.

FIGO. Federation Internationale de Gynecologie et Obstetrique (International Federation of Gynecology and Obstetrics).

filgrastim. Also known as Neupogen, a biological agent class of chemotherapy.

flare. Common side effects of hormonal anticancer drugs.

flow cytometry. A process that examines individual cells as they pass through a complex detector system; can measure the extent of growth and aggressiveness of a malignant tumor.

floxuridine. Also known as FUDR or Fluorodeoxyuridine, an antimetabolite class of chemotherapy drug.

fludaribine. Also known as FLUDARA, an antimetabolite class of chemotherapy drug.

Fluorodeoxyuridine. (*see* floxuridine)

Fluoxymesterol. Also known as Halotestin, an anticancer hormone, biological agent chemotherapy drug.

flutamide. Also known as Eulexin, an anticancer hormonal agent chemotherapy drug.

folate. A B vitamin. (*see* Leucovorin)

folinic acid. (*see* Leucovorin)

free radical. A molecule capable of adding or removing an electron from a human cell and thus damaging the cell. Free radicals can damage healthy cells. They are also used by some chemotherapy drugs and radiation therapies to damage tumor cells.

fungicide. (*see* pesticide)

gemcitabine. Also known as Gemzar, an antimetabolite class of chemotherapy drug.

Gemzar. (*see* gemcitabine)

glioma. A nervous system tumor.

glucose. Sugar, blood sugar in humans.

goserelin. Also known as Zoladex, an anticancer hormonal agent chemotherapy drug.

granulocyte. A kind of white blood cell.

graft versus host disease. A condition following bone marrow transplants when the transplanted marrow cells attack the body's cells.

growth factors. Naturally occurring chemicals and drugs simulating these chemicals that, in the bone marrow, stimulate the production of blood cells.

growth hormone. A hormone secreted by the pituitary gland that stimulates growth in tissues of the body that are capable of growing.

harvesting. A surgical procedure in which bone marrow is removed.

hematopoiesis. Formation of new red blood cells.

hematologist. Physician who studies and treats blood disorders.

hematology. A blood test that examines white blood cells, red blood cells, and platelets.

hepatic. Relating to the liver.

hepatobiliary. Relating to the liver, gall bladder, and biliary ducts that deliver bile to the small intestine.

hepatoma. Also known as hepatocellular carcinoma, a kind of liver cancer.

hepatotoxic. Toxic to the liver.

herbicide. (*see* pesticide)

herpes. A family of viruses including mouth sores, genital herpes, and Epstein-Barr virus.

Hexamethylmelamine. (*see* altretamine)

Hodgkin's disease. A kind of cancer affecting the lymph nodes, spleen, liver, and sometimes other organs.

homeopathic medicine. A therapy using very weak solutions to stimulate the body's immune response.

hormone. A chemical formed in one part of the body that travels through the blood to another part of the body where it stimulates a particular function.

Hydrea. (*See* hydroxyurea)

hydrocodone. A pain-killing drug. An analgesic.

hydromorphone. A pain-killing drug. An analgesic.

hydroxyurea. Also known as Hydrea, an antimetabolite class of chemotherapy drug.

hypercalcemia. Excess calcium in the blood.

hypertension. High blood pressure.

hyperthermia. Body temperature above normal.

hypervitaminosis A. A condition resulting from excess dosages of vitamin A with a variety of symptoms, including interference with liver function.

hypocalcemia. Low blood calcium.

hypotension. Low blood pressure.

Idamyicin. (*See* idarubicin)

idarubicin. Also known as Idamycin, an antitumor antibiotic class of chemotherapy drug.

Ifex. (*See* ifosfamide)

ifosfamide. Also know as Ifex, an alkylating agent class of chemotherapy drug.

immune system. The white blood cells and the organs that manufacture and regulate them including the bone marrow, spleen, and thymus and lymph glands.

immune system suppression. (*see* bone marrow suppression)

immunoglobulin. A class of proteins in the body that attack and eliminate antigens such as infectious agents. They include IgA, IgD, IgE, IgG, and IgM, each with a distinctive role.

infection. The growth of an organism in the body where it does not belong or at levels greater than normal.

infertility. The inability to reproduce.

insecticide. (*see* pesticide)

insulin. A hormone created by the pancreas that facilitates the storage and utilization of energy molecules from foods, including blood sugar and amino acids. Inadequate insulin can cause increased levels of blood sugar and diabetes. Too much insulin or inappropriate secretion can cause low blood sugar, hypoglycemia.

interferons. A class of naturally occurring biological substances (and the drugs that simulate them) that regulate cell reproduction and have many other functions. We are still learning about interferons.

interleukins. A class of biological substances (and the drugs that simulate them) that stimulate the immune system.

ions. A particle that has an electrical charge, either plus or minus.

irinotecan. A plant-derived class of chemotherapy drugs.

ischemia. The loss of blood flow to a part of the body or organ.

Islet cells. Cells in the pancreas.

Katz index of independence activities. A functional assessment used to determine an elderly person's status and ability to function with the daily activities of life.

Leucovorin. The physiologically active form of the B vitamin folic acid. It is used as a chemotherapeutic agent as well as a "rescue" following drugs that deplete the body's folic acid. Such drugs include methotrexate.

leukemia. A kind of cancer affecting the normal production of white blood cells.

leukopenia. A condition where the body has too few white blood cells.

leukoplakia. The formation of white patches or spots in the mouth. They can be precancerous.

leuprolide. Also known as Lupron, an anticancer hormone, biological agent chemotherapy drug.

levamisole. Also known as Ergamisol, a biological agent class of chemotherapy drug.

Live cell analysis. A controversial test where a drop of blood is observed under a dark field microscope to determine the existence of and potential treatment for cancer.

lomustine. Also known as CCNU, an alkylating agent class of chemotherapy.

L-PAM. (*see* melphalan)

L-Sarcolysin. (*see* melphalan)

lymphocyte. A kind of white blood cell.

lymphedema. Swelling of the arm or leg due to surgical removal of lymph nodes.

lymphoma. A kind of cancer involving the lymph system including lymph glands.

lymphorecticuloma. Also known as Hodgkin's disease, the most common cancer of the lymphatic system.

MABCDP. A combination of the drugs methotrexate, doxorubicin, bleomycin, cyclophosphamide, dactinomycin, and cisplatin.

magnetic resonance imaging (MRI). Radiographic technique that creates a magnetic field in the body and then measures how the body parts disrupt that field.

MAID. A combination of the drugs mesna, doxorubicin, ifosfamide, and dacarbazine.

malignancy. Cancer.

malignant effusion. Fluid in the body containing malignant cells.

malnutrition. Inadequate nutrition for maintaining normal function of the body.

mechlorethamine. Also known as Mustargen, an alkylating agent class of chemotherapy drug.

melanoma. A particularly virulent kind of skin cancer.

melphalan. Also known as L-PAM, an alkylating agent class of chemotherapy drug.

mentation. Ability to comprehend and process information.

mercaptopurine. Also known as Purinethol, an antimetabolite class of chemotherapy drug.

Mesna. An antioxidant drug used to protect the urinary tract from toxicity with certain alkylating agents.

metastatic disease. Growth of cancer at a site distant from the primary tumor.

methotrexate. Also known as Folex, an antimetabolite chemotherapy agent.

micrometastases. Small, free-floating tumor cells.

micronutrient. A nutrient that is required by the body for normal function but is only necessary in small amounts.

mineral. A naturally occurring element from the earth, in our case one needed for human nutrition.

mitomycin. Also known as mitomycin C and Mutamycin, an antitumor antibiotic class of chemotherapy.

mitotane. Pesticide derivative used as chemotherapy, principally for the treatment of adrenal tumors.

mitoxantrone. Also known as Novantrone, an antitumor antibiotic class of chemotherapy drug.

mobilization. Beginning of bone marrow transplant procedure, in which a drug is administered to generate more bone marrow cells. These cells are then removed or "harvested" for use later.

MOPP. A combination of the drugs mechlorethamine, vincristine, procarbazine, and prednisone.

morphine. A pain-killing drug.

MRI. (*see* magnetic resonance imaging)

mucositis. Reversible mouth sores resulting from some chemotherapy agents.

multiple interaction pathways. Ensuring that all conventional and nonconventional treatments work together in cases of multiple cancers.

mutation. Cancer cells that have changed their character so that they respond differently to a treatment.

M-VAC. A combination of the drugs methotrexate, vinblastine, doxorubicin, and cisplatin.

MVP. A combination of the drugs cisplatin, mitomycin C, and vinblastine.

myeloma. A kind of cancer composed of cells that are normally found in the bone marrow.

myelosuppression. (*see* bone marrow suppression)

myoclonus. Twitching or spasm of muscles.

myopathy. Any disease of skeletal muscles.

naturopathic physicians. Most broadly trained nonconventional providers.

nephritis. Inflammation of the kidney.

neuroendocrine system. The combined nervous system and glands that control the secretion of hormones.

neuropathy.   Any disease of the nerves.

neurotoxicity.   Poisonous to the nervous system.

neutropenia.   Low levels of certain white blood cells known as neutrophils.

nitrosurea.   A subcategory of the alkylating agent class of chemotherapy drugs, which includes carmustine, lomustine, semustine, and streptozocin.

nodes negative.   Meaning that the tumor spread is not detectable in lymph nodes.

non-Hodgkin's lymphoma.   A kind of lymphoma that does not have the Reed-Sternberg cells found in Hodgkin's disease.

non-ionizing radiation.   The magnetic field that surrounds power lines, electrical wires, and any other electrical conductor carrying current.

nutrient.   A substance that the body gets from the diet used to maintain normal function.

nutrition.   All of the processes of taking in, breaking down, absorbing, and utilizing the substances in the diet necessary for normal growth, repair, and maintenance of the body.

obesity.   Excess weight that can interfere with normal health and body function.

octeotride.   A biological agent class of chemotherapy drug.

oncologist.   Physician who specializes in cancer care.

osteosarcoma.   A malignancy of immature bone tissue.

osteopathic physician.   Doctor trained similarly to a medical doctor but also providing manipulation of the spine and extremities.

ovary.   A female gonad responsible for producing the ova or egg as well as a complex set of hormones.

oxycodone.   A pain-killing drug. An analgesic.

ozone.   A form of oxygen in which three oxygen molecules are formed together instead of the normal two found in air. Ozone is used therapeutically and can also be considered air pollution in excess.

paclitaxel.   Also known as Taxol, a plant-derived class of chemotherapy drug.

pain tools.   Questionnaires to help diagnose pain.

pancreas.   An organ that has many functions, including production of digestive enzymes and control of blood sugar.

papillary carcinoma.   Common, slow-growing form of thyroid tumor.

parasympathetic nervous system.   That part of the nervous system that allows us to rest and relax.

PE.   A combination of the drugs cisplatin and etoposide.

PEB.   A combination of the drugs cisplatin, etoposide, and bleomycin.

pentostatin.   Also known as NIPENT, an antimetabolite class of chemotherapy drug.

pericarditis.   Inflammation of the sac surrounding the heart.

peripheral neuropathy.   Numbness of the hands and feet.

peripheral stem cell transplant.   A kind of bone marrow transplant that replaces immature cells rather than marrow cells.

peritoneum.   The membrane surrounding the inside of the abdomen and pelvis.

pesticide.   Chemicals used to kill insects and other organisms. Normally used in agriculture, some are associated with certain cancers.

PET scan.   (*see* positron emission tomography)

pharmacognosy.   The science of the medicinal use of botanicals (herbs).

pharmacology.   The science of drugs and their actions and interactions.

platelet.   Cells formed in the bone marrow responsible, in part, for the ability of blood to clot.

pleura.   The membrane that surrounds the lungs.

pleural effusion.   Fluid inside the pleura.

plicamycin.   Also known as Mithracin, an antitumor antibiotic class of chemotherapy.

pneumonia.   Inflammation of the lungs.

positron emission tomography.   Also known as a PET scan, a procedure that observes gamma rays emitted by the body following administration of an isotope.

positive lymph node.   Indication that cancer cells have been found in a lymph node. This is an indication that they have spread from the primary site.

Prednisone.   A steroid drug.

pressor.   Food that should be avoided when using drugs that have monoamine oxidase–inhibiting actions.

procarbazine. Also known as Matulane and MIH, an alkylating agent class of chemotherapy agent.

ProMACE-CytaBOM. A chemotherapy drug combination.

prostaglandin. A class of fats in the body involved in a number of actions and effects including inflammation response, blood vessel constriction or dilation (in other words increasing or decreasing blood flow), and reduced platelet aggregation (in other words reduced clotting ability).

prostate gland. A gland in males surrounding the urethra (the tube that connects the urinary bladder to the penis). This gland contributes to the seminal fluid that carries sperm.

protected zone. The time period when and that part of the body where conventional cancer treatment is doing its work.

protein. A class of complex compounds found in foods that also serve in the body as enzymes, hormones, immunoglobulins, and other functions.

pruritis. Itching.

pulmonary. Concerning the lungs.

pulmonary edema. Fluid in the lungs.

radiation. Energy transmitted by invisible waves through space. In radiation therapy, also known as radiotherapy, waves that are powerful enough to knock an electron off atoms is used to damage tumor cells.

radiation oncologist. Physician who provides radiation therapy.

radiotherapy. (*see* radiation)

radon. A colorless radioactive gas. It is used in radiation therapy and can also be found in nature.

Raynaud's phenomenon. Intermittent attacks of reduced blood flow to the hands and feet, which results in them being cold, often with numbness and pain. It is usually relieved by heat.

RDA. (*see* Daily Recommended Value)

Recommended Daily Allowance. Also known as RDA. (*see* Daily Recommended Value)

renal. Pertaining to the kidneys.

rescues. Treatments designed to undo toxicity of a prior treatment.

retina. The lining at the back of the eye where the image is focused. The retina converts the image of light into a signal that is sent to the brain.

retinoic acid. Also known as cis-retinoic acid and 13-cis-retinoic acid. A drug similar to vitamin A; used as cancer chemotherapy.

retinoid. A substance that has chemical activity similar to vitamin A.

salivary gland. Glands surrounding the mouth that produce saliva, which is responsible for lubrication and pre-digestion of food.

sarcoma. Tumors arising from connective tissue and other origins such as muscle, bone, and skin.

sargramostim. Also known as Leukine and Prokine, a biological agent class of chemotherapy drug.

Schwann cells. Cells in the nervous system that are the source of the myelin insulator around nerve cells that keeps them from short-circuiting.

seizure. A nervous system event where loss of consciousness, loss of muscle control, convulsions, or other nervous system malfunction occurs.

sentinel node biopsy. Procedure in which one or a few lymph nodes are removed for diagnosis.

sepsis. Infection in the blood.

SMAC. Shorthand for blood tests that include a number of blood chemistry tests. Also known as blood screens.

sputum. Matter from the lungs that is spit out through the mouth.

staging. A way tumors are classified with respect to how far they have progressed and their potential for responding to treatment. (*See also* TNM)

stem cell. A precursor cell. In the bone marrow, these are the cells that create or precede the cells produced for the blood.

steroid. A broad group of chemicals found in the human body and in nature. Steroids include many human hormones.

streptozocin. An alkylating agent class of chemotherapy drug.

succussing. Method of preparing homeopathic solutions.

sundowning. Confusion in the elderly in new surroundings, which usually worsens at night.

sympathetic nervous system. That part of the nervous system that responds to crisis. Also known as the fight-or-flight response.

tamoxifen. An antiestrogenic class of hormonal agent chemotherapy drug.

Taxol. (*see* paclitaxel)

temozolide. An alkylating agent class of chemotherapy drug.

teniposide. Also known as Vumon, a plant-derived chemotherapy drug.

therapeutic window. Also known as the therapeutic index. The range of dosage of medicine that provides an acceptable result. The lower limit is the minimum dose that has a desired therapeutic effect. The maximum is the dose beyond which side effects are unacceptable.

thioguanine. Also known as 6-TG, an antimetabolite class of chemotherapy drug.

thiotepa. An alkylating agent class of chemotherapy drug.

thorax. That part of the anatomy between the neck and the abdomen also known as the chest.

thrombocytopenia. Decreased number of platelets in the blood.

thyroid. A gland in the neck that regulates metabolic rate in the body as well as calcium deposition in bone.

TNM. A system for staging cancer progress based on tumor size and character, lymph node involvement, and distant metastasis.

total parenteral nutrition. Also known as TPN, a source of nutrition administered intravenously.

transurethral resection. A surgical procedure where the surgeon enters through the urethra.

treatment response. In studies, data describing cases where the cancer regressed when a particular treatment was used.

tumor markers. Substances in the blood that indicate malignant growth.

ultrasound. A technique using sound to provide a picture of what is happening inside the body.

urinalysis. The examination of urine for a variety of properties, chemicals, and other content.

urinary tract. The organs and pathways that carry urine, starting with the kidneys, each connected by a ureter to a common urinary bladder, which in turn empties into a single urethra that carries urine from the body.

uterus. A hollow, muscular organ in females where the fertilized egg normally implants and develops.

VAB-6. A combination of the drugs vinblastine, cyclophosphamide, dactinomycin, bleomycin, and cisplatin.

VACD. A combination of the drugs vincristine, doxorubicin, cyclophosphamide, and dactinomycin.

Vanderbilt regime. A combination of chemotherapy drugs.

VATH. A combination of the drugs vinblastine, doxorubicin, thiotepa, and fluoxymesterone.

VBMCP. A combination of chemotherapy drugs.

vinblastine. Also known as Velban and Velsar, a plant-derived chemotherapy agent.

vincristine. Also known as Oncovin, a plant-derived chemotherapy agent.

vinorelbine. Also known as Navelbine, a plant-derived chemotherapy agent.

vitamin. A substance found in food that is necessary for human function and cannot be manufactured by the body.

Whipple procedure. Complex surgery for pancreatic cancer that involves removal of the lower part of the stomach, a section of the small intestine, and part of the pancreas.

X ray. High speed electromagnetic vibrations that travel in waves. X rays cannot penetrate all parts of the body equally so that, when they are delivered to one side of the body and a photographic plate is on the other side of the body, the surviving X rays hitting the plate form a picture of the organs and structure in the body. X rays are an ionizing form of radiation, which means that they are capable of dislodging an electron from the atoms they hit and thus forming free radicals.

INDEX

ABCM, 152–153
Abdominal discomfort from biological agents, 79–80
Ability to function, changes in, 271–274, 282
Ablative oophorectomy, 113
Absorption problems
    for alkylating agents, 72
    for antimetabolics, 77
    for antitumor antibiotics, 75
    for plant-derived agents, 83
    preventing, 6–7
    from vitamin C, 232
ABVD, 139–140
Accessibility. *See* Availability
Acid/alkaline cleansing diet, 178
Acid foods
    alkylating agents and, 73
    biological agents and, 80
    hormonal agents and, 82
    nausea and vomiting and, 98
Aconitum napellus (monkshood), 267–268
Activities of Daily Living (ADL) index, 242
Acupuncture and Oriental medicine, 178–179, 266
Acupuncturists, 41. *See also* Nonconventional providers
Acute lymphoblastic leukemia (ALL). *See* Leukemias
Acute myeloid leukemia (AML). *See* Leukemias
Adaptogens, 226
Addiction
    to marijuana, 211
    to vitamin B$_6$, 231
Adenocarcinoma, 158. *See also* Pancreatic cancer
ADL (*Katz index of independence Activities of Daily Living*), 242
Admitting privileges at hospitals, 33
Adrenal cancer, 108–109
    alternative therapies for, 109
    conventional therapies for, 108–109
    diagnosis, 108
    risk factors to avoid, 257
Adriamycin. *See* Doxorubicin (Adriamycin)
Age. *See* Children; Elderly people
Agitation from opioid drug painkillers, 270
Aihara macrobiotic teachings, 210
Aircraft, travel by, 254–255

Air pollution, 253–254
AJCC TNM system of staging, 106
ALA (alpha-linolenic acid), 196. *See also* Essential fatty acids
Alcohol
    cancer prevention and, 256
    liver toxicity and, 103, 307
    vitamin deficiency and, 261
Aldesleukin, 78, 79, 80
Alkaline/acid cleansing diet, 178
Alkaloids, 172
Alkeran. *See* Melphalan
Alkylating agents, 70–74. *See also* Chemotherapy; *specific agents*
    cancers treated by, 70
    cautions when combining with natural treatments, 72–74
    common agents, 71
    overview, 70
    side effects, 71–72
Alkylglycerols, 179–180
ALL (acute lymphoblastic leukemia). *See* Leukemias
Allergic response
    alternative therapies for, 101, 277
    alternative therapies to avoid, 101
    to antimetabolics, 77
    to docetaxel and paclitaxel, 83
    overview, 100–101
Allium sativum (garlic), 104, 199–200
Allogenic bone marrow transplant, 90
Aloe, 180
Alpha-linolenic acid (ALA), 196. *See also* Essential fatty acids
Alternative medical doctors, 41. *See also* Nonconventional providers
Alternative osteopathic doctors, 41. *See also* Nonconventional providers
Alternative therapies. *See also* Choosing treatments; Combination treatment plan; Nonconventional providers; *specific types of alternative therapies*
    for adrenal cancer, 109
    allergic response and, 101
    for attacking tumor cells, 170
    benefits of, 2–3
    bone marrow suppression and, 97
    botanical medicines, 172–174

Alternative therapies, *continued*
    for breast cancer, 118–119
    for carcinoid tumors, 120–121
    choosing a provider first, 38–39
    choosing treatments, 55–66
    for colon and rectal cancer, 123–124
    combinations and miscellaneous substances, 175
    combination treatment plan, 105–108
    conventional provider selection and, 29–30, 36–37
    distrust by conventional providers, 2
    enzymes, 174–175
    for esophageal cancer, 126–127
    for genitourinary cancers, 129
    for gliomas, 131–132
    for gynecological cancers, 134–135
    hair loss and, 102
    heart toxicity and, 100
    for Hodgkin's disease, 140–141
    hormones, 175
    for immune system stimulation, 170
    for immune system support, 169
    kidney and urinary tract toxicity and, 99
    for leukemia, 142–143
    for liver, gallbladder, and biliary cancer, 145
    liver toxicity and, 104
    for lung cancer, 150
    lung toxicity and, 103
    mouth sores and, 101
    for myelomas, 70, 74, 151–153
    nausea and vomiting and, 98
    nerve damage (numbness of hands and feet) and, 102–103
    for non-cancer health problems, 172
    for non-Hodgkin's lymphoma, 156
    noninterference principle, 4–5
    nonsterile, risks from, 9–10
    nutritionals, 174
    objectives, 168–169
    for pancreatic cancer, 158–159
    for physical function compensation, 273
    prayer, 294
    procedures, 176–177
    proprietary treatments, 175–176
    protected zone and, 5–6
    quality of life and, 3, 277–278
    for reducing conventional therapy side effects, 3,
        171–172, 276
    for reducing immune system workload, 171
    for reducing tumor side effects, 171
    for sarcomas, 162
    for skin cancer, 164–165
    types of, 172–177
    visualization, 294–295
    warning, 177
Althea officinalis (marshmallow root), 98, 99, 212
Altretamine, 71, 74
Aluminum foil, 250
American Biologics, 180
American Joint Committee on Cancer TNM system of staging, 106
Amino acids
    asparaginase absorption and, 77
    melphalan absorption and, 72
Aminoglutethimide, 81

AML (acute myeloid leukemia). *See* Leukemias
Amygdalus persica (laetrile), 208–209
Analysis as evidence for treatments, 58
Ananas comosus (bromelain), 185
Anecdotal evidence, 57–58
Anemia. *See also* Bone marrow suppression
    from alkylating agents, 71–72
    defined, 96
    from interleukins, 79
    from lapachol, 220
    overview, 96–97
    from zinc, 235
Angelica, 181
Antacids and esophageal cancer, 126
Antiangiogenesis, 226
Antibiotics
    astragalus, 183
    barberry, 183
    bromelain, 185
    burdock, 186
    colloidal silver, 190
    echinacea, 193
    garlic, 200
    monkshood, 267
    Oregon grape, 217
    valerian, 269
    wintergreen, 269
    zinc, 235
Antidepressants and carcinoid tumors, 120
Antihistamine, chaparral as, 187
Anti-inflammatory drugs, nonsteroidal, and antimetabolics, 77
Anti-inflammatory natural therapies
    antimetabolics and, 77
    chaparral, 187
    chlorella, 188
    essential fatty acids, 195
    turmeric, 269
Antimetabolites, 76–77. *See also* Chemotherapy; *specific antimetabolites*
Antineoplastin Therapy, 181
Antioxidants
    adrenal cancer and, 109
    alkylating agent absorption and, 72
    beta-carotene, 150, 184–185, 261
    botanicals as, 173
    breast cancer and, 119
    in burdock, 186
    in chaparral, 187
    coenzyme Q10, 189
    colon and rectal cancer and, 123
    common antioxidants, 303
    doxorubicon interference by, 8
    esophageal cancer and, 126
    in Essiac tea, 197
    flavonoids, 198–199
    genitourinary cancers and, 129
    germanium, 200
    gliomas and, 131–132
    in grapes, 202
    in green tea, 202
    gynecological cancers and, 134
    head and neck cancers and, 138

for heart toxicity, 99–100
Hodgkin's disease and, 140
ionizing radiation and, 255
in kampo, 208
leukemia and, 142
liver, gallbladder, and biliary cancer and, 145
for lung cancer, 150
lung cancer and, 150
for lung toxicity, 103
in milk thistle, 214
myeloma and, 153
for nerve damage (numbness of hands and feet), 102, 103
non-Hodgkin's lymphoma and, 156
oxygen treatments and, 218–219
pancreatic cancer and, 158–159
in pau d'arco, 219
plant-derived agent absorption and, 83
in red clover, 223
for reducing immune system workload, 171
sarcomas and, 162
selenium, 225
skin cancer and, 164
turmeric, 269
vitamin A, 9, 104, 230–231, 261
vitamin B$_6$, 231, 261
vitamin C, 98, 101, 231–232, 261
vitamin E, 100, 233–234
zinc, 235
Antitumor actions
of acupuncture and oriental medicines, 178
of alkylglycerols, 179
of aloe, 180
of American Biologics, 180
of angelica, 181
of arginine, 181
of aspirin, 182
of astragalus, 182
avoiding interference with, 7–8
of barberry, 183
of beet root, 183
of beta-carotene, 184
of bromelain, 185
of burdock, 185
of calcium, 186
of Cancell, 187
of Carnivora, 187
of chaparral, 187
of chlorella, 188
of chromium, 188
of coenzyme Q10, 189
of Coley's Toxins, 190
of colonic therapy, 190
of copper, 191
of cottonseed oil, 191
of DHEA, 192
of echinacea, 193
of enzyme balancing, 193–194
of essential fatty acids, 195
of Essiac tea, 197
of exercise, 197–198
of flavonoids, 198–199
of garlic, 199

of germanium, 200
of goldenseal, 201
of Gonzalez program, 201
of green tea, 202
of homeopathy, 203
hormonal agents and, 82
of Hoxsey formula, 204
of hydrotherapy, 204
of hyperthermia, 205
of inositol, 206
of iodine, 207
of Issels' Whole Body Therapy, 207
of kampo, 208
of laetrile, 208
of manipulation, 210
of massage, 212
of melatonin, 213
of mistletoe, 215
of molybdenum, 215
of mushrooms, 216
of noni, 216
of Oregon grape, 217
of oxygen treatments, 217–218
of pancreatic enzyme, 219
of pau d'arco, 219
of PC-SPES, 220
of phytoestrogens, 221
of qigong, 223
of red clover, 223
of rosemary, 224
of saw palmetto, 224
of selenium, 225
of shark cartilage, 226
of Siberian ginseng, 226
of tellurium, 227
of tetterwort, 228
of tolpa torf preparation (TTP), 229
of turmeric, 229
of Venus's-flytrap, 230
of vitamin A, 230
of vitamin B$_6$, 231
of vitamin C, 231–232
of vitamin D, 232–233
of vitamin E, 233
of vitamin K, 234
of wheatgrass, 234
of zinc, 235
Antitumor antibiotics, 74–75. See also Chemotherapy; specific antibiotics
Antiviral ganciclovir for gliomas, 131
Anxiety
from melatonin, 213
from Siberian ginseng, 227
Appearance, changes in, 274, 285
Appetite loss
from alkylating agents, 72
from chaparral, 188
improving, 286–288
from radiation therapy, 86
from vitamin A, 230
from vitamin D, 233
from zinc, 235

Ara-C. *See* Cytarabine
Arctium lappa (burdock), 185–186, 196, 204
Arginine, 181–182
Ascorbic acid. *See* Vitamin C
Asparaginase, 76, 77, 142
Aspirin
    antimetabolics and, 77
    overview, 182
    surgery safety issue, 9
Astragalus, 182–183
Astrocytomas. *See* Gliomas
Athletes and nutritional deficiencies, 261
Attitude and quality of life, 276–277, 278
Auricularia auricula (wood ear mushrooms), 216
Autologous bone marrow transplant, 90
Availability
    of medical specialists, 34
    of nonconventional providers, 45, 48

Bacillus Calmette-Guerin (BCG), 78, 79, 80
Backup coverage
    for medical specialist, 33
    for nonconventional provider, 47
Bacterial chemotherapy agents, 78
Barberry, 183, 204
Basal cell carcinoma, 163, 164. *See also* Skin cancer
Basic tool kit, 11–23
    decision-making process, 12–15
    getting a second opinion, 15–19
    miscellaneous tips, 22–23
    understanding diagnostic tests, 19–22
BCG (bacillus Calmette-Guerin), 78, 79, 80
BCNU. *See* Carmustine (BCNU)
Beet root, 98, 183–184
Bends, the, 218
BEP for genitourinary cancers, 128
Berberis aquifolia (Oregon grape), 217
Berberis vulgaris (barberry), 183, 204
Beta-carotene. *See also* Vitamin A
    for lung cancer, 150
    oral contraceptives and deficiency, 261
    overview, 184–185
    synthetic (trans-) vs. natural (cis-), 184, 185
Beta vulgaris (beet root), 98, 183–184
BiCNU. *See* Carmustine (BCNU)
Bile production stimulation, beet root for, 184
Biliary cancer, 143–145
    alternative therapies for, 145
    conventional therapies for, 144–145
    diagnosis, 143–144
    risk factors to avoid, 259
Biofeedback, 271, 292
Biological agents, 77–80. *See also* Chemotherapy;
    specific agents
Biopsy, diagnostic, 21, 87–88
Bladder cancer. *See also* Genitourinary cancers
    chemotherapy for, 70, 129
    vitamin B$_6$ for, 231
Bladder irritation from BCG, 79
Bleeding disorders. *See also* Blood clotting
    from alkylating agents, 72

garlic and, 200
    red clover and, 223
    vitamin E and, 233
Blenoxane. *See* Bleomycin
Bleomycin, 74
    ABVD, 139–140
    for genitourinary cancers, 128
    for Hodgkin's disease, 139–140
    lung damage from, 75
    MABCDP, 161
    for non-Hodgkin's lymphoma,
      155–156
    PEE and BEP, 128
    Pro-mACE-CytaBOM, 155
    for sarcomas, 161
    side effects avoided with, 74–75
    VAB-6, 128
    Vanderbilt regime, 155–156
Blood chemistries test, 20–21
Blood clotting. *See also* Bleeding disorders
    bromelain for preventing, 185
    EFAs and, 195
    from stimulating factors, 79
    vitamin K and, 234
Blood-sugar metabolism
    aspirin and, 182
    burdock for lowering, 186
    chromium and, 188
    garlic for, 200
    hyperthermia safety issue, 205
    problems from biological agents, 80
Blood tests, 20–21
Blurred vision from vitamin A, 230
BMI (bone marrow irradiation), 84, 91. *See also*
    Radiation therapy
Board-certification for medical specialists, 35–36
Bone cancer. *See also* Sarcomas
    chemotherapy for, 76
    osteosarcoma, 159, 161
Bone damage, manipulation safety issue, 211
Bone loss
    osteoporosis, 261
    from zinc, 235
Bone marrow irradiation (BMI), 84, 91. *See also*
    Radiation therapy
Bone marrow stimulants
    barberry, 183
    DHEA, 192
    goldenseal, 201
    green tea, 202
    Oregon grape, 217
Bone marrow suppression
    by alkylating agents, 71–72
    alternative therapies for, 97
    alternative therapies to avoid, 97
    by antimetabolics, 76
    by antitumor antibiotics, 74
    by biological agents, 79
    overview, 96–97
    by plant-derived agents, 83
    by vitamin C, 232

Bone marrow toxicity, 73. *See also* Organstress or toxicity
Bone marrow transplants
 for leukemia, 141
 for non-Hodgkin's lymphoma, 154
 overview, 90–91
 as rescues, 92
Botanical medicines. *See also* Herbs
 aloe, 180
 angelica, 181
 for appetite and digestion, 287
 astragalus, 182–183
 barberry, 183
 beet root, 98, 183–184
 bromelain, 185
 burdock, 185–186
 chaparral, 104, 187–188
 chlorella, 188
 cottonseed oil, 191–192
 diuretics, 301
 echinacea, 193
 elderly people and, 241–242
 garlic, 104, 199–200
 goldenseal, 104, 201
 green tea, 202
 laetrile, 208–209
 list of, 173–174
 marijuana, 211–212
 marshmallow root, 98, 99, 212
 milk thistle, 214
 mistletoe, 215
 mushrooms, 216
 noni, 216–217
 Oregon grape, 217
 overview, 172–173
 pain-killing herbs, 266–270
 pau d'arco, 219–220
 red clover, 223
 rosemary, 224
 saw palmetto, 224–225
 Siberian ginseng, 226–227
 tetterwort, 104, 228
 tolpa torf preparation (TTP), 229
 turmeric, 229
 Venus's-flytrap, 187, 230
 wheatgrass, 234–235
Brachytherapy, 84. *See also* Radiation therapy
Brain function, reduced, 273–274
Brain tumors, 70. *See also* Gliomas
Breast calcifications, 118
Breast cancer, 110–119
 alternative therapies for, 118–119
 chemotherapy for, 70, 74, 76, 114–117
 conventional therapies for, 112–117
 diagnosis, 110–112
 inflammatory, 112
 obesity and, 257
 phytoestrogen safety issue, 221
 radiation therapy for, 114
 risk factors to avoid, 257–258
 rosemary for, 224
 surgery for, 113

Breathing problems
 from monkshood, 268
 from opioid drug painkillers, 270
 from tetterwort, 228
Bromelain, 185
Bronchitis, bromelain for, 185
Bryony, 267
Buckthorn bark in Hoxsey formula, 204
Burdock, 185–186, 196, 204
Burns
 from moxibustion, 179
 from radiation therapy, 86
Burzynski Treatment, 181
Busulfan, 71, 73
B vitamins
 antimetabolics and, 77
 B_1, 261
 B_6, 231, 261
 B_{12}, 261
 B_{17} (laetrile), 208–209
 folate or folic acid, 77, 101, 261
 for hair loss, 101, 102
 heavy exercise and deficiency, 261
 for nausea and vomiting, 98
 overview, 186

CA
 for breast cancer, 114
 for gynecological cancers, 134
Cactus and heart toxicity, 100
CAE for lung cancer, 148
Caffeine
 alkylating agents and, 73
 antimetabolics and, 77
 biological agents and, 80
 cancer risk and, 257
 foods and medications containing, 299
 in green tea, 202
 nerve damage (numbness of hands and feet) and, 102, 103
CAF for breast cancer, 115
Caisse, Rene, 196
Calcifications, breast, 118
Calcium, 186–187, 261
Calmette-Guerin bacillus (BCG), 78, 79, 80
Camellia sinensis (green tea), 202
Camptothecan drugs
 for colon and rectal cancer, 123
 irinotecan, 82, 83, 123, 158
 for pancreatic cancer, 158
 topotecan, 82, 83
 toxicity of, 83
Cancell, 187
Cancer Lifeline, 278, 297
Cancer prevention, 247–262. *See also* Immune system support
 angelica for, 181
 beet root for, 184
 carcinogens in the environment, 253–255
 diet and, 249–253, 257, 260–261
 green tea for, 202
 immune system support, 260–262
 ionizing radiation and, 255

Cancer prevention, *continued*
  lifestyle and, 256–257, 261–262
  other benefits of, 262
  reducing external risk factors, 248–257
  selenium for, 225
  unique risk factor reduction strategies, 257–260
  vitamin D for, 232–233
Cancer recurrence, 244–245
Cancer risk. *See also* Cancer prevention;
    Risk factors
  from alkylating agents, 72
  from DHEA, 192
  from radiation therapy, 86
  reducing external risk factors, 248–257
  unique risk factor reduction strategies, 257–260
Cannabis sativa (marijuana), 211–212
CA plus Taxol for breast cancer, 114–115
Capsicum frutescens (cayenne), 267
Carboplatin, 71
  CEV, 149
  for gynecological cancers, 133
  for lung cancer, 147, 148, 149
  nerve damage from, 74
  PJ, 148
Carcinogens in the environment, 253–255
Carcinoid tumors, 119–121
  alternative therapies for, 120–121
  conventional therapies for, 120
  risk factors to avoid, 258
Cardiac toxicity. *See* Heart toxicity
Carmustine (BCNU), 71
  for gliomas, 131
  liver stress from, 73
  for myeloma, 152–153
  VBMCP, 152
  VMCP/VBAP plus ABCM, 152–153
Carnivora, 187
Cascara amarga in Hoxsey formula, 204
CAT (computerized axial tomography) scans, 20
CAV for lung cancer, 148–149
Cayenne, 267
CCNU (lomustine), 71, 73
CeeNU (lomustine), 71, 73
Celandine (tetterwort), 104, 228
Certification for medical specialists, 35–36
Cerubidine (daunorubicin), 74, 141, 142
Cervical cancer, 70, 133. *See also* Gynecological cancers
CEV for lung cancer, 149
CF for head and neck cancers, 137
CG1 and CG2 for lung cancer, 149
Chaparral, 104, 187–188
Chelation therapy, 41
Cheledonium majus (tetterwort), 104, 228
Chemicals
  environmental, 253–254
  in foods, 252
  occupational risks, 257
Chemotherapy, 69–84. *See also* Conventional therapies;
    Side effects
  for adrenal cancer, 109
  alkylating agents, 70–74

antimetabolites, 76–77
antitumor antibiotics, 74–75
biological agents, 77–80
for bladder cancer, 70, 129
blood cells and, 27
for breast cancer, 70, 74, 76, 114–117
for carcinoid tumors, 120
children's tolerance for, 238–239
for colon and rectal cancer, 123
combination treatments, 84
elderly people and, 241–242
for esophageal cancer, 125
for genitourinary cancers, 128–129
for gliomas, 130–131
for gynecological cancers, 133–134
for head and neck cancers, 70, 76, 136–137
for Hodgkin's disease, 70, 139–140
hormonal agents, 80–82
interference with, 7–8
for leukemia, 70, 74, 76, 78, 141–142
for liver, gallbladder, and biliary cancer, 76, 145
for lung cancer, 74, 76, 147–150
for melanomas, 70, 164
for myelomas, 70, 74, 151–153
for non-Hodgkin's lymphoma, 70, 154–156
overview, 69
for pain control, 266
for pancreatic cancer, 76, 157, 158
plant-derived agents, 82–83
for pre-surgical debulking, 91–92
radiation therapy with, 92
for sarcomas, 74, 160–161
for skin cancer, 164
for testicular cancer, 70, 128
treatment choices, 62–63
variety of, 69–70
Chest pain, from tetterwort, 228
Children, 237–241
  calcium toxicity in, 186
  communication issues, 239
  parents' issues, 240–241
  psychological issues, 239–240
  teenagers and vitamin deficiencies, 261
  tolerance for treatment, 238–239
Chiropractors, 40. *See also* Nonconventional providers
Chlorambucil, 71, 73, 142
Chlorella, 188
Cholecalciferol. *See* Vitamin D
Cholesterol reduction, garlic for, 200
Choosing health care providers, 25–53
  conventional medical specialists, 26–37
  importance of, 26
  nonconventional providers, 37–51
Choosing treatments, 55–66
  evaluating potential solutions, 15
  evidence for therapies, 56–58, 68
  key questions, 63–64
  objectives, 61–64
  other statistics, 60–61
  quality of life issues, 62, 66
  questions for providers, 64–65

statistics and complementary cancer therapies, 61
survival statistics, 58–60
CHOP for non-Hodgkin's lymphoma, 154
Chromium, 188–189, 261
Chronic diseases and nutritional deficiency, 261
Chronic lymphocytic leukemia (CLL). *See* Leukemias
Chronic myeloid leukemia (CML). *See* Leukemias
Cis-beta carotene. *See also* Beta-carotene; Vitamin A
    for lung cancer, 150
    trans-beta carotene vs., 184, 185
Cisplatin, 71
    for breast cancer, 115
    CF, 137
    CG1 and CG2, 149
    DC1, 115
    DHAP, 155
    for esophageal cancer, 125
    for genitourinary cancers, 128–129
    for gliomas, 131
    for gynecological cancers, 134
    for head and neck cancers, 137
    for lung cancer, 148, 149–150
    MABCDP, 161
    for melanoma, 164
    M-VAC, 129
    MVP, 149
    nerve damage from, 74
    for non-Hodgkin's lymphoma, 155
    PE, 149–150
    PEE and BEP, 128
    PFL, 137
    for sarcomas, 161
    VAB-6, 128
Cis-retinoic acid for gynecological cancers, 134
Citrullus (watermelon) and liver toxicity, 104
Cladribine, 76, 142
Clark (Hulda), 189
Cleansing diet, 178
Cleansing herbs, nausea and vomiting and, 98
Clear margin, 89
CLL (chronic lymphocytic leukemia). *See* Leukemias
CMF for breast cancer, 115
CML (chronic myeloid leukemia). *See* Leukemias
Coenzyme Q10, 99–100, 189
Coffee. *See* Caffeine
Coley's Toxins, 190
Colloidal silver, 190
Colon and rectal cancer, 121–124
    alternative therapies for, 123–124
    calcium for preventing, 186
    conventional therapies for, 122–123
    diagnosis, 121–122
    garlic for, 199–200
    obesity and, 257
    risk factors to avoid, 258
Colonic therapy, 190–191
Colostomy, 122
Combinations and miscellaneous substances
    alkylglycerols, 179–180
    aspirin, 9, 77, 182
    Essiac tea, 196–197

Hoxsey formula, 203–204
kampo, 207–208
list of, 175
shark cartilage, 226
Combination treatment plan, 105–108
    concurrent health problems, 107
    conventional oncology treatment, 107
    diagnostic information, 106
    factors to consider, 105–106
    health history, 107
    personal needs and objectives, 108
    previous oncology treatments, 107
    warning, 177
Communication
    about pain and discomfort, 264, 284
    children's issues, 239
    by medical specialists, 28
    by nonconventional providers, 43
Complications. *See also* Side effects
    reducing risk of, 9–10
Computerized axial tomography (CAT) scans, 20
Conclusive scientific testing, 57
Conflicting information, 12–13, 39
Confusion, from *Sho-Saiko-To* in kampo, 208
Connections
    medical specialists' need for, 29, 35
    nonconventional providers' need for, 44
Constipation
    from calcium, 187
    colon and rectal cancer and, 123
    colonic therapy for, 190
    from opioid drug painkillers, 270
    from vitamin D, 233
Contaminants in Oriental herbs, 179
Contraceptives and vitamin deficiencies, 261
Conventional medical specialists. *See* Medical specialists
Conventional therapies. *See also* Chemotherapy; Choosing
    treatments; Combination treatment plan; Radiation
    therapy; Side effects; Surgery
    for adrenal cancer, 108–109
    for breast cancer, 112–117
    for carcinoid tumors, 120
    choosing treatments, 55–66
    for colon and rectal cancer, 122–123
    combination treatment plan, 105–108
    difficulties with information, 1–2
    distrust of natural medicine in, 2
    for esophageal cancer, 125
    for genitourinary cancers, 127–129
    for gliomas, 130–131
    for gynecological cancers, 132–134
    for Hodgkin's disease, 139–140
    for leukemia, 141–142
    for liver, gallbladder, and biliary cancer, 144–145
    for lung cancer, 147–150
    minimizing side effects, 275
    for non-Hodgkin's lymphoma, 154–156
    noninterference principle, 4–5
    for pancreatic cancer, 157–158
    for physical function compensation, 273
    protected zone for, 5–6

Conventional therapies, *continued*
    quality of life and, 275–277
    for sarcomas, 160–161
    scientific evidence for, 56–58, 68
    for skin cancer, 163–164
    types of, 68–69
Convulsions from goldenseal, 201
Coping. *See* Pain and discomfort; Stress; Support systems
Copper, 191, 235
CoQ10, 99–100, 189
Coriolus mushrooms, 216
Cosmegen. *See* Dactinomycin
Cosmic radiation, 255
Cottonseed oil, 191–192
Coumarin in red clover, 223
Counseling
    for attitude adjustment, 278, 285
    for children, 240
    for depression, 280
    for parents, 241
    as support system, 297
Credibility of nonconventional providers, 44
Cultural needs, accommodating, 34, 48
Curcuma longa (turmeric), 229, 269
"Cure for All Cancers" (Clark), 189
CVP for non-Hodgkin's lymphoma, 155
Cyanide poisoning from laetrile, 209
Cyclophosphamide (Cytoxan), 71
    appetite loss from, 73
    for breast cancer, 114–115, 117
    CA, 114, 134
    CAE, 148
    CAF, 115
    CA plus Taxol, 114–115
    CAV, 148–149
    CHOP, 154
    CMF, 115
    CVP, 155
    DC2, 115
    for genitourinary cancers, 128
    for gynecological cancers, 134
    for leukemia, 142
    for lung cancer, 148–149
    MABCDP, 161
    for myeloma, 152–153
    for non-Hodgkin's lymphoma, 154–156
    Pro-mACE-CytaBOM, 155
    for sarcomas, 161
    TAC, 117
    VAB-6, 128
    VACD, 161
    Vanderbilt regime, 155–156
    VBMCP, 152
    VMCP/VBAP plus ABCM, 152–153
Cytadren (aminoglutethimide), 81
Cytarabine, 76
    DHAP, 155
    gastrointestinal problems from, 77
    for leukemia, 141, 142
    for non-Hodgkin's lymphoma, 155
    Pro-mACE-CytaBOM, 155

Cytosar-U. *See* Cytarabine
Cytosine arabinoside. *See* Cytarabine
Cytoxan. *See* Cyclophosphamide (Cytoxan)

Dacarbazine, 71
    ABVD, 139–140
    appetite loss from, 73
    for Hodgkin's disease, 139–140
    MAID, 160
    for melanoma, 164
    for sarcomas, 160
Dactinomycin, 74
    for genitourinary cancers, 128
    liver stress from, 75
    MABCDP, 161
    for sarcomas, 161
    side effects avoided with, 75
    VAB-6, 128
    VACD, 161
Dairy foods
    cancer risk and, 251
    nausea and vomiting and, 98
Daunorubicin, 74, 141, 142
DC1 and DC2 for breast cancer, 115
DCF (pentostatin), 76, 77, 142
DD for breast cancer, 115–116
Debulking, pre-surgical, 91–92
Decadron (dexamethasone), 151–152, 155
Decision-making process, 12–15
    conflicting information, 12–13
    step 1: defining the problem, 13–14
    step 2: deciding on objectives, 14–15
    step 3: evaluating potential solutions, 15
    tip: write it down, 13
Defining the problem, 13–14
Dehydration
    from colonic therapy, 190
    dry mouth from echinacea, 193
    eye dryness from retinoids, 80
    from hydrotherapy, 205
    from hyperthermia, 205
    from tetterwort, 228
Dehydroepiandrosterone (DHEA), 192
Depression
    from biological agents, 80
    cayenne for, 267
    conventional therapies for, 280
    from failure to thrive, 280–282
    from hormonal agents, 81
    from opioid drug painkillers, 270
    from radiation therapy, 86
    from Siberian ginseng, 227
DES (diethylstilbestrol), 81, 82
Detoxification
    hydrotherapy for, 204
    Kelley Nutritional Metabolic Therapy for, 208
    wheatgrass for, 234–235
Dexamethasone (Decadron), 151–152, 155
DF for breast cancer, 116
DGLA (dihommogamma linolenic acid), 196. *See also* Essential fatty acids

DHA (docasahexaenoic acid), 196. *See also* Essential fatty acids
DHAP for non-Hodgkin's lymphoma, 155
DHEA (dehydroepiandrosterone), 192
Diabetes
   hydrotherapy safety issue, 205
   hyperthermia safety issue, 205
   nutritional deficiencies and, 261
Diagnosis
   for adrenal cancer, 108
   for breast cancer, 110–112
   of children, 237–238
   for colon and rectal cancer, 121–122
   combination treatment plan and, 106
   for esophageal cancer, 124–125
   for gliomas, 130
   for gynecological cancers, 132
   for head and neck cancers, 135–136
   for Hodgkin's disease, 139–140
   for leukemia, 141–142
   for liver, gallbladder, and biliary cancer, 143–144
   for lung cancer, 146–147
   for myeloma, 151
   for non-Hodgkin's lymphoma, 154
   for pancreatic cancer, 157
   for sarcomas, 159–160
   for skin cancer, 162–163
Diagnostic tests, 19–22
   blood tests, 20–21
   diagnostic biopsy, 21, 87–88
   flow cytometry, 21
   lymph node biopsy, 21, 88
   need for second opinion, 16–17
   partially correct diagnosis, 16–17
   radiography, 19–20
   reading your reports, 22–23
   tumor grade, 21, 87
   understanding, 22–23
Diarrhea
   from alkylating agents, 72
   from aloe, 180
   from antimetabolics, 76, 77
   from beet root, 184
   from biological agents, 79
   from bryony, 267
   from cayenne, 267
   colon and rectal cancer and, 123
   from milk thistle, 214
   from plant-derived agents, 83
   from tetterwort, 228
   from vitamin A, 230
   from vitamin C, 232
   from vitamin D, 233
Dictionaries, medical, 23
Diet. *See also* Appetite loss; Foods; Nutritional issues
   accommodating needs, 34, 48
   caffeine-containing foods, 299
   cancer prevention and, 249–253, 257
   diuretic foods, 301
   immune system support and, 260–261
   improving diet and appetite, 286–288

pressors, 305
   raw fruits and vegetables, 73, 98
Dietary therapies
   acid/alkaline cleansing diet, 178
   grape cure, 202
   macrobiotic diet, 209–210
Diethylstilbestrol, 81, 82
Dietitians, 42. *See also* Nonconventional providers
Digestive aids
   botanicals, 287
   bromelain, 185
   burdock, 186
   cayenne, 267
   marshmallow root, 212
   Oregon grape, 217
   peppermint, 268
Digestive enzymes
   enzyme balancing, 193–195
   esophageal cancer and, 126
Digestive process and absorption, 6–7
Digestive tract cancer, 76, 199–200
Dihommogamma linolenic acid (DGLA), 196. *See also* Essential fatty acids
Dionaea muscipula (Venus's-flytrap), 187, 230
Discomfort. *See* Pain and discomfort
Discovery of cancer, issues arising from, 1–2
Dissatisfaction with your provider, 52–53
Diterpene-based drugs, 83. *See also* Docetaxel; Paclitaxel (Taxol)
Diuretics
   alkylating agents and, 73
   antitumor antibiotics and, 75
   biological agents and, 80
   burdock, 186
   kidney and urinary tract toxicity and, 99
   list of, 301
   pentostatin and, 77
Dizziness
   from biological agents, 80
   from laetrile, 209
   from monkshood, 268
   from opioid drug painkillers, 270
   from *Sho-Saiko-To* in kampo, 208
Docasahexaenoic acid (DHA), 196. *See also* Essential fatty acids
Docetaxel, 82
   allergic response to, 83
   for breast cancer, 115–116, 117
   DC1, 115
   DC2, 115
   DD, 115–116
   DF, 116
   DV, 116
   nerve damage from, 83
   TAC, 117
Dong quai (angelica), 181
Dosages. *See also specific treatments*
   cancer recurrence and, 245
   for children, 238
   for the elderly, 241–242
   therapeutic window, 241

Doxorubicin (Adriamycin), 74
   ABVD, 139–140
   antioxidant interference with, 8
   for breast cancer, 114–117
   CA, 114, 134
   CAE, 148
   CAF, 115
   CA plus Taxol, 114–115
   CAV, 148–149
   DD, 115–116
   for genitourinary cancers, 129
   for gynecological cancers, 134
   for Hodgkin's disease, 139–140
   for leukemia, 142
   for lung cancer, 148–149
   MABCDP, 161
   MAID, 160
   M-VAC, 129
   for myeloma, 151–153
   for non-Hodgkin's lymphoma, 154, 155
   for pancreatic cancer, 158
   PD1 and PD2, 116–117
   Pro-mACE-CytaBOM, 155
   for sarcomas, 160–161
   TAC, 117
   VACD, 161
   VAD, 151–152
   VD, 117
   VMCP/VBAP plus ABCM, 152–153
Drowsiness from vitamin A, 230
Drug interactions. See Interference, avoiding
Dry mouth from echinacea, 193
DTIC. See Dacarbazine
Dukes' staging system, 121–122
DV for breast cancer, 116

Ears
   hearing damage from alkylating agents, 74
   ringing from wintergreen, 269
Echinacea, 193
Edema (swelling)
   from stimulating factors, 79
   from vitamin A, 230
EFAs. See Essential fatty acids
Eicosapentaenoic acid (EPA), 196. See also Essential fatty acids
Elderly people, 241–243, 261
Electromagnetic fields (EMF), 256
Eleuterococcus senticosus (Siberian ginseng), 226–227
Elimination organ stress. See Organ stress or toxicity
Elixir lactate of pepsin, 204
ELSPAR (asparaginase), 76, 77, 142
EMF (electromagnetic fields), 256
Endometrial cancer, 133, 257. See also Gynecological cancers
Endoxan. See Cyclophosphamide (Cytoxan)
Enemas (colonic therapy), 190–191
Engraftment of bone marrow, 91
Environment
   carcinogens in, 253–255
   ionizing radiation, 255
   issues for the elderly, 242–243
   living situation and quality of life, 278–279

non-ionizing radiation, 255–256
   occupations and cancer risk, 257
Enzyme balancing, 193–195
Enzyme treatments
   enzyme balancing, 193–195
   list of, 175
   overview, 174
   pancreatic enzyme, 219
EPA (eicosapentaenoic acid), 196. See also Essential fatty acids
Ephedra
   alkylating agents and, 73
   antimetabolics and, 77
   biological agents and, 80
   nerve damage (numbness of hands and feet) and, 102, 103
Epirubicin, 74, 149
EPO, 78
Epoetin, 78
Epogen, 78
Ergamisol (levamisole), 79, 123
Erratic pulse, from Sho-Saiko-To in kampo, 208
Erythropoietin, 78
Esophageal cancer, 124–127
   alternative therapies for, 126–127
   conventional therapies for, 125
   diagnosis, 124–125
   molybdenum and, 215
   risk factors to avoid, 258
Essential fatty acids
   for bone marrow suppression, 97
   for kidney and urinary tract toxicity, 99
   for nerve damage (numbness of hands and feet), 102
   overview, 195–196
Essiac tea, 196–197
Estrogen-blocking by green tea, 202
Etoposide, 82
   CAE, 148
   CEV, 149
   for leukemia, 142
   for lung cancer, 148, 149–150
   for non-Hodgkin's lymphoma, 155–156
   PE, 149–150
   Pro-mACE-CytaBOM, 155
   Vanderbilt regime, 155–156
Eulexin (flutamide), 81
Eurixor (mistletoe), 215
Evaluating health care providers. See Choosing health care providers
Evaluating potential solutions. See Choosing treatments
Evers therapy, 197
Evidence
   for conventional therapies, 56–58, 68
   for natural therapies, 168
   survival statistics, 58–60, 63, 66
   treatment response statistics, 60–61
Ewing's sarcoma, 161. See also Sarcomas
Exercise
   for cancer prevention, 257
   for immune system support, 260–261
   maintaining flexibility, 284
   maintaining muscle mass, 282–284

for nerve damage (numbness of hands and feet), 102, 103
nutritional deficiencies and, 261
overview, 197–198
qigong, 222–223
Experience requirements. *See* Training, skill, and experience requirements
Exploratory surgery, 88
External beam, 84. *See also* Radiation therapy
Eye dryness from retinoids, 80

Facility of nonconventional providers, 45
Failure to thrive, 279–289
diet and appetite improvement, 286–288
emotional, psychological, and spiritual considerations, 280–282
lifestyle considerations, 288–289
physical considerations, 282–285
Family, support from, 295–296
Family health history, 107
Fatigue
from biological agents, 80
from radiation therapy, 86
from vitamin B_6, 231
Feedback to providers, 51
Fertility and antimetabolics, 76–77
Fever
bryony for, 267
from monkshood, 268
"Fight-or-flight system," 281, 292–293
Filgrastim, 78
Financial difficulties, 279
Fish, 250
5-Fluorouracil. *See* Fluorouracil (5-FU)
5-FU. *See* Fluorouracil (5-FU)
5-FUDR (floxuridine), 76, 77, 145
5-HTP and carcinoid tumors, 120
Flare, from hormonal agents, 81
Flavonoids, 198–199
Flexibility, maintaining, 284
Flow cytometry, 21
Floxuridine, 76, 77, 145
Fludarabine phosphate, 76, 142
FLUDARA (fludarabine phosphate), 76, 142
Flu-like symptoms as side effects, 79
Fluorodeoxyuridine (floxuridine), 76, 77, 145
Fluorouracil (5-FU), 76
for breast cancer, 115, 116, 117
CAF, 115
CF, 137
CMF, 115
for colon and rectal cancer, 123
DF, 116
diarrhea from, 77
for esophageal cancer, 125
for head and neck cancers, 137
for liver, gallbladder, and biliary cancer, 145
for pancreatic cancer, 158
PFF1 and PFF2, 117

PFL, 137
for skin cancer, 164
VF, 117
Fluoxymesterol, 81, 82
Flutamide, 81
Flying in airplanes, 254–255
Foil for cooking, 250
Folate
alcohol abuse and deficiency, 261
elderly people and deficiency, 261
mouthwash for mouth sores, 101
oral contraceptives and deficiency, 261
smoking and deficiency, 261
teenagers and deficiency, 261
Folex. *See* Methotrexate
Folic acid and antimetabolics, 77
Food allergies
cravings and, 252–253
nutritional deficiency and, 261
Foods. *See also* Appetite loss; Diet; Nutritional issues; Nutritionals
acid, 73, 80, 82, 98
caffeine-containing, 299
chemicals in, 252
diuretics, 301
pressors, 305
raw fruits and vegetables, 73, 98
rich, 73, 80, 82, 98
vegetables for cancer prevention, 249–250
Fotumestine, 71
Fox glove and heart toxicity, 100
Free radical creation
by alkylating agents, 70
by copper, 191
by doxorubicin, 8
by oxygen treatments, 218
by pau d'arco, 219
by plant-derived agents, 83
by radiation therapy, 85
Friends, support from, 295–296
Fruits, raw, 73, 98
FUDR (floxuridine), 76, 77, 145
Functional abilities, changes in, 271–274, 282
Fungicides
burdock, 186
garlic, 200

Gallbladder cancer, 143–145
alternative therapies for, 145
conventional therapies for, 144–145
diagnosis, 143–144
risk factors to avoid, 259
Gamma linolenic acid (GLA), 196. *See also* Essential fatty acids
Ganoderma lucidum (reishi mushrooms), 216
Ganzheitstherapie (Issels' Whole Body Therapy), 207
Garlic, 104, 199–200
Garlic breath from selenium, 255
Gastrointestinal problems
alkylating agents and, 71, 72–73
from antimetabolics, 77
from antitumor antibiotics, 75

Gastrointestinal problems, *continued*
  from beet root, 184
  from bryony, 267
  from chaparral, 188
  from echinacea, 193
  from hormonal agents, 82
  from pancreatic enzyme, 219
  from peppermint, 269
  from selenium, 255
  from vitamin C, 232
  from wintergreen, 269
Gaultheria procumbens (wintergreen), 269–270
G-CSF, 78
Gemcitabine, 76, 149, 158
Gemzar (gemcitabine), 76, 149, 158
Gender as limitation on finding providers, 32, 46
Gene therapy for gliomas, 131
Genetic testing, 106
Genitourinary cancers, 127–129
  alternative therapies for, 129
  bladder cancer, 70, 129, 231
  conventional therapies for, 127–129
  diagnosis, 127
  prostate cancer, 220, 224–225
  renal cell carcinoma, 127, 128
  risk factors to avoid, 258
  testicular cancer, 70, 128
Geographical limitations on finding providers, 31–32, 46
Germanium, 200
Gerson, Max, 201
Gerson therapy, 190, 201
Ginseng, Siberian, 226–227
GLA (gamma linolenic acid), 196. *See also* Essential fatty acids
Glioblastomas. *See* Gliomas
Gliomas, 130–132. *See also* Brain tumors
  alternative therapies for, 131–132
  conventional therapies for, 130–131
  diagnosis, 130
  risk factors to avoid, 258
GM-CSF (sargramostim), 79, 80
Goals
  choosing a medical specialist and, 29
  choosing a nonconventional provider and, 44
  combination treatment plan and, 108
  for combined therapy, 4
  in decision-making process, 14–15
  maximum treatment, palliation, or no treatment,
    62–64
  for nonconventional therapies, 168–169
  quality of life and, 62, 66
  treatment objectives, 61–64
Goldenseal, 104, 201
Gonzalez program, 201
Goserelin acetate, 81
Gossypium species (cottonseed oil), 191–192
Grades. *See* Staging
Grape cure, 202
Green tea, 202
Grifola frondosa (maitake mushrooms), 216
Guilt, parents', 240–241
Gut feelings, importance of, 18

Gynecological cancers, 132–135
  alternative therapies for, 134–135
  cervical, 70, 133
  conventional therapies for, 132–134
  diagnosis, 132
  endometrial, 133, 257
  ovarian, 70, 76, 132, 133
  risk factors to avoid, 258
  uterine, 133

Hahnemann, Samuel, 202
Hair loss
  from alkylating agents, 71, 74
  alternative therapies for, 102
  alternative therapies to avoid, 102
  from antimetabolics, 76
  from antitumor antibiotics, 74, 75
  overview, 101–102
  from plant-derived agents, 83
  from retinoids, 80
  from selenium, 255
  from vitamin A, 230
Hairy cell leukemia. *See* Leukemias
Halotestin (fluoxymesterol), 81, 82
Harvesting bone marrow, 91
Headache
  biofeedback for controlling, 292
  from biological agents, 79, 80
  from echinacea, 193
  from laetrile, 209
  from retinoids, 80
  from stimulating factors, 79
  from vitamin A, 230
Head and neck cancers, 135–138
  alternative therapies for, 137–138
  chemotherapy for, 70, 76, 136–137
  diagnosis, 135–136
  radiation therapy for, 136
  risk factors to avoid, 258–259
  surgery for, 136
Health care providers. *See also* Medical specialists;
    Nonconventional providers
  choosing medical specialists, 26–37
  choosing nonconventional providers, 37–51
  dissatisfaction with, 52–53
  guidelines for working with, 51–52
  importance of, 26
  qualifications for second opinion provider, 17–18
  questions to ask about treatments, 64–65
Health history, 107
Hearing damage from alkylating agents, 74
Heart disease, hyperthermia safety issue, 205
Heart-stimulating herbs, 100
Heart toxicity. *See also* Organ stress or toxicity
  alternative therapies for, 100
  alternative therapies to avoid, 100
  from antitumor antibiotics, 74, 75
  from aspirin, 182
  from biological agents, 79
  overview, 99–100
Hematologists, 27. *See also* Medical specialists

Hematology test, 20–21
Herbs. *See also* Botanical medicines
    allergic response and, 103
    diuretics, 301
    liver toxicity and, 104, 307
    lung toxicity and, 103
    pain-killing, 266–270
Herpes and arginine, 182
Herpes simplex thymidine kinase, 131
Hexametheylmelamine (altretamine), 71, 74
High blood pressure
    garlic for, 200
    hydrotherapy and, 205
    from procarbazine and pressors, 74
    from stimulating factors, 79
    valerian for, 269
High-fat diets, 261
Hippocrates, 199
Histories of personal and family health, 107
Hodgkin's disease, 138–141
    alternative therapies for, 140–141
    chemotherapy for, 70, 139–140
    diagnosis, 139
    radiation therapy for, 139
    risk factors to avoid, 259
Home-health and -hospice care, 242
Homeopaths, 42–43. *See also* Nonconventional providers
Homeopathy, 202–203
Hormonal agents, 80–82. *See also* Chemotherapy; *specific agents*
Hormone regulators, 78
Hormones
    cancer risk and, 257
    carcinoid tumor secretion of, 119
    DHEA, 192
    list of, 175
    melatonin, 213–214
    overview, 175
    phytoestrogens, 82, 175, 181, 220, 221–222
Hospice care, 242
Hospital admitting privileges, 33
Hospitalization and nutritional deficiency, 261
Hot flashes, 80, 81
Hoxsey formula, 203–204
Huang qi (astragalus), 182–183
Hulda Clark "Cure for All Cancers," 189
Hydrastis canadensis (goldenseal), 104, 201
Hydrazine sulfate, 288
Hydrea (hydroxyurea), 76, 137, 142
Hydrogen peroxide treatment, 217–219
Hydrotherapy, 204–205
Hydroxydaunorubicin. *See* Doxorubicin (Adriamycin)
Hydroxyurea, 76, 137, 142
Hyperbaric oxygen treatment, 217–219
Hypertension. *See* High blood pressure
Hyperthermia, 205–206, 239
Hypervitaminosis A, 230–231
Hypervitaminosis D, 233
Hypnosis for pain relief, 271
Hypothermia treatments and
        children, 239
Hysterectomy, 133

IAT (immuno-augmentive therapy), 206
Ice packs and hair loss, 102
Idamycin (idarubicin), 74, 141
Idarubicin, 74, 141
Ideal conventional provider, 30–31
IE for sarcomas, 161
Ifex. *See* Ifosfamide
Ifosfamide, 71
    IE, 161
    liver stress from, 73
    MAID, 160
    for sarcomas, 160, 161
IL-2 (aldesleukin), 78, 79, 80
IL-3, 79
IL-4, 79
IL-10, 79
Immune stimulants
    alkylating agents and, 73
    astragalus, 183
    bone marrow suppression and, 97
    Coley's Toxins, 190
    echinacea, 193
    Essiac tea, 197
    inositol, 206
    Issels' Whole Body Therapy, 207
    kampo, 208
    natural medicines as, 170
    saw palmetto, 224
Immune-suppressing drugs, 170
Immune suppression from echinacea, 193
Immune system
    copper and, 191
    reducing workload of, 171
    vitamin D and, 233
    weakened, risk from natural therapies and, 10
Immune system support
    American Biologics for, 180
    essential fatty acids for, 195
    Gonzalez program for, 201
    hydrotherapy for, 204
    immuno-augmentive therapy (IAT) for, 206
    Issels' Whole Body Therapy for, 207
    lifestyle considerations, 261–262
    Livingston therapy for, 209
    natural medicines for, 169
    nutritional considerations, 260–261
    overview, 169, 260–262
    Revici therapy for, 224
    714X therapy for, 225
Immuno-augmentive therapy (IAT), 206
Improvement, lack of. *See* Failure to thrive
Incomplete or partially correct diagnosis, 16–17
Independence of second opinion provider, 17–18
Indian hemp (marijuana), 211–212
Indigestion. *See* Gastrointestinal problems
Infection
    as acupuncture risk, 179
    BCG symptoms, 79
    chemotherapy for, 78
    from nonsterile natural therapies, 9–10
Infectious diseases and nutritional deficiency, 261

Inflammatory breast cancer, 112
Inositol, 206
Insomnia. *See also* Sleep
    dealing with, 288
    from green tea, 202
    from Siberian ginseng, 227
Insurance coverage
    for medical specialists, 35
    for nonconventional providers, 48–49
    for second opinions, 16
Interactions. *See* Interference, avoiding
Interference, avoiding
    with antitumor actions, 7–8
    controlling organ stress, 8–9
    preventing absorption problems, 6–7
    principles, 4–5, 6
    protected zone and, 5–6
    reducing risk of complications, 9–10
Interferons, 79
    for colon and rectal cancer, 123
    for gynecological cancers, 134
    for leukemia, 142
    for liver, gallbladder, and biliary cancer, 145
    for melanoma, 164
    for myeloma, 152
    overview, 78
    side effects, 79
    VBMCP plus interferon, 152
Interleukins, 78, 79
Internet, inaccurate information on, 12
Interviewing
    medical specialists, 32–37
    nonconventional providers, 46–50
Intravenous (IV) infusion of bone marrow, 91
Iodine, 207
Ionizing radiation, 255
Ipe roxo (pau d'arco), 219–220
Irinotecan, 82
    for colon and rectal cancer, 123
    diarrhea from, 83
    for pancreatic cancer, 158
Iron, zinc and, 235
Irritability
    from Siberian ginseng, 227
    from vitamin A, 230
Irritable bowel syndrome, 123
Iscador (mistletoe), 215
Islet cell carcinoma, 158. *See also* Pancreatic cancer
Isotretinoin. *See* Retinoids
Issels' Whole Body Therapy, 207
IV (intravenous) infusion of bone marrow, 91

Jargon, understanding, 23
Jaundice history and liver toxicity, 103
Joint pain from molybdenum, 215
Journal keeping, 22
Juicing, nausea and vomiting and, 98
Jurisdiction of nonconventional providers' licensing, 49
Juzen-Taino-To in kampo, 207–208

Kampo, 207–208
Kaposi's sarcoma, 78. *See also* Sarcomas

Katz index of independence Activities of Daily Living
    (ADL), 242
Kelley Nutritional Metabolic Therapy, 190, 208
Ketoconazole, 81, 82
Kidney cancer. *See* Genitourinary cancers; Renal cell carcinoma
Kidney stress or toxicity. *See also* Organ stress or toxicity
    from alkylating agents, 73
    alternative therapies for, 99
    alternative therapies to avoid, 99
    from antimetabolics, 77
    from antitumor antibiotics, 75
    from biological agents, 79, 80
    from garlic, 200
    overview, 98–99
    from pentostatin, 77
Kushi macrobiotic teachings, 210

Laetrile, 208–209
LA (linolenic acid), 196. *See also* Essential fatty acids
Lapachol, 220
Larrea tridentata (chaparral), 104, 187–188
Laryngeal cancer. *See* Head and neck cancers
L-Asparaginase (asparaginase), 76, 77, 142
Laxatives
    alkylating agent absorption and, 72
    barberry, 183
    bryony, 267
    mother's wort, 268
Lentinan edodes (shiitake mushrooms), 216
Leonurus cardiaca (mother's wort), 268
Leucovorin, 76
    for breast cancer, 117
    for colon and rectal cancer, 123
    for head and neck cancers, 137
    for leukemia, 142
    for liver, gallbladder, and biliary cancer, 145
    for non-Hodgkin's lymphoma, 155–156
    PFF1 and PFF2, 117
    PFL, 137
    Pro-mACE-CytaBOM, 155
    side effects avoided with, 76
    Vanderbilt regime, 155–156
Leukemias, 141–143
    alternative therapies for, 142–143
    chemotherapy for, 70, 74, 76, 78, 141–142
    diagnosis, 141
    radiation therapy for, 141
    risk factors to avoid, 259
Leukeran (chlorambucil), 72, 73, 142
Leukine (sargramostim), 79, 80
Leukopenia, 96–97. *See also* Bone marrow suppression
Leuprolide, 81
Leustatin (cladribine), 76, 142
Levamisole, 79, 123
Licensed massage therapists, 41–42. *See also*
    Nonconventional providers
Licensing of nonconventional providers, 40–43, 49–50, 51
Licorice root
    hormonal agents and, 82
    in Hoxsey formula, 204
    for nausea and vomiting, 98
Life root and liver toxicity, 104

Lifestyle issues. *See also* Exercise; Quality of life; Stress;
  Support systems
    adjusting for treatments, 276
    for cancer prevention, 256–257
    failure to thrive, 288–289
    for immune support, 261–262
Light sensitivity from retinoids, 80
Lily-of-the-valley, 100
Linolenic acid (LA), 196. *See also* Essential fatty acids
Lip inflammation from retinoids, 80
Live cell therapy, 209
Liver cancer, 143–145
    alternative therapies for, 145
    chemotherapy for, 76, 145
    conventional therapies for, 144–145
    diagnosis, 143–144
    garlic for, 199–200
    risk factors to avoid, 259
Liver stress or toxicity. *See also* Organ stress or toxicity
    from alkylating agents, 73
    alternative therapies for, 104
    alternative therapies to avoid, 104
    from antimetabolics, 77
    from antitumor antibiotics, 75
    from biological agents, 80
    from chaparral, 188
    common stressors, 307
    from floxuridine, 77
    from garlic, 200
    from hormonal agents, 82
    hyperthermia safety issue, 205
    milk thistle for, 214
    overview, 103–104
    from plant-derived agents, 83
    from tetterwort, 228
    from vinorelbine, 83
    from vitamin A, 9, 230
    vitamin K and, 234
Liver tonics
    barberry, 183
    peppermint, 268
Living situation. *See also* Environment
    issues for the elderly, 242–243
    quality of life and, 278–279
Livingston therapy, 209
Location as limitation on finding providers, 31–32, 46
Lomustine, 71, 73
Loss of appetite. *See* Appetite loss
Loss of weight. *See* Weight loss
Low blood pressure
    from goldenseal, 201
    hydrotherapy and, 205
    from milk thistle, 214
Low heart rate from milk thistle, 214
Low-microbial diet hygiene for mouth sores, 101
Low temperature from monkshood, 268
L-PAM. *See* Melphalan
L-Sarcolysin. *See* Melphalan
Lumpectomy, 113
Lung cancer, 146–150
    alternative therapies for, 150
    chemotherapy for, 74, 76, 147–150

diagnosis, 146
    radiation therapy for, 147
    risk factors to avoid, 259
    surgery for, 147
Lung damage from antitumor antibiotics, 75
Lung toxicity, 79, 103. *See also* Organ stress or toxicity
Lupron (leuprolide), 81
Lymphedema
    alternative therapies for, 118–119
    from lymph node biopsy, 88
Lymph nodes
    biopsy, 21, 88
    breast cancer and, 112
    combination treatment plan and, 106
    TNM staging system and, 106
Lymphomas
    chemotherapy for, 70, 74, 76
    non-Hodgkin's, 70, 153–156, 259
Lymphoreticuloma. *See* Hodgkin's disease

MABCDP for sarcomas, 161
Macrobiotic diet, 209–210
Magnesium deficiency from diabetes, 261
Magnetic resonance imaging (MRI), 20
MAID for sarcomas, 160
Maitake mushrooms (*Grifola frondosa*), 216
Malignant melanomas. *See* Melanomas
Manipulation, 210–211, 277
MAO (monoamine oxidase) inhibitors, 305
Marijuana, 211–212
Marshmallow root, 98, 99, 212
Massage, 212–213
Massage therapists, 41–42. *See also* Nonconventional providers
Mastectomy, 113
Matulane. *See* Procarbazine
Maximum treatment vs. palliation, 62–64
Meat, 250–251
Mechlorethamine, 71
    for Hodgkin's disease, 140
    liver stress from, 73
    MOPP, 139, 140
Medical centers, connections with, 35
Medical doctors, alternative, 41. *See also* Nonconventional
    providers
Medical oncologists. *See also* Medical specialists
    need for, 27
    overview, 27
    second opinion from, 17–18
Medical records, reading, 22–23
Medical specialists, 26–37. *See also* Choosing treatments
    dissatisfaction with, 52–53
    guidelines for working with, 51–52
    ideal provider, 30–31
    interviewing, 32–37
    making the selection, 31–33
    qualities to look for, 28–30
    questions to ask, 33–37
    second opinion from, 17–18
    types of, 27–28
    willingness to work with nonconventional providers, 29–30,
      36–37
Megace (megestrol acetate), 81, 82, 134

Megastrol acetate, 81, 82, 134
Melanomas. *See also* Skin cancer
    chemotherapy for, 70, 164
    overview, 163
    surgery for, 164
Melatonin, 213–214
Melphalan, 71
    amino acids and absorption of, 72
    for melanoma, 164
    mouth sores from, 73
    MP, 151
    for myeloma, 151, 152–153
    phenylalanine interference with, 7
    VBMCP, 152
    VMCP/VBAP plus ABCM, 152–153
Menadione. *See* Vitamin K
Menstrual flow increase, mother's wort for, 268
Mental clouding from opioid drug painkillers, 270
Mental function, reduced, 273–274
Mentha piperita (peppermint), 268–269
Mercaptopurine, 76, 131, 142
Mesna, 160, 161
Meta-analysis as evidence for treatments, 58
Metabolic treatment (Kelley Nutritional Metabolic Therapy), 190, 208
Metastatic disease
    breast cancer and, 112, 114
    combination treatment plan and, 106
    defined, 89
    micrometastases, 89
    surgery, 89, 109, 113
    surgical control of, 89
Metastatic spread of cancer
    lymph node biopsy for determining, 21
    TNM staging system and, 106
Methotrexate, 76
    for breast cancer, 115
    CMF, 115
    diarrhea from, 77
    for genitourinary cancers, 129
    for leukemia, 142
    MABCDP, 161
    M-VAC, 129
    for non-Hodgkin's lymphoma, 155–156
    Pro-mACE-CytaBOM, 155
    for sarcomas, 161
    Vanderbilt regime, 155–156
Micrometastases, 89
Mifepristone, 81, 82
MIH. *See* Procarbazine
Milk thistle, 214
Minerals
    for bone marrow suppression, 97
    colonic therapy and deficiencies, 190
    deficiencies, 261
    for hair loss, 101, 102
    hydrotherapy and deficiencies, 205
    hyperthermia and deficiencies, 205
    for nerve damage (numbness of hands and feet), 102
Mistletoe, 215
Mithracin (plicamycin), 74, 75, 83

Mitomycin C, 74
    for breast cancer, 116
    for colon and rectal cancer, 123
    for lung cancer, 149
    lung damage from, 75
    MVP, 149
    organ stress from, 75
    plus vinblastine, 116
Mitoxantrone, 74, 141
Mobilization of bone marrow, 90–91
Molybdenum, 215
Monkshood, 267–268
Monoamine oxidase inhibitors, 305
MOPP for Hodgkin's disease, 139, 140
Morinda citrifolia (noni), 216–217
Mother's wort, 268
Mouth sores
    from alkylating agents, 71, 73
    alternative therapies for, 101
    alternative therapies to avoid, 101
    from antimetabolics, 76
    from antitumor antibiotics, 74, 75
    overview, 101
    from plant-derived agents, 83
Moving elderly people, 242–243
Moxibustion, 179
MP for myeloma, 151
MRI (magnetic resonance imaging), 20
MTX. *See* Methotrexate
Multiple myeloma, 70
Multiple tumor types, 244
Muscle mass, maintaining, 282–284
Mushrooms, 216
Mustargen. *See* Mechlorethamine
Mutamycin. *See* Mitomycin C
Mutation of cancer cells, 245
Muyleran (busulfan), 71, 73
M-VAC for genitourinary cancers, 129
MVP for lung cancer, 149
Myelomas, 150–153
    alternative therapies for, 153
    chemotherapy for, 70, 74, 151–153
    diagnosis, 151
    multiple, 70
    risk factors to avoid, 259

Nasal cancer. *See* Head and neck cancers
Natural therapies. *See* Alternative therapies
Naturopathic physicians, 40. *See also* Nonconventional providers
Nausea and vomiting
    acupuncture for, 179
    alkylating agent absorption and, 72
    from alkylating agents, 71
    alternative therapies for, 98
    alternative therapies to avoid, 98
    from antimetabolics, 77
    from antitumor antibiotics, 74, 75
    from biological agents, 79
    from bryony, 267
    from cayenne, 267
    from chaparral, 188

from cytarabine, 77
from hormonal agents, 82
from laetrile, 209
from opioid drug painkillers, 270
Oregon grape for, 217
overview, 97–98
peppermint for, 268
from radiation therapy, 86
from retinoids, 80
from tetterwort, 228
from vitamin A, 230
from vitamin C, 232
from vitamin D, 233
Navelbine. *See* Vinorelbine
Neck cancer. *See* Head and neck cancers
Needs (nonmedical)
    accommodating, 34, 48
    combination treatment plan and, 108
Neosar. *See* Cyclophosphamide (Cytoxan)
Nerve damage
    from alkylating agents, 74
    alternative therapies for, 102–103
    alternative therapies to avoid, 103
    from antimetabolics, 77
    overview, 102–103
    from plant-derived agents, 83
Nerve deadening procedures, 270
Neupogen, 78
NIPENT (pentostatin), 76, 77, 142
Nizoral (ketoconazole), 81, 82
Nodes negative tumors, 21
Nodes positive tumors, 21
Nolvadex (tamoxifen), 82, 83, 164
Nonconventional providers., 37–51. *See also*
    Choosing treatments
Nonconventional providers
    choosing before selecting natural therapies,
        38–39
    conventional provider's willingness to work with, 29–30,
        36–37
    dissatisfaction with, 52–53
    guidelines for working with, 51–52
    interviewing, 46–50
    licensing of, 40–43, 49–50, 51
    making the selection, 45–47
    qualities to look for, 43–45
    questions to ask, 47–50
    types of, 39–43
    willingness to work with medical
        specialists, 50
Nonconventional therapies. *See* Alternative therapies
Non-Hodgkin's lymphoma, 153–156
    alternative therapies for, 156
    chemotherapy for, 70, 154–156
    conventional therapies for, 154–156
    diagnosis, 154
    radiation therapy for, 154
    risk factors to avoid, 259
Noni, 216–217
Noninterference, principle of, 4–5
Non-ionizing radiation, 255–256
Nonsterile medicines, risks from, 9–10

Nosebleeds from retinoids, 80
Nose cancer. *See* Head and neck cancers
Novantrone (mitoxantrone), 74, 141
Numbness of hands and feet. *See also* Nerve damage
    from alkylating agents, 74
    alternative therapies for, 102–103
    alternative therapies to avoid, 103
    overview, 102–103
Numbness of skin, from monkshood, 268
Nurses, 42. *See also* Nonconventional providers
Nutritional issues. *See also* Appetite loss
    accommodating dietary needs, 34, 48
    acid foods, 73, 80, 82, 98
    caffeine-containing foods, 299
    chemicals in foods, 252
    dairy foods, 98, 251
    diet and cancer prevention, 249–253, 257
    diuretic foods, 301
    for immune support, 260–261
    pain, 271
    for pregnant women, 243–244
    pressors, 305
    raw fruits and vegetables, 73, 98
    rich foods, 73, 80, 82, 98
Nutritional metabolic therapy, 190, 208
Nutritionals
    for appetite improvement, 287–288
    arginine, 181–182
    beta-carotene, 150, 184–185
    B vitamins, 77, 98, 101, 102, 186
Nutritionals, *countinued*
    calcium, 186–187
    children's issues, 238–239
    chromium, 188–189
    coenzyme Q10, 99–100, 189
    copper, 191
    deficiencies, 261
    essential fatty acids, 97, 99, 102, 195–196
    flavonoids, 198–199
    germanium, 200
    inositol, 206
    iodine, 207
    list of, 174
    molybdenum, 215
    overview, 174
    selenium, 225
    tellurium, 227
    vitamin A, 9, 104, 230–231
    vitamin B_6, 231
    vitamin C, 98, 101, 231–232
    vitamin D, 232–233
    vitamin E, 100, 233–234
    vitamin K, 104, 234
    zinc, 235
Nutritionists, 42. *See also* Nonconventional providers

Obesity and cancer risk, 257
Objectives
    choosing a medical specialist and, 29
    choosing a nonconventional provider and, 44
    combination treatment plan and, 108
    for combined therapy, 4

Objectives, *continued*
  in decision-making process, 14–15
  maximum treatment, palliation, or no treatment, 62–64
  for nonconventional therapies, 168–169
  quality of life and, 62, 66
  treatment objectives, 61–64
Occupations and cancer risk, 257
Octeotride, 79, 80
Off-gassing, 254
Office of Technology Assessment, 56, 68
"Off label" drug use, 68
Older people, 241–243, 261
Omega-3 DHA fatty acids, 99. *See also* Essential fatty acids
Omega-6 fatty acids. *See* Essential fatty acids
Oncologists. *See also* Medical specialists
  medical, 17–18, 27
  need for, 27
  qualifications for, 17–18
  radiation, 28
Oncovin. *See* Vincristine
Opioid drug painkillers, 270
Oral contraceptives and vitamin deficiencies, 261
Oral oxygen inhalation, 217–219
Orange skin from beta-carotene, 185
Oregon grape, 217
Organizations, cancer support, 297
Organ stress or toxicity. *See also* Heart toxicity; Kidney stress or
    toxicity; Liver stress or toxicity; Side effects; Toxicity;
    Urinary tract stress or toxicity
  alkylating agents and, 72, 73
  antimetabolics and, 77
  antitumor antibiotics and, 75
  bone marrow toxicity, 73
  common liver stressors, 307
  controlling, 8–9
  from hormonal agents, 82
  lung toxicity, 79, 103
  from plant-derived agents, 83
  rescue drugs for, 92
Oriental medicine and acupuncture, 178–179, 266
Osteopathic doctors, alternative, 41. *See also* Nonconventional
    providers
Osteoporosis and nutritional deficiencies, 261
Osteosarcoma, 159, 161. *See also* Sarcomas
Ostomy, 122
Ovarian ablation, 113
Ovarian cancer. *See also* Gynecological cancers
  chemotherapy for, 70, 76
  surgery for, 132, 133
Over-the-counter pain relievers and liver toxicity, 103
Oxygen treatments, 217–219
Ozone treatment, 217–219

Paclitaxel (Taxol), 82
  allergic response to, 83
  for breast cancer, 114–115, 116–117
  CA plus Taxol, 114–115
  carboplatin plus Taxol, 133, 147
  cisplatin plus Taxol, 134, 148
  for gynecological cancers, 133–134
  for lung cancer, 147–148
  nerve damage from, 83

PD1 and PD2, 116–117
PFF1 and PFF2, 117
PJ, 148
Pain and discomfort, 264–271
  biofeedback for, 271, 292
  chemotherapy for, 266
  communicating about, 264, 284
  deadening the pain, 266–271
  during acupuncture, 179
  hypnosis for, 271
  importance of controlling, 284–285
  from manipulation, 277
  manipulation for, 210
  nutrition and, 271
  pain-killing drugs, 270
  pain-killing herbs, 266–270
  pain-numbing procedures, 270–271
  pain relievers and liver toxicity, 103
  pain tools, 264
  radiation therapy for, 265–266
  removing the source, 265–266
  surgery for, 265
Palladium in Poly MVA, 222
Palliation vs. maximum treatment, 62–64
Pancreatic cancer, 156–159
  alternative therapies for, 158–159
  chemotherapy for, 76, 158
  coffee intake and, 257
  conventional therapies for, 157–158
  diagnosis, 157
  risk factors to avoid, 260
Pancreatic enzyme, 219
Paraplatin. *See* Carboplatin
Parasympathetic nervous system, 292–293
Parents' issues, 240–241
Partially correct diagnosis, 16–17
Pathogens in nonsterile natural therapies, 9–10
Pathology and combination treatment plan, 106
Pau d'arco, 219–220
PC-SPES, 220
PD1 and PD2 for breast cancer, 116–117
Peach tree (laetrile), 208–209
PEE for genitourinary cancers, 128
PE for lung cancer, 149–150
Pentostatin, 76, 77, 142
Peppermint, 268–269
Peripheral neuropathy. *See* Nerve damage; Numbness of hands
    and feet
Peripheral stem cell transplants
  for breast cancer, 113
  for leukemia, 141
  overview, 90–91
  as rescues, 92
Personal health history, 107
PET (positron emission tomography) scans, 20
PFF1 and PFF2 for breast cancer, 117
PFL for head and neck cancers, 137
Pharmacognosy, 172–173
Phenylalanine, melphalan interference by, 7
Phylloquinone. *See* Vitamin K
Physical function, reduced, 272–273, 282
Physician's assistants, 42. *See also* Nonconventional providers

Phytoestrogens
  in angelica, 181
  defined, 175
  hormonal agents and, 82
  overview, 221–222
  in PC-SPES, 220
  in red clover, 223
Phytonadione. *See* Vitamin K
Pill strategies
  for children, 238
  for digestive problems, 277
Pineapple (bromelain), 185
PJ for lung cancer, 148
Plant-derived agents, 82–83. *See also* Chemotherapy;
    specific agents
Plant hormones, hormonal agents and, 82
Platinol. *See* Cisplatin
Plicamycin, 74, 75, 83
Podophyllotoxins, 83. *See also* Etoposide; Teniposide
Pokeweed root in Hoxsey formula, 204
Polarity therapy, 222
Poly MVA, 222
Poria mushrooms (*Wolfporia cocos*), 216
Positive attitude, 276–277, 278
Positron emission tomography (PET) scans, 20
Potassium iodide in Hoxsey formula, 204
Potential solutions, evaluating. *See* Choosing treatments
Prayer, 294
Prednisone
  CHOP, 154
  CVP, 155
  for Hodgkin's disease, 140
  MOPP, 139, 140
  MP, 151
  for myeloma, 151, 152–153
  for non-Hodgkin's lymphoma, 154–156
  Pro-mACE-CytaBOM, 155
  Vanderbilt regime, 155–156
  VBMCP, 152
  VMCP/VBAP plus ABCM, 152–153
Pregnancy safety issues
  for aloe, 180
  for aspirin, 182
  for cottonseed oil, 192
  for flavonoids, 199
  for hyperthermia, 205
  for polarity therapy, 222
Pregnant women with cancer, 243–244
Pressors, 74, 305
Pre-surgical debulking, 91–92
Preventing cancer. *See* Cancer prevention
Prickly ash bark in Hoxsey formula, 204
Principle of noninterference, 4–5
Principles for avoiding undesirable interactions,
    6–10
  avoiding interfering with antitumor actions, 7–8
  controlling organ stress, 8–9
  preventing absorption problems, 6–7
  reducing risk of complications, 9–10
Prioritizing
  health complaints, 275
  objectives, 14–15

Procarbazine, 71
  appetite loss from, 73
  for Hodgkin's disease, 140
  liver stress from, 73
  MOPP, 139, 140
  mouth sores from, 73
  pressors and high blood pressure attacks, 74
Procedures (alternative)
  acupuncture and Oriental medicine, 178–179
  colonic therapy, 190–191
  exercise, 102, 103, 197–198
  homeopathy, 202–203
  hydrotherapy, 204–205
  hyperthermia, 205–206
  list of, 176–177
  manipulation, 210–211, 277
  massage, 212–213
  oxygen treatments, 217–219
  polarity therapy, 222
  prayer, 294
  qigong, 222–223
  therapeutic touch, 228
  visualization, 294–295
Procedures, pain-numbing, 270–271
Processing organ stress. *See* Organ stress or toxicity
Progress of other health issues, 274–275
Prokine (sargramostim), 79, 80
Proleukin (aldesleukin), 78, 79, 80
Pro-mACE-CytaBOM for non-Hodgkin's lymphoma, 155
Proof of effectiveness
  for conventional therapies, 56–58, 68
  for natural therapies, 168
  survival statistics, 58–60, 63, 66
  treatment response statistics, 60–61
Proprietary treatments
  American Biologics, 180
  Antineoplastin Therapy, 181
  Cancell, 187
  Carnivora, 187
  Clark, 189
  Coley's Toxins, 190
  colloidal silver, 190
  Evers therapy, 197
  Gerson therapy, 190, 201
  Gonzalez program, 201
  immuno-augmentive therapy (IAT), 206
  Issels' Whole Body Therapy, 207
  Kelley Nutritional Metabolic Therapy, 190, 208
  list of, 176
  live cell therapy, 209
  Livingston therapy, 209
  overview, 175–176
  PC-SPES, 220
  Poly MVA, 222
  Revici therapy, 224
  714X therapy, 225
Prostate cancer, 220, 224–225. *See also* Genitourinary cancers
Prostate problems from aspirin, 182
Protected zone, 5–6, 72
Psychological issues in children, 239–240
Psychosocial issues for the elderly, 242–243
Purinethol (mercaptopurine), 76, 131, 142

Purple coneflower (echinacea), 193
Pyridoxine (vitamin B_6), 231, 261

Qigong, 222–223
Qualifications
    for medical specialists, 28–37
    for nonconventional providers, 43–45
    for second opinion provider, 17–18
Quality of life, 263–289. *See also* Failure to thrive
    attitude and, 276–277, 278
    changes in appearance, 274, 285
    conventional treatments' impact, 275–277
    failure to thrive, 279–289
    financial issues, 279
    importance of, 263
    living situation and, 278–279
    manipulation for, 211
    muscle mass and, 282
    natural medicine for maintaining, 3
    nonconventional treatments' impact, 277–278
    pain and discomfort, 264–271
    progress of other health issues, 274–275
    reduced functional abilities, 271–274, 282
    treatment choice and, 62, 66
Questions
    accessibility of providers for, 34, 48
    to ask about treatments, 64–65
    for conventional medical specialists, 33–37
    for determining the best treatment, 63–64
    for nonconventional providers, 47–50

Radiation
    ionizing, 255
    non-ionizing, 255–256
Radiation oncologists, 28, 85, 86. *See also* Medical specialists
Radiation therapy, 84–86. *See also* Conventional therapies; Side effects
    for breast cancer, 114
    chemotherapy with, 92
    for colon and rectal cancer, 123
    for esophageal cancer, 125
    for genitourinary cancers, 128
    for gliomas, 130
    for gynecological cancers, 133
    for head and neck cancers, 136
    for Hodgkin's disease, 139
    interference with, 7–8
    for leukemia, 141
    for liver, gallbladder, and biliary cancer, 145
    for lung cancer, 147
    for non-Hodgkin's lymphoma, 154
    overview, 69, 84–86
    for pain control, 265–266
    for pancreatic cancer, 157, 158
    for pre-surgical debulking, 91–92
    for sarcomas, 160
    side effects, 86, 125
    skin cancer and, 164
    with surgery, 85–86
    vitamin E with, 233
Radiography, 19–20
Ragwort and liver toxicity, 104

Rashes from retinoids, 80
Raw fruits and vegetables
    alkylating agent interaction with, 73
    nausea and vomiting and, 98
Reading diagnostic reports, 22–23
Records, medical, reading, 22–23
Recreational drugs and liver toxicity, 103
Rectal cancer. *See* Colon and rectal cancer
Recurrence of cancer, 244–245
Red clover, 204, 223
Reduced functional abilities, 271–274, 282
Reducing stress, 262
Referrals
    for medical specialists, 31
    for nonconventional providers, 45–46
Regression, treatment statistics for, 60, 61
Reishi mushrooms (*Ganoderma lucidum*), 216
Religious needs, accommodating, 34, 48
Relocating elderly people, 242–243
Renal cell carcinoma, 127, 128. *See also* Genitourinary cancers
Reports, diagnostic, reading, 22–23
Requirements. *See* Choosing health care providers; Qualifications
Rescue drugs, 92
Research institutions, connections with, 35
"Rest-and-relax" system, 292–293
Restlessness from opioid drug painkillers, 270
Retinoids, 79
    liver stress from, 80
    organ stress from, 80
    overview, 77
    side effects, 80
Revici therapy, 224
Rhabdomyosarcoma, 161. *See also* Sarcomas
Rheum palmatum (turkey rhubarb) in Essiac tea, 196
Rich foods
    alkylating agents and, 73
    biological agents and, 80
    hormonal agents and, 82
    nausea and vomiting and, 98
Ringing ears from wintergreen, 269
Risk factors. *See also* Cancer prevention; Cancer risk
    dietary issues, 249–253
    environmental carcinogens, 253–255
    ionizing radiation, 255
    lifestyle issues, 256–257
    non-ionizing radiation, 255–256
    overview, 248–249
    reducing external risk factors, 248–257
    unique risk factor reduction strategies, 257–260
Rosemary, 224
Rumex actosella (sheep sorrel) in Essiac tea, 196

Saline mouthwash for mouth sores, 101
Salivary gland cancer. *See* Head and neck cancers
Sandostatin (octeotride), 79, 80
Sarcomas, 159–162
    alternative therapies for, 162
    chemotherapy for, 74, 160–161
    conventional therapies for, 160–161
    diagnosis, 159–160

Kaposi's, 78
risk factors to avoid, 260
Sargramostim, 79, 80
Saw palmetto, 224–225
Scientific evidence
  for conventional therapies, 56–58, 68
  for natural therapies, 168
  survival statistics, 58–60, 63, 66
  treatment response statistics, 60–61
Secondhand smoke, 254
Second opinions, 15–19
  getting satisfaction, 18–19
  importance of, 15–17
  obtaining, 17–18
Sedatives
  monkshood, 267
  opioid drug painkillers, 270
  valerian, 269
  wintergreen, 269
Seizures from hydrotherapy, 205
Selecting health care providers. *See* Choosing health care
    providers
Selecting treatments. *See* Choosing treatments
Selenium, 225
Senecio and liver toxicity, 104
Seniors, 241–243, 261
Sentinel node biopsies, 88
Serenoa repens (saw palmetto), 224–225
Serotonin-affecting drugs and supplements, carcinoid
    tumors and, 120
714X therapy, 225
Sex as limitation on finding providers, 32, 46
Shark cartilage, 226
Sheep sorrel in Essiac tea, 196
Shellfish, 250
Shiitake mushrooms (*Lentinan edodes*), 216
Shi-Un-Kou in kampo, 207–208
Shock
  of cancer discovery, 1
  from tetterwort, 228
Sho-Saiko-To in kampo, 207–208
Siberian ginseng, 226–227
Side effects. *See also* Organ stress or toxicity; Pain and discom-
    fort; Toxicity; *specific symptoms*
  of alkylating agents, 71–72
  of antimetabolites, 76–77
  of antitumor antibiotics, 74–75
  asking about, 65
  of biological agents, 79–80
  of botanicals, 173
  complications, reducing risk of, 9–10
  fears about, 93–95
  of hormonal agents, 81
  limiting, 9
  of natural medicine, 277–278
  natural medicine for, 3, 171–172
  of natural therapies, 168
  of opioid drug painkillers, 270
  overview, 95–104
  of plant-derived agents, 83
  of radiation therapy, 86, 125
  reducing, 3, 171–172, 275–276

symptoms without treatment vs., 64
treatment choice and, 63–64, 65, 66
of tumors, reducing, 171
W.H.O. ratings for chances of, 95–96
Siezures from hydrotherapy, 205
Silybum marianum (milk thistle), 214
Silymarin, 214
Simonton, O. Carl, 292
6-mercaptopurine (mercaptopurine), 76, 131, 142
6-MP (mercaptopurine), 76, 131, 142
6-TG (thioguanine), 76, 142
6-thioguanine, 76, 142
Skill requirements. *See* Training, skill, and experience
    requirements
Skin cancer, 162–165
  alternative therapies for, 164–165
  conventional therapies for, 163–164
  diagnosis, 162–163
  melanomas, 70, 163, 164
  risk factors to avoid, 260
Skin color change
  from beta-carotene, 185
  from selenium, 255
Skin conditions from vitamin A, 230
Skin sensitivity from angelica, 181
Sleep. *See also* Insomnia
  cancer prevention and, 257
  disturbances from melatonin, 213
  problems with, 288
  rosemary and, 224
Slippery elm bark in Essiac tea, 196
Smoking
  secondhand smoke, 254
  turmeric and, 229
  vitamin deficiency and, 261
Social life, maintaining, 279
Somatostatin analogue (octeotride), 79, 80
Special cases
  children, 237–241
  elderly people, 241–243
  multiple tumor types, 244
  pregnant women, 243–244
  recurrence of cancer, 244–245
Specialists. *See* Medical specialists
Speculative cancer advice, 39
Spread of cancer. *See also* Metastatic disease
  biopsy safety issues, 87
  lymph node biopsy for determining, 21, 88
  massage and, 212–213
  TNM staging system and, 106
Squamous cell carcinoma, 163. *See also* Skin cancer
Staff of nonconventional providers, 45
Staging
  for adrenal cancer, 108
  for breast cancer, 110–112
  for colon and rectal cancer, 121–122
  combination treatment plan and, 106
  for esophageal cancer, 124–125
  for gliomas, 130
  for gynecological cancers, 132
  for head and neck cancers, 135–136
  for Hodgkin's disease, 139–140

Staging, *continued*
  incorrect diagnosis of, 17
  for liver, gallbladder, and biliary cancer, 143–144
  for lung cancer, 146–147
  for myeloma, 151
  for non-Hodgkin's lymphoma, 154
  for pancreatic cancer, 157
  for sarcomas, 159–160
  for skin cancer, 162–163
  TNM system, 106
Statistics. *See also* Survival statistics
  survival, 58–60, 63, 66
  treatment response, 60–61
Stem cell transplants. *See* Peripheral stem cell transplants
Steroid hormones for leukemia, 142
Stiffness from zinc, 235
Stillingia in Hoxsey formula, 204
Stimulants. *See also* Caffeine; Ephedra
  alkylating agents and, 73
  cayenne, 267
  nerve damage (numbness of hands and feet) and,
    102, 103
  Siberian ginseng, 226–227
Stimulating factors, 78, 79
Stomach bleeding from aspirin, 182
Stomach cancer
  chemotherapy for, 74
  garlic for, 199–200
  risk factors to avoid, 260
Stomach discomfort. *See* Gastrointestinal problems
Strategies (alternative)
  acid/alkaline cleansing diet, 178
  grape cure, 202
  list of, 177
  macrobiotic diet, 209–210
Streptozocin, 71
  for gliomas, 131
  liver stress from, 73
  for pancreatic cancer, 158
Stress. *See also* Organ stress or toxicity
  biofeedback for reducing, 292
  importance of reducing, 262
  living with, 292–294
  on parents with sick children, 238, 240–241
  removing stressors, 288–289
  sympathetic nervous system and, 281
Stressors, 288–289
Succussing, 42
Sugar, 250, 286
Suggestion as evidence for treatments, 58
Suggestive but nonconclusive scientific testing, 57
Sundowning, 243
Supplements. *See* Nutritionals
Support systems. *See also* Quality of life
  Cancer Lifeline, 278, 297
  cancer support groups, 296–297
  cancer support organizations, 297
  counseling, 297
  family and friends, 295–296
  for financial difficulties, 279
  maintaining social life, 279
Surgeons, 27. *See also* Medical specialists

Surgery. *See also* Conventional therapies
  for adrenal cancer, 109
  bone marrow and peripheral stem cell transplants, 90–91
  for breast cancer, 113
  for carcinoid tumors, 120
  for colon and rectal cancer, 122
  controlling related tumor problems, 89–90
  diagnostic biopsy, 21, 87–88
  diagnostic exploration, 88
  for esophageal cancer, 125
  for genitourinary cancers, 127
  for gliomas, 130
  for gynecological cancers, 133
  for head and neck cancers, 136
  for Hodgkin's disease, 139
  for liver, gallbladder, and biliary cancer, 145
  for lung cancer, 147
  metastatic disease control, 89
  nutritional deficiency and, 261
  overview, 69, 86
  for pain control, 265
  for pancreatic cancer, 157, 158
  pre-surgical debulking, 91–92
  radiation therapy with, 85–86
  for sarcomas, 160
  for skin cancer, 164
  tumor removal, 88–89
Survival statistics
  evaluating, 59–60
  muscle mass and, 282
  for no treatment, 63
  treatment choice and, 59, 60, 63, 66
  usefulness of, 60
  withholding of, 58–59
Survival tool kit. *See* Basic tool kit
Swedish massage, 213
Swelling (edema)
  from stimulating factors, 79
  from vitamin A, 230
Sympathetic nervous system, 281, 292–293
Symptoms. *See also* Pain and discomfort; Side effects;
    Toxicity
  children's' communication about, 239
  elderly people's communication about, 242

*T*abebuia (pau d'arco), 219–220
Taber's Cyclopedic Medical Dictionary, 23
Tabloid (thioguanine), 76, 142
TAC for breast cancer, 117
Taheebo (pau d'arco), 219–220
Tamoxifen, 81, 82, 164
Taste changes from cancer treatment, 286
Taxol. *See* Paclitaxel (Taxol)
Taxotere. *See* Docetaxel
TBI (total body irradiation), 84, 91. *See also* Radiation
    therapy
Tea, green, 202
Teenagers and vitamin deficiencies, 261
Tellurium, 227
Temozolide, 71
Temperature treatments
  children and, 239

hyperthermia, 205–206, 239
hypothermia, 239
Teniposide, 82
Teratogens, flavonoids as, 199
Terminology, understanding, 23
Testicular cancer, 70, 128. *See also* Genitourinary cancers
Testimonials, 58
Tests, diagnostic. *See* Diagnostic tests
Tetterwort, 104, 228
Thera-cys (bacillus Calmette-Guerin or BCG), 78, 79, 80
Therapeutic touch, 228
Therapeutic window, 241
Thioguanine, 76, 142
Thiotepa, 71
    appetite loss from, 73
    diarrhea from, 73
Thriving, lack of. *See* Failure to thrive
Throat cancer. *See* Head and neck cancers
Thrombocytopenia, 79, 96–97. *See also* Bone marrow
    suppression
Thyroid cancer, 74, 260
Thyroid function reduction
    from biological agents, 79
    from iodine, 207
Thyroid problems from aspirin, 182
TICE (bacillus Calmette-Guerin or BCG), 78, 79, 80
Tingling skin from monkshood, 268
TNM system of staging, 106. *See also* Staging
Tobacco
    chewing, 252
    smoking, 229, 254, 261
Tolerance for treatment
    in children, 238–239
    in the elderly, 241–242
Tolpa torf preparation (TTP), 229
Tool kit, basic. *See* Basic tool kit
Tooth decay from selenium, 255
Topotecan, 82, 83
Total body irradiation (TBI). *See also* Radiation therapy
    with bone marrow or peripheral stem cell transplants, 84, 91
    for non-Hodgkin's lymphoma, 154
Toxicity. *See also* Organ stress or toxicity; Pain and discomfort;
        Side effects
    of acupuncture and Oriental medicine, 179
    of alkylglycerols, 180
    of aloe, 180
    of angelica, 181
    of arginine, 181
    of aspirin, 182
    of astragalus, 183
    of barberry, 183
    of beet root, 183
    of beta-carotene, 184–185
    of bromelain, 185
    of bryony, 267
    of burdock, 186
    of calcium, 186–187
    of cayenne, 267
    of chaparral, 188
    of chlorella, 188
    of chromium, 189
    of coenzyme Q10, 189

    of colonic therapy, 190
    of copper, 191
    of cottonseed oil, 192
    of DHEA, 192
    of echinacea, 193
    of enzyme balancing, 194–195
    of essential fatty acids, 195
    of Essiac tea, 197
    of exercise, 198
    of flavonoids, 199
    of garlic, 200
    of germanium, 200
    of goldenseal, 201
    of green tea, 202
    of homeopathy, 203
    of Hoxsey formula, 204
    of hydrotherapy, 205
    of hyperthermia, 205
    of inositol, 206
    of iodine, 207
    of kampo, 208
    of laetrile, 209
    of manipulation, 211
    of marijuana, 211
    of marshmallow root, 212
    of massage, 212–213
    of melatonin, 213
    of milk thistle, 214
    of mistletoe, 215
    of molybdenum, 215
    of monkshood, 268
    of mushrooms, 216
    of noni, 217
    of Oregon grape, 217
    of oxygen treatments, 218
    of pancreatic enzyme, 219
    of pau d'arco, 220
    of PC-SPES, 220
    of peppermint, 269
    of phytoestrogens, 221
    of qigong, 223
    of red clover, 223
    of rosemary, 224
    of saw palmetto, 225
    of selenium, 225
    of shark cartilage, 226
    of Siberian ginseng, 227
    of tellurium, 227
    of tetterwort, 228
    of tolpa torf preparation (TTP), 229
    of turmeric, 269
    of valerian, 269
    of Venus's-flytrap, 230
    of vitamin A, 230–231
    of vitamin B_6, 231
    of vitamin C, 232
    of vitamin D, 233
    of vitamin E, 233
    of vitamin K, 234
    of wheatgrass, 235
    of wintergreen, 269
    of zinc, 235

Training, skill, and experience requirements
    for medical specialists, 28
    for nonconventional providers, 40–43, 44, 45, 50
    for second opinion provider, 17
Trans-beta carotene vs. cis-beta carotene, 184, 185. *See also*
        Beta-carotene
Trauma in children, 239–240
Travel, 254–255
Treatment choice. *See* Choosing treatments
Tremella mushrooms, 216
Tretinoin. *See* Retinoids
Trifolium pratense (red clover), 204, 223
Tryptophan and carcinoid tumors, 120
TTP (tolpa torf preparation), 229
Tumor cell attack by natural therapies, 170
Tumor grade, 21, 87
Tumor markers
    blood tests for, 20–21
    for breast cancer, 112
    combination treatment plan and, 106
Tumor removal, 88–89. *See also* Surgery
Turkey rhubarb in Essiac tea, 196
Turmeric, 229, 269
2-CDA (cladribine), 76, 142
2-Chlorodeoxyadenosine (cladribine), 76, 142
Tylenol and liver toxicity, 103

*U*lmus fulva (slippery elm bark) in Essiac tea, 196
Ultrasound, 20
Upset stomach. *See* Gastrointestinal problems
Urinary tract stress or toxicity. *See also* Organ stress or toxicity
    from alkylating agents, 73
    alternative therapies for, 99
    alternative therapies to avoid, 99
    from antitumor antibiotics, 75
    from BCG, 79
    from biological agents, 80
    overview, 98–99
    from pentostatin, 77
Urination, excessive, from vitamin D, 233
Uterine cancer, 133. *See also* Gynecological cancers

*V*AB-6 for genitourinary cancers, 128
Vaccines
    for breast cancer, 113
    for melanoma, 164
VACD for sarcomas, 161
VACD plus IE for sarcomas, 161
VAD for myeloma, 151–152
Valerian, 269
Vanderbilt regime, 155–156
VBAP for myeloma, 152–153
VBMCP for myeloma, 152
VD for breast cancer, 117
Vegetables
    for cancer prevention, 249–250
    raw, 73, 98
Vegetarianism and vitamin deficiencies, 261
Velban. *See* Vinblastine
Velsar. *See* Vinblastine
Venus's-flytrap, 187, 230
VePesid. *See* Etoposide

VF for breast cancer, 117
Vinblastine, 83
    ABVD, 139–140
    for breast cancer, 116
    for genitourinary cancers, 128–129
    for Hodgkin's disease, 139–140
    for lung cancer, 149
    for melanoma, 164
    mitomycin C plus, 116
    M-VAC, 129
    MVP, 149
    nerve damage from, 83
    VAB-6, 128
Vinca alkaloids, 83. *See also* Vinblastine; Vincristine;
        Vinorelbine
Vincasar PFS. *See* Vincristine
Vincristine, 83
    CAV, 148–149
    CVP, 155
    for Hodgkin's disease, 140
    for leukemia, 142
    for lung cancer, 148–149
    MOPP, 139, 140
    for myeloma, 151–153
    nerve damage from, 83
    for non-Hodgkin's lymphoma, 154–156
    Pro-mACE-CytaBOM, 155
    side effects avoided by, 83
    VAD, 151–152
    Vanderbilt regime, 155–156
    VMCP/VBAP plus ABCM, 152–153
Vinorelbine, 83
    for breast cancer, 116, 117
    DV, 116
    liver stress from, 83
    for lung cancer, 148
    nerve damage from, 83
    VD, 117
    VF, 117
Viscum album (mistletoe), 215
Vision blurring from vitamin A, 230
Visits, scheduling, 295–296
Visualization, 294–295
Vitamin A. *See also* Beta-carotene
    deficiency, 261
    liver stress from, 9, 307
    liver toxicity and, 104
    overview, 230–231
Vitamin A analogues. *See* Retinoids
Vitamin B$_1$ deficiency, 261
Vitamin B$_6$
    deficiency, 261
    overview, 231
Vitamin B$_{12}$ deficiency, 261
Vitamin B$_{17}$ (laetrile), 208–209
Vitamin C
    deficiency, 261
    mouth sores and, 101
    nausea and vomiting and, 98
    overview, 231–232
Vitamin D
    calcium toxicity and, 187

deficiency, 261
overview, 232–233
Vitamin E
for heart toxicity, 100
overview, 233–234
smoking and deficiency, 261
Vitamin K
liver toxicity and, 104, 307
overview, 234
Vitamins
for bone marrow suppression, 97
deficiencies, 190, 261
for nerve damage (numbness of hands and feet), 102
VMCP/VBAP plus ABCM for myeloma, 152–153
Voice box cancer. *See* Head and neck cancers
Vomiting. *See* Nausea and vomiting
Vumon, 82

Water
cancer risk and, 251–252
for kidney and urinary tract toxicity, 99
Watermelon and liver toxicity, 104
Weakness from opioid drug painkillers, 270

Weight loss
from alkylating agents, 72
improving diet and appetite, 286–288
maintaining muscle mass, 282–284
Wheatgrass, 234–235
Whipple procedure, 158
Whole Body Therapy, Issels,' 207
W.H.O. (World Health Organization) ratings for side effects, 95–96
Wintergreen, 269–270
Wolfporia cocos (poria mushrooms), 216
Wood ear mushrooms (*Auricularia auricula*), 216
World Health Organization (W.H.O.) ratings for side effects, 95–96
Writing
in decision-making process, 13
journal keeping, 22

X-rays, 255

Zanosar. *See* Streptozocin
Zinc, 235
Zoladex (goserelin acetate), 81

ABOUT THE AUTHOR

Dan Labriola is a practicing naturopathic physician and founder of the Northwest Natural Health-Specialty Care Clinic in Seattle. A former faculty member at Bastyr University, he consults for a number of area hospitals. For more than a decade, he has specialized in the appropriate use of alternative care therapies for patients using conventional medical treatments for cancer and other chronic diseases, and was one of the first alternative care physicians to treat patients in a hospital environment. He has also seen patients in consultation with many major hospital centers such as Columbia-Presbyterian Medical Center, Mayo Clinic, M.D. Anderson Cancer Center, the Northwest Prostate Institute, and others.

Dr. Labriola is a graduate of Syracuse University and Bastyr University. He is a member of the Cancer Lifeline Medical Advisory Committee and the Hepatitis Education Project Board of Directors. He was the first Special Advisor to the Secretary and Department of Health for Alternative and Complementary Medicine and Chair of the Naturopathic Advisory Committee for the state of Washington Department of Health, president of the Washington Association of Naturopathic Physicians, and a member of the state of Washington Health Personnel Resource Plan. In late 1999, the prestigious, peer-reviewed journal *Oncology* published an article co-authored by Dr. Labriola about combining natural therapies with conventional therapies.

Dr. Labriola provides training and information for M.D.s, pharmacists, alternative care providers, and the public. He conducts clinical seminars and does training for several organizations, including the University of Washington School of Medicine, University of Washington Medical Center Cancer Center, Washington State Medical Association, Fred Hutchinson Cancer Research Center, Children's Hospital and Medical Center of Seattle, Seattle Society of Hospital Pharmacists, Drug Information Association, Cancer Research Center of Hawaii, and many more.

Before becoming a naturopathic physician, Dr. Labriola was a licensed mechanical and aerospace engineer, a commercial and experimental pilot and a flight instructor, and president of two aviation-related companies. He also plays classical and jazz piano, enjoys motorcycles, and writes novels.